m
la

STAT!

A Quick-Reference Guide

medical
language
STAT!
A Quick-Reference Guide

Susan M. Turley
MA (Educ.), BSN, RN, RHIT, CMT

James F. Allen, Jr.
RN, BSN, MBA/HCM, JD

PEARSON
Prentice
Hall

Upper Saddle River, New Jersey 07458

Library of Congress Cataloging-in-Publication Data

Turley, Susan M.
  Medical language STAT! : a quick-reference guide / Susan M. Turley, James Allen Jr.
    p. ; cm.
  Abridged version of: Medical language / Susan Turley. c2007.
  ISBN-13: 978-0-13-501956-6
  ISBN-10: 0-13-501956-7
  1. Medicine--Terminology--Handbooks, manuals, etc. I. Allen, James (James F.) II. Turley, Susan M. Medical language. III. Title.
  [DNLM: 1. Terminology as Topic--Problems and Exercises. W 18.2 T941mg2009]
  R123.T872 2009
  610.1'4--dc22
                                    2008014525

Notice: The authors and publisher of this volume have taken care that the information and technical recommendations contained herein are based on research and expert consultation, and are accurate and compatible with the standards generally accepted at the time of publication. Nevertheless, as new information becomes available, changes in clinical and technical practices become necessary. The reader is advised to carefully consult manufacturers' instruction and information material for all supplies and equipment before use, and to consult with a health care professional as necessary. This advice is especially important when using new supplies or equipment for clinical purposes. The authors and publisher disclaim all responsibility for any liability, loss, injury, or damage incurred as a consequence, directly or indirectly, of the use and application of any of the contents of this volume.

Publisher: Julie Levin Alexander
Publisher's Assistant: Regina Bruno
Executive Editor: Mark Cohen
Development Editor: Melissa Kerian
Assistant Editor: Nicole Ragonese
Managing Production Editor: Patrick Walsh
Production Liaison: Christina Zingone
Production Editor: Katie Boilard
Manufacturing Manager: Ilene Sanford
Manufacturing Buyer: Pat Brown
Creative Design Director: Christy Mahon
Senior Art Director: Maria Guglielmo
Director of Marketing: Karen Allman

Executive Marketing Manager: Katrin Beacom
Marketing Specialist: Michael Sirinides
Marketing Assistant: Lauren Castellano
Medical Illustrator: Anita Impagliazzo
Manager, Cover Visual Research & Permissions: Karen Sanatar
Composition: Pine Tree Composition, Inc.
Printer/Binder: Bind-Rite Graphics
Cover Printer: Phoenix Color Corp.
Cover Image: Getty Images, Inc./Allsport Photography

Pearson Education Ltd., London
Pearson Education Singapore, Pte. Ltd.
Pearson Education Canada, Inc.
Pearson Education–Japan
Pearson Education Australia PTY, Limited
Pearson Education North Asia, Ltd., Hong Kong
Pearson Educación de Mexico, S.A. de C.V.
Pearson Education Malaysia, Pte. Ltd.
Pearson Education, Upper Saddle River, New Jersey

10 9 8 7 6 5 4 3
978-0-13-501956-6
0-13-501956-7

The authors wish to dedicate this quick-reference
guide to our families, who supported us throughout
this project with their love and understanding.
Without their support, the process would have been
much more difficult and time-consuming.

THANKS!
Susan and Jim

CONTENTS

WELCOME TO
Medical Language STAT!

Medical Language STAT! is your new quick-reference guide to medical language.

Sometimes you need access to medical language information quickly—at the tip of your fingers. This is what *Medical Language STAT!* can do for you.

Handy to carry and easy to use whether you are a health care student in school or a health care professional on the job, *Medical Language STAT!* will quickly become your newest and best source of quick information.

The contents of *Medical Language STAT!* are drawn from the comprehensive, best-selling textbook *Medical Language*, but *Medical Language STAT!* also contains its own unique features!

Medical Language STAT! provides you with a quick and easy way to look up essential information related to medical language. Using this guide, you will be able to quickly

- Break down and build medical words
- Look up medical word parts and their definitions
- Locate medical word and phrase definitions
- Identify medical word synonyms
- Define medical abbreviations, acronyms, and symbols
- Analyze laboratory tests, values, and their meaning
- Classify drugs by drug category, therapeutic action, and drug name
- Distinguish between sound-alike medical words
- Review full-color illustrations of the anatomy of body systems.

This quick-reference guide works hard for you, so that you can concentrate on medical language in your studies or on the job. **Enjoy!**

ACKNOWLEDGMENTS

The authors wish to acknowledge Mark Cohen, Executive Editor for Health Professions at Pearson/Prentice Hall, for his expertise, creative insights, support, professionalism, and enthusiasm for *Medical Language STAT!* We also wish to thank Melissa Kerian, Development Editor, for expertly overseeing the details for this reference book.

The authors also wish to express their sincere thanks to medical illustrator Anita Impagliazzo for the use of her uniquely original anatomical medical illustrations that first appeared in the textbook *Medical Language* (Pearson/Prentice Hall, 2007).

We also wish to acknowledge the many teachers and students who will utilize this reference book. From the original concept all the way through to the final production, we kept you in mind, and our focus was on how to best meet your needs.

ABOUT THE AUTHORS

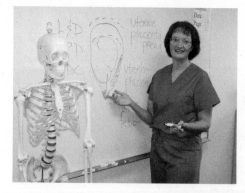

Susan M. Turley, MA (Educ.), BSN, RN, RHIT, CMT, is an adjunct professor in the School of Health Professions, Wellness, and Physical Education at Anne Arundel Community College in Arnold, Maryland, where she has taught medical terminology, human diseases, medical transcription, pharmacology, and medical office procedures. She is also the author of *Medical Language* (Pearson/Prentice Hall) and the fourth edition of *Understanding Pharmacology for Health Professionals* (Pearson/Prentice Hall).

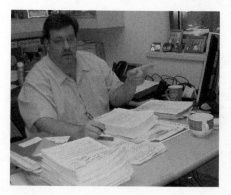

James F. Allen, Jr., RN, BSN, MBA/HCM, JD, is an adjunct professor in the Community Health Services Education Department at Lansing Community College, Lansing, Michigan, where he teaches health law & ethics, medical terminology, pharmacology–allied health, and pathophysiology.

medical
language
STAT!
A Quick-Reference Guide

Introduction to Medical Language

Break Down and Build Medical Words

This section provides an introduction to the essentials of medical language. It consists of four parts.

PART A: MEDICAL WORD PARTS AND CHARACTERISTICS

The characteristics of medical word parts are listed to explain how to break down medical words into word parts.

PART B: BUILDING MEDICAL WORDS

The building of medical words is reviewed to show how medical word parts are put together.

PART C: ANALYZING AND DEFINING MEDICAL WORDS

The rules associated with analyzing and defining medical words are provided to help you to learn quickly the meaning of a medical word.

PART D: MEDICAL WORD SINGULAR AND PLURAL NOUNS

There are specific rules for making medical word singular nouns into plural nouns. These rules are provided here to help you turn a singular noun into a plural noun.

PART A: MEDICAL WORD PARTS AND CHARACTERISTICS

Medical language is composed of medical words. Each medical word is composed of word parts. Word parts are the puzzle pieces that, when fit together, make up medical words. There are only three different kinds of word parts: combining forms, suffixes, and prefixes.

Characteristics of a Combining Form

- Every medical word contains a combining form.
- A combining form is the foundation of a medical word and gives the word its medical meaning.
- Sometimes a medical word contains two or more combining forms, one right after the other.
- Prefixes and suffixes modify the meaning of the combining form.
- A combining form is the first word part if there is no prefix. Otherwise, the combining form is positioned in the middle of a medical word between the prefix and the suffix.
- A combining form always ends with a hyphen to show that it is a word part, not a complete word. The hyphen is deleted when the combining form joins with a suffix.
- A combining form contains two parts: a root and a combining vowel (see Figure 1-1 ■). The root contains the medical meaning. The combining vowel allows the combining form to join with another word part. The root is separated from the combining vowel by a forward slash (/). The combining vowel is at the end of the combining form.

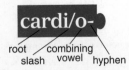

Figure 1-1 ■ Combining form. A combining form is the foundation of a medical word. A combining form contains a root, a combining vowel, a forward slash that separates the root from the combining vowel, and a hyphen at the end to show that the combining form is a word part, not a complete word. The combining form *cardi/o-* means *heart*.

Characteristics of a Suffix

- Every medical word contains a suffix.
- A suffix can be a single letter or a group of letters.
- A suffix cannot be the foundation of a medical word.
- A suffix is always positioned at the end of a medical word. Occasionally, a medical word contains two suffixes, one right after the other.
- A suffix attaches to the end of a combining form and modifies its meaning.
- A suffix always begins with a hyphen to show that it is a word part, not a complete word. The hyphen is deleted when the suffix joins the combining form (see Figure 1-2 ■).

Figure 1-2 ■ Suffix. A suffix always begins with a hyphen to show that it is a word part, not a complete word. The hyphen is deleted when the suffix joins the combining form. The suffix *-al* means *pertaining to.*

Characteristics of a Prefix

- Not every medical word contains a prefix. It is an optional word part.
- A prefix can be a single letter or a group of letters.
- A prefix cannot be the foundation of a medical word.
- When present, a prefix is always positioned at the beginning of a medical word. Occasionally, a medical word has two prefixes, one right after the other.
- A prefix attaches to the beginning of a combining form and modifies its meaning.
- A prefix always ends with a hyphen to show that it is a word part, not a complete word. The hyphen is deleted when the prefix joins the combining form (see Figure 1-3 ■).

Figure 1-3 ■ Prefix. A prefix always ends with a hyphen to show that it is a word part, not a complete word. The hyphen is deleted when the prefix joins the combining form. The prefix *peri-* means *around.*

If all three word parts are present in a medical word, their order is as follows: prefix, combining form, and then suffix (see Figure 1-4 ■).

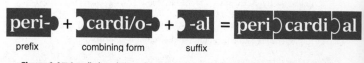

prefix   combining form   suffix

Figure 1-4 ■ A medical word. This prefix, combining form, and suffix can be combined to form a medical word. This medical word means *pertaining to around the heart.*

PART B: BUILDING MEDICAL WORDS

Combining Forms and Suffixes

Medical words are like puzzles, and their word parts are like the pieces of the puzzle. To build a medical word, you must put the word part puzzle pieces together in the correct way.

Follow these two simple rules for joining a combining form to a suffix to build a medical word.

1. If the suffix begins with a vowel, delete the combining vowel from the combining form. Delete the slash and hyphen from the combining form, delete the hyphen from the suffix, and then join the two word parts (see Figure 1-5 ■).

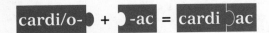

Figure 1-5 ■ Combining form plus a suffix that begins with a vowel. The combining form *cardi/o-* plus the suffix *-ac* equals the medical word *cardiac*. *Cardiac* means *pertaining to the heart.*

2. If the suffix begins with a consonant, keep the combining vowel on the combining form (see Figure 1-6 ■).

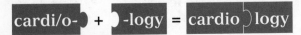

Figure 1-6 ■ Combining form plus a suffix that begins with a consonant. The combining form *cardi/o-* plus the suffix *-logy* equals the medical word *cardiology*. *Cardiology* means *study of the heart.*

Prefixes, Combining Forms, and Suffixes

Follow these two simple rules for joining a prefix to a combining form with suffix to make a medical word.

1. Delete the hyphen from the prefix (see Figure 1-7 ■). (*Note:* Some medical words, but not all, keep the hyphen if the last letter of the prefix is the same as the first letter of the combining form.)

2. Join the prefix to the beginning of the combining form.

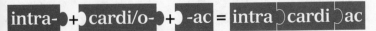

Figure 1-7 ■ Prefix plus a combining form plus a suffix. The prefix *intra-* plus the combining form *cardi/o-* plus the suffix *-ac* equals the medical word *intracardiac*. *Intracardiac* means *pertaining to within the heart.*

PART C: ANALYZING AND DEFINING MEDICAL WORDS

Combining Forms and Suffixes

When you analyze something, you break it into smaller pieces that are easier to understand. When you analyze a medical word, you break it into its component word parts. In order to define a medical word, you must first define each word part by giving its medical meaning. The meanings of all the word parts are then combined to give the definition of the entire medical word.

Follow these three simple rules to define a medical word that contains a combining form and a suffix.

1. Define each word part.

2. Then put the definitions of the word parts in order, beginning with the definition of the suffix, followed by the definition of the combining form.

3. Add small connecting words to make a correct and complete definition.

Example: To define the word *cardiac,* define the meaning of the suffix -ac (pertaining to) and then the meaning of the combining form *cardi/o-* (heart). Then put the definitions in order, beginning with the definition of the suffix. *Cardiac* means *pertaining to the heart.*

Analyzing and Defining Medical Words: Prefixes, Combining Forms, and Suffixes

Follow these three simple rules to define a medical word that contains a prefix, combining form, and a suffix.

1. Define each word part.

2. Put the definitions of the word parts in order, beginning with the suffix, followed by the prefix, and then the combining form.

3. Add small connecting words to make a correct and complete definition.

Example: To define the word *pericardial,* define the meaning of the suffix -*al* (pertaining to), then the meaning of the prefix *peri-* (around), and then the meaning of the combining form *cardi/o-* (heart). Then put the definitions in order, beginning with the definition of the suffix. *Pericardial* means *pertaining to around the heart.*

PART D: MEDICAL WORD SINGULAR AND PLURAL NOUNS

Because medical language contains so many Latin and Greek words, it is important to know how to make the plural forms of Latin and Greek nouns. The Latin and Greek languages had rules that governed how plural nouns were formed, and those rules still apply today.

Singular and Plural Noun Endings

Category	Singular Ending	How to Form the Plural	Example
Latin noun (feminine)	-a	Change -a to -ae	vertebra → vertebrae
Latin noun (masculine)	-us	Change -us to -i	nucleus → nuclei
Latin noun (neuter)	-um	Change -um to -a	atrium → atria bacterium → bacteria
Latin noun (other)	-is	Change -is to -es	diagnosis → diagnoses testis → testes
	-ex, -ix	Change -ex or -ix to -ices	helix → helices apex → apices
Greek noun	-nx	Change -nx to -nges	phalanx → phalanges
	-on	Change -on to -a	ganglion → ganglia
	-oma	Change -oma to -omata	carcinoma → carcinomata

Latin feminine, masculine, and neuter nouns have rules that govern the pronunciation of their singular and plural forms.

Pronunciation Guide for Latin Singular and Plural Nouns

Latin Feminine Singular	Latin Feminine Plural	Medical Meaning
bursa (BER-sah)	bursae (BER-see)	fluid-filled sac under a tendon
scapula (SKAP-yoo-lah)	scapulae (SKAP-yoo-lee)	shoulder blade
vertebra (VER-teh-brah)	vertebrae (VER-teh-bree)	bone in the spinal column

Latin Masculine Singular	Latin Masculine Plural	Medical Meaning
bronchus (BRONG-kus)	bronchi (BRONG-kigh)	air tube leading to the lung
musculus (MUS-kyoo-lus)	musculi (MUS-kyoo-lie)	Latin word for *muscle*

Latin Neuter Singular	Latin Neuter Plural	Medical Meaning
atrium (AA-tree-um)	atria (AA-tree-ah)	upper chamber of the heart
bacterium (bak-TEER-ee-um)	bacteria (bak-TEER-ee-ah)	microscopic disease-causing cell

Medical Word Parts and Definitions

Look Up Medical Word Parts and Their Definitions

Medical language is composed of medical words. Each medical word is composed of word parts. Each medical word part has a definition(s). Knowing what the medical word parts are and what their definitions are will assist you in understanding medical words quickly.

This section provides medical word parts commonly used in medical language. This section consists of two parts.

PART A: MEDICAL WORD PARTS AND DEFINITIONS

An alphabetical listing of medical word parts with their definitions is provided so that you can find quickly what a medical word part means.

PART B: DEFINITIONS AND MEDICAL WORD PARTS

An alphabetical listing in which the definition of the word part is provided first so that you can easily find what medical word parts go with that definition.

PART A: MEDICAL WORD PARTS AND DEFINITIONS

Word Part	Definition(s) of Word Part
A	
a-	away from; without
ab-	away from
abdomin/o-	abdomen
ablat/o-	take away; destroy
-able	able to be
abort/o-	stop prematurely
abras/o-	scrape off
absorpt/o-	absorb or take in
-ac	pertaining to
access/o-	supplemental or contributing part
accommod/o-	to adapt
acetabul/o-	acetabulum (hip socket)
acid/o-	acid (low pH)
acous/o-	hearing; sound
acr/o-	extremity; highest point
acromi/o-	acromion
actin/o-	rays of the sun
act/o-	action
acu/o-	needle; sharpness
-acusis	hearing
acus/o-	the sense of hearing
ad-	toward
-ad	toward; in the direction of
addict/o-	surrender to; be controlled by
-ade	action; process
aden/o-	gland
adhes/o-	to stick to
adip/o-	fat
adjuv/o-	giving help or assistance
adnex/o-	accessory connecting parts
adolesc/o-	the beginning of being an adult
adrenal/o-	adrenal gland
adren/o-	adrenal gland
affect/o-	state of mind; mood; to have an influence on
affer/o-	bring toward the center
agglutin/o-	clumping; sticking
aggreg/o-	crowding together
ag/o-	to lead to
agon/o-	causing action

Word Part	Definition(s) of Word Part
agor/a-	open area or space
-al	pertaining to
albin/o-	white
albumin/o-	albumin
alges/o-	sensation of pain
-algia	painful condition
alg/o-	pain
align/o-	arranged in a straight line
aliment/o-	food; nourishment
-alis	pertaining to
alkal/o-	base (high pH)
allerg/o-	allergy
all/o-	other; strange
alveol/o-	alveolus (air sac)
ambly/o-	dimness
ambulat/o-	walking
amnes/o-	forgetfulness
amni/o-	amnion (fetal membrane)
-amnios	amniotic fluid
amputat/o-	to cut off
amput/o-	to cut off
amygdal/o-	almond shape
amyl/o-	carbohydrate; starch
an-	without; not
-an	pertaining to
ana-	apart from; excessive
anabol/o-	building up
analy/o-	to separate
anastom/o-	unite two tubular structures
-ance	state of
ancill/o-	servant; accessory
-ancy	state of
andr/o-	male
aneurysm/o-	aneurysm (dilation)
angin/o-	angina
angi/o-	blood vessel; lymphatic vessel
anis/o-	unequal
ankyl/o-	fused together; stiff
an/o-	anus
ant-	against
-ant	pertaining to
antagon/o-	oppose or work against
ante-	forward; before
anter/o-	before; front part
anthrac/o-	coal

Word Part	*Definition(s) of Word Part*
anti-	against
anxi/o-	fear; worry
aort/o-	aorta
apher/o-	withdrawal
aphth/o-	ulcer
apic/o-	apex (tip)
apo-	away from
appendic/o-	appendix
appendicul/o-	limb; small attached part
append/o-	small structure hanging from a larger structure; appendix
appercept/o-	fully perceived
aque/o-	watery substance
-ar	pertaining to
arachn/o-	spider; spider web
-arche	a beginning
areol/o-	small area around the nipple
-arian	pertaining to a person
-aris	pertaining to
arteri/o-	artery
arteriol/o-	arteriole
arter/o-	artery
arthr/o-	joint
articul/o-	joint
-ary	pertaining to
asbest/o-	asbestos
ascit/o-	ascites
-ase	enzyme
aspir/o-	to breathe in; to suck in
asthm/o-	asthma
astr/o-	starlike structure
-ate	composed of; pertaining to
-ated	pertaining to a condition; composed of
atel/o-	incomplete
ather/o-	soft, fatty substance
atheromat/o-	fatty deposit or mass
athet/o-	without position or place
-atic	pertaining to
-ation	a process; being or having
-ative	pertaining to
-ator	person or thing that produces or does
-atory	pertaining to
atri/o-	atrium (upper heart chamber)

Word Part	Definition(s) of Word Part
attenu/o-	weakened
-ature	system composed of
audi/o-	the sense of hearing
audit/o-	the sense of hearing
augment/o-	increase in size or degree
aur/i-	ear
auricul/o-	ear
auscult/o-	listening
aut/o-	self
autonom/o-	independent; self-governing
axill/o-	axilla (armpit)
axi/o-	axis

B

bacteri/o-	bacterium
balan/o-	glans penis
bar/o-	weight
basil/o-	base of an organ
bas/o-	basic (alkaline); base of a structure
behav/o-	activity or manner of acting
bi-	two
bil/i-	bile; gall
bilirubin/o-	bilirubin
bi/o-	life; living organisms; living tissue
-blast	immature cell
blast/o-	immature; embryonic
blephar/o-	eyelid
-body	a structure or thing
botul/o-	sausage
brachi/o-	arm
brachy-	short
brady-	slow
bronchi/o-	bronchus
bronchiol/o-	bronchiole
bronch/o-	bronchus
brux/o-	to grind the teeth
buccinat/o-	cheek
bucc/o-	cheek
bulb/o-	like a bulb
bunion/o-	bunion
burs/o-	bursa

C

cac/o-	bad; poor
calcane/o-	calcaneus (heel bone)

Word Part	Definition(s) of Word Part
calc/i-	calcium
calcific/o-	hard from calcium
calc/o-	calcium
calcul/o-	stone
calic/o-	calix
cali/o-	calix
calor/o-	heat
cancell/o-	lattice structure
cancer/o-	cancer
candid/o-	*Candida* (a yeast)
can/o-	resembling a dog
capill/o-	hairlike structure; capillary
capn/o-	carbon dioxide
capsul/o-	capsule (enveloping structure)
carb/o-	carbon atoms
carbox/y-	carbon monoxide
carcin/o-	cancer
card/i-	heart
cardi/o-	heart
cari/o-	caries (tooth decay)
carot/o-	stupor; sleep
carp/o-	wrist
cartilagin/o-	cartilage
cata-	down
catabol/o-	breaking down
catheter/o-	catheter
caud/o-	tail; lower part of the body
caus/o-	burning
cavit/o-	hollow space
cav/o-	hollow space
cec/o-	cecum (first part of large intestine)
-cele	hernia
celi/o-	abdomen
cellul/o-	cell
-centesis	procedure to puncture
centr/o-	center; dominant part
cephal/o-	head
-cephalus	head
-ceps	head
-cere	waxy substance
cerebell/o-	cerebellum (posterior part of the brain)
cerebr/o-	cerebrum (largest part of the brain)
cervic/o-	neck; cervix
cheil/o-	lip

Word Part	Definition(s) of Word Part
chem/o-	chemical; drug
chez/o-	to pass feces
chir/o-	hand
chlor/o-	chloride
cholangi/o-	bile duct
chol/e-	bile; gall
cholecyst/o-	gallbladder
choledoch/o-	common bile duct
cholesterol/o-	cholesterol
chol/o-	bile; gall
chondri/o-	little granule
chondr/o-	cartilage
chori/o-	chorion (fetal membrane)
chorion/o-	chorion (fetal membrane)
choroid/o-	choroid (middle layer around the eye)
chrom/o-	color
chron/o-	time
cid/o-	killing
cili/o-	hairlike structure
cin/e-	movement
circa-	about
circulat/o-	movement in a circular route
circul/o-	circle
circum-	around
cirrh/o-	yellow
cis/o-	to cut
-clast	cell that breaks down substances
claudicat/o-	limping pain
claustr/o-	enclosed space
clavicul/o-	clavicle (collar bone)
clav/o-	clavicle (collar bone)
-cle	small thing
cleid/o-	clavicle (collar bone)
clinic/o-	medicine
clon/o-	rapid contracting and relaxing; identical group derived from one
-clonus	condition of rapid contracting and relaxing
-cnemius	leg
coagul/o-	clotting
coarct/o-	pressed together
cocc/o-	spherical bacterium
-coccus	spherical bacterium
coccyg/o-	coccyx (tail bone)
cochle/o-	cochlea (of the inner ear)

Word Part	Definition(s) of Word Part
cognit/o-	thinking
coit/o-	sexual intercourse
coll/a-	fibers that hold together
-collis	condition of the neck
col/o-	colon (part of large intestine)
colon/o-	colon (part of large intestine)
colp/o-	vagina
comat/o-	deep unconsciousness
comminut/o-	break into minute pieces
communic/o-	impart; transmit
compens/o-	counterbalance; compensate
compress/o-	press together
compromis/o-	exposed to danger
compuls/o-	drive or compel
con-	with
concept/o-	to conceive or form
concuss/o-	violent shaking or jarring
conduct/o-	carrying; conveying
conform/o-	having the same scale or angle
congenit/o-	present at birth
congest/o-	accumulation of fluid
coni/o-	dust
conjug/o-	joined together
conjunctiv/o-	conjunctiva
con/o-	cone
constip/o-	compacted feces
constrict/o-	drawn together; narrowed
construct/o-	to build
contin/o-	hold together
contra-	against
contract/o-	pull together
contus/o-	bruising
converg/o-	coming together
convuls/o-	seizure
copr/o-	feces; stool
corne/o-	cornea (of the eye)
cor/o-	pupil (of the eye)
coron/o-	encircling structure
corpor/o-	body
cortic/o-	cortex (outer region)
cosmet/o-	attractive; adorned
cost/o-	rib
crani/o-	cranium (skull)
-crasia	a mixing
-crine	a thing that secretes

Word Part	Definition(s) of Word Part
crin/o-	secrete
-crit	separation of
cry/o-	cold
crypt/o-	hidden
cubit/o-	elbow
culd/o-	cul-de-sac
cusp/o-	projection; point
cutane/o-	skin
cut/i-	skin
cyan/o-	blue
cycl/o-	ciliary body of the eye; cycle; circle
cyst/o-	bladder; fluid-filled sac; semisolid cyst
-cyte	cell
cyt/o-	cell

D

dacry/o-	lacrimal sac; tears
-dactyly	condition of fingers or toes
de-	reversal of; without
dec/i-	one tenth
decidu/o-	falling off
defici/o-	lacking; inadequate
degluti/o-	swallowing
delt/o-	triangle
delus/o-	false belief
dem/o-	people; population
dendr/o-	branching structure
densit/o-	density
dent/i-	tooth
dentit/o-	eruption of teeth
dent/o-	tooth
depend/o-	to hang onto
depress/o-	press down
derm/a-	skin
-derma	skin
dermat/o-	skin
derm/o-	skin
desicc/o-	to dry up
-desis	procedure to fuse together
dextr/o-	right
di-	two
dia-	complete; completely through
diabet/o-	diabetes
diaphore/o-	sweating
diaphragmat/o-	diaphragm

Word Part	Definition(s) of Word Part
diaphys/o-	shaft of a bone
diastol/o-	dilating
-didymis	testes (twin structures)
didym/o-	testes (twin structures)
dietet/o-	foods; diet
diet/o-	foods; diet
differentiat/o-	being distinct or specialized
different/o-	being distinct; different
digest/o-	break down food; digest
digit/o-	digit (finger or toe)
dilat/o-	dilate; widen
dipl/o-	double
dips/o-	thirst
dis-	away from
disk/o-	disk
dissect/o-	to cut apart
dissemin/o-	widely scattered throughout the body
distent/o-	distended; stretched
dist/o-	away from the center or point of origin
diverticul/o-	diverticulum
donat/o-	give as a gift
dors/o-	back; dorsum; uppermost part
-dose	measured quantity
dos/i-	dose
-drome	a running
duc/o-	bring or move
-duct	duct (tube)
duct/o-	bring or move; a duct
du/o-	two
duoden/o-	duodenum (first part of small intestine)
dur/o-	dura mater
dynam/o-	power; movement
dyn/o-	pain
dys-	painful; difficult; abnormal

E

e-	without; out
-eal	pertaining to
ec-	out; outward
ecchym/o-	blood in the tissues
ech/o-	echo (sound wave)
eclamps/o-	a seizure
-ectasis	condition of dilation
ectat/o-	dilation
ecto-	outermost; outside

Word Part	Definition(s) of Word Part
-ectomy	surgical excision
ectop/o-	outside of a place
-ed	pertaining to
-edema	swelling
edentul/o-	without teeth
-ee	person who is the object of an action
efface/o-	do away with; obliterate
effer/o-	go out from the center
effus/o-	a pouring out
ejaculat/o-	to expel suddenly
-elasma	platelike structure
elast/o-	flexing; stretching
electr/o-	electricity
elimin/o-	expel; remove
-elle	little thing
em-	in
-ema	condition
emaci/o-	to make thin
embol/o-	embolus (occluding plug)
embryon/o-	embryo; immature form
-emesis	vomiting
emet/o-	to vomit
-emia	condition of the blood; substance in the blood
-emic	pertaining to blood or a substance in the blood
emiss/o-	to send out
emot/o-	moving; stirring up
emulsific/o-	droplets of fat suspended in a liquid; particles suspended in a solution
en-	in; within; inward
-ence	state of
encephal/o-	brain
-encephaly	condition of the brain
-ency	condition of being
endo-	innermost; within
-ent	pertaining to
enter/o-	intestine
-entery	condition of the intestine
enucle/o-	to remove the kernal or nucleus
enur/o-	to urinate in
-eon	one who performs
eosin/o-	eosin (acidic red dye)
ependym/o-	lining membrane
epi-	upon; above
epilept/o-	seizure

Word Part	Definition(s) of Word Part
epiphys/o-	growth area at the end of a long bone
episi/o-	vulva (female external genitalia)
-er	person or thing that produces or does
erect/o-	to stand up
erg/o-	activity; work
-ergy	activity; process of working
erupt/o-	breaking out
-ery	process of
erythemat/o-	redness
erythr/o-	red
-esis	condition
es/o-	inward
esophag/o-	esophagus
esthes/o-	sensation; feeling
esthet/o-	sensation; feeling
estr/a-	female
estr/o-	female
ethm/o-	sieve
-etic	pertaining to
eti/o-	cause of disease
-ety	condition; state
etym/o-	word origin
eu-	normal; good
ex-	out; away from
exacerb/o-	increase; provoke
excis/o-	to cut out
excori/o-	to take out skin
excret/o-	removing from the body
exhibit/o-	showing
ex/o-	away from; external; outward
explorat/o-	to search out
express/o-	communicate
extens/o-	straightening
extern/o-	outside
extra-	outside of
extrins/o-	on the outside
exud/o-	oozing fluid

F	
faci/o-	face
factiti/o-	artificial; contrived
fallopi/o-	fallopian tube
fasci/o-	fascia
fec/o-	feces; stool

Word Part	Definition(s) of Word Part
femor/o-	femur (thigh bone)
fer/o-	to bear
ferrit/o-	iron
ferr/o-	iron
fertil/o-	able to conceive a child
fet/o-	fetus
fibrill/o-	muscle fiber; nerve fiber
fibrin/o-	fibrin
fibr/o-	fiber
fibul/o-	fibula (lower leg bone)
filtrat/o-	filtering; straining
filtr/o-	filter
fiss/o-	splitting
fixat/o-	to make stable or still
flatul/o-	flatus (gas)
flex/o-	bending
fluor/o-	fluorescence
-flux	flow
foc/o-	point of activity
foli/o-	leaf
follicul/o-	follicle (small sac)
foramin/o-	foramen (opening into a cavity or channel)
forens/o-	court proceedings in criminal law
-form	having the form of
format/o-	structure; arrangement
fove/o-	small, depressed area
fract/o-	break up
fratern/o-	close association or relationship
-frice	thing that produces friction
front/o-	front
fruct/o-	fruit
fulgur/o-	spark of electricity
fund/o-	fundus (part farthest from the opening)
fundu/o-	fundus (part farthest from the opening)
fung/o-	fungus
fus/o-	pouring
G	
galact/o-	milk
ganglion/o-	ganglion
gangren/o-	gangrene
gastr/o-	stomach
gemin/o-	twins; set or group
-gen	that which produces
-gene	gene

Word Part	Definition(s) of Word Part
gene/o-	gene
gener/o-	production; creation
genit/o-	genitalia
gen/o-	arising from; produced by
germin/o-	embryonic tissue
ger/o-	old age
gestat/o-	from conception to birth
gest/o-	from conception to birth
gigant/o-	giant
gingiv/o-	gums
glandul/o-	gland
glen/o-	socket of a joint
-glia	substance that holds things together
gli/o-	substance that holds things together
glob/o-	shaped like a globe; comprehensive
globul/o-	shaped like a globe
glomerul/o-	glomerulus
gloss/o-	tongue
glott/o-	glottis (of the larynx)
gluc/o-	glucose (sugar)
glycer/o-	glycerol (sugar alcohol)
glyc/o-	glucose (sugar)
glycos/o-	glucose (sugar)
gnos/o-	knowledge
gonad/o-	gonads (ovaries and testes)
goni/o-	angle
gon/o-	seed (ovum or spermatozoon)
-grade	going
-graft	tissue for implant or transplant
-gram	a record or picture
granul/o-	granule
-graph	instrument used to record
graph/o-	record
-graphy	process of recording
-gravida	pregnancy
gustat/o-	the sense of taste
gynec/o-	female; woman

H

habilitat/o-	give ability
halit/o-	breath
hallucin/o-	imagined perception
hal/o-	breathe
hebe/o-	youth
hec/o-	habitual condition of the body

Word Part	Definition(s) of Word Part
hedon/o-	pleasure
helic/o-	a coil
hemat/o-	blood
hemi-	one half
hem/o-	blood
hemoglobin/o-	hemoglobin
hemorrh/o-	a flowing of blood
hemorrhoid/o-	hemorrhoid
hepat/o-	liver
heredit/o-	genetic inheritance
hered/o-	genetic inheritance
herni/o-	hernia
heter/o-	other
hex/o-	habitual condition of the body
hidr/o-	sweat
hil/o-	hilum (indentation in an organ)
hirsut/o-	hairy
histi/o-	tissue
home/o-	same
hom/i-	man
horizont/o-	boundary between the earth and sky
hormon/o-	hormone
humer/o-	humerus (upper arm bone)
hyal/o-	clear, glasslike substance
hydatidi/o-	fluid-filled vesicles
hydr/o-	water; fluid
hygien/o-	health
hy/o-	U-shaped structure
hyper-	above; more than normal
hypn/o-	sleep
hypo-	below; deficient
hypophys/o-	pituitary gland
hyster/o-	uterus (womb)

I

-ia	condition; state; thing
-iac	pertaining to
-ial	pertaining to
-ian	pertaining to
-ias	condition
-iasis	state of; process of
-iatic	pertaining to a state or process
iatr/o-	physician; medical treatment
-iatry	medical treatment

Word Part	Definition(s) of Word Part
-ic	pertaining to
-ical	pertaining to
-ician	a skilled professional or expert
-ics	knowledge; practice
icter/o-	jaundice
ict/o-	seizure
-id	resembling; source or origin
-ide	chemically modified structure
idi/o-	unknown; individual
-ie	a thing
-il	a thing
-ile	pertaining to
ile/o-	ileum (third part of small intestine)
ili/o-	ilium (hip bone)
-ility	having the quality of
illus/o-	false perception
im-	not
-immune	immune response
immun/o-	immune response
impact/o-	wedged in
implant/o-	placed within
in-	in; within; not
-in	a substance
incarcer/o-	to imprison
incis/o-	to cut into
incud/o-	incus (anvil-shaped bone)
induct/o-	a leading in
-ine	substance pertaining to
infarct/o-	area of dead tissue
infect/o-	disease within
infer/o-	below
inflammat/o-	redness and warmth
infra-	below; beneath
-ing	doing
inguin/o-	groin
inhibit/o-	block; hold back
inject/o-	insert or put in
insemin/o-	plant a seed
insert/o-	to put in or introduce
inspect/o-	looking at
insulin/o-	insulin
insul/o-	island
integument/o-	skin
integu/o-	to cover

Word Part	Definition(s) of Word Part
inter-	between
intern/o-	inside
interstiti/o-	spaces within tissue
intestin/o-	intestine
intra-	within
intrins/o-	on the inside
intussuscep/o-	to receive within
invas/o-	to go into
involut/o-	enlarged organ returns to normal size
iodin/o-	iodine
iod/o-	iodine
-ion	action; condition
-ior	pertaining to
-ious	pertaining to
irid/o-	iris (colored part of the eye)
ir/o-	iris (colored part of the eye)
ischi/o-	ischium (hip bone)
isch/o-	keep back; block
-ism	process; disease from a specific cause
-ist	one who specializes in
-istic	pertaining to
-istry	process related to the specialty of
-isy	condition of inflammation
-ite	thing that pertains to
-itian	a skilled professional or expert
-itic	pertaining to
-ition	condition of having
-itis	inflammation of
-ity	state; condition
-ium	a chemical element; a structure
-ive	pertaining to
-ix	a structure
-ization	process of making, creating, or inserting
-ize	affecting in a particular way
-izer	thing that affects in a particular way

J

jejun/o-	jejunum (middle part of small intestine)
jugul/o-	jugular (throat)

K

kal/i-	potassium
kary/o-	nucleus
kel/o-	tumor

Word Part	Definition(s) of Word Part
kerat/o-	cornea (of the eye); hard, fibrous protein
ket/o-	ketones
keton/o-	ketones
-kine	movement
-kinesis	condition of movement
kines/o-	movement
kin/o-	movement
klept/o-	to steal
kyph/o-	bent; humpbacked

L	
labi/o-	lip; labium
laborat/o-	workplace; testing place
labyrinth/o-	labyrinth (in the inner ear)
lacer/o-	a tearing
lacrim/o-	tears
lact/i-	milk
lact/o-	milk
-lalia	condition of speech
lamin/o-	lamina (flat area on the vertebra)
lapar/o-	abdomen
laryng/o-	larynx (voice box)
later/o-	side
lei/o-	smooth
lenticul/o-	lens (of the eye)
lent/o-	lens (of the eye)
-lepsy	seizure
leuk/o-	white
lev/o-	left
lex/o-	word
ligament/o-	ligament
ligat/o-	to tie up or bind
limb/o-	edge; border
lingu/o-	tongue
lipid/o-	lipid (fat)
lip/o-	lipid (fat)
-lith	stone
lith/o-	stone
lob/o-	lobe of an organ
locat/o-	a place
loc/o-	in one place
log/o-	word; the study of
-logy	the study of
lord/o-	swayback

Word Part	Definition(s) of Word Part
luc/o-	clear and shining
lumb/o-	lower back; area between the ribs and pelvis
lumin/o-	lumen (opening)
lun/o-	moon
-ly	going toward
lymph/o-	lymph; lymphatic system
ly/o-	break down; separate; dissolve
-lysis	abnormal condition; process of breaking down or dissolving
lys/o-	break down or dissolve
-lyte	dissolved substance

M	
macr/o-	large
macul/o-	small area or spot
magnet/o-	magnet
mal-	bad; inadequate
-malacia	condition of softening
malac/o-	softening
malign/o-	intentionally causing harm; cancer
malle/o-	malleus (hammer-shaped bone)
malleol/o-	malleolus
mamm/a-	breast
mamm/o-	breast
mandibul/o-	mandible (lower jaw)
-mania	condition of frenzy
man/o-	thin
manu/o-	hand
masset/o-	chewing
mastic/o-	chewing
mast/o-	breast; mastoid process
mastoid/o-	mastoid process
matur/o-	mature
maxill/o-	maxilla (upper jaw)
mediastin/o-	mediastinum
medic/o-	physician; medicine
medi/o-	middle
medull/o-	medulla (inner region)
meg/a-	large
megal/o-	large
-megaly	enlargement
melan/o-	black
melen/o-	black
meningi/o-	meninges

Word Part	Definition(s) of Word Part
mening/o-	meninges
menisc/o-	meniscus (crescent-shaped cartilage)
men/o-	month
menstru/o-	monthly discharge of blood
-ment	action; state
ment/o-	mind; chin
mesenter/o-	mesentery
mesi/o-	middle
meso-	middle
meta-	after; subsequent to; transition; change
metabol/o-	change; transformation
-meter	instrument used to measure
metri/o-	uterus (womb)
metr/o-	measurement; uterus (womb)
-metry	process of measuring
micr/o-	small; one millionth
micturi/o-	making urine
mid-	middle
-mileusis	process of carving
mineral/o-	mineral; electrolyte
mi/o-	lessening
mit/o-	threadlike structure
mitr/o-	structure like a miter (tall hat with 2 points)
mitt/o-	to send
mon/o-	one; single
morbid/o-	disease
morb/o-	disease
morph/o-	shape
mort/o-	death
mot/o-	movement
-motor	thing that produces movement
muc/o-	mucus
mucos/o-	mucous membrane
mult/i-	many
muscul/o-	muscle
mutat/o-	to change
myc/o-	fungus
mydr/o-	widening
myelin/o-	myelin
myel/o-	bone marrow; spinal cord; myelin
my/o-	muscle
myop/o-	near

Word Part	Definition(s) of Word Part
myos/o-	muscle
myring/o-	tympanic membrane (eardrum)
myx/o-	mucus-like substance

N

narc/o-	stupor; sleep
nas/o-	nose
-nate	born
nat/o-	birth
nause/o-	nausea
necr/o-	death
ne/o-	new
nephr/o-	kidney; nephron
nerv/o-	nerve
neur/o-	nerve
neutr/o-	not taking part
nid/o-	nest; focus
-nine	pertaining to a single chemical substance
noct/o-	night
nod/o-	node (knob of tissue)
nodul/o-	small, knobby mass
non-	not
norm/o-	normal; usual
nuch/o-	neck; nape of neck
nucle/o-	nucleus (of a cell or an atom)
nucleol/o-	nucleolus
null/i-	none
nutri/o-	nourishment
nutriti/o-	nourishment

O

obes/o-	fat
obsess/o-	besieged by thoughts
obstetr/o-	pregnancy and childbirth
obstip/o-	severe constipation
obstruct/o-	blocked by a barrier
occipit/o-	occiput (back of the head)
occlus/o-	close against
ocul/o-	eye
odont/o-	tooth
odyn/o-	pain
-oid	resembling
-ol	chemical substance
-ole	small thing

Word Part	Definition(s) of Word Part
olfact/o-	the sense of smell
olig/o-	scanty
olisthe/o-	slipping
-olisthesis	abnormal condition and process of slipping
-oma	tumor; mass
-omatosis	abnormal condition of multiple tumors or masses
oment/o-	omentum
om/o-	tumor; mass
omphal/o-	umbilicus; navel
-on	a substance; structure
onc/o-	tumor; mass
-one	chemical substance
onych/o-	nail
o/o-	ovum (egg)
oophor/o-	ovary
operat/o-	perform a procedure; surgery
ophidi/o-	snake
ophthalm/o-	eye
-opia	condition of vision
opportun/o-	well timed; taking advantage of an opportunity
oppos/o-	forceful resistance
-opsy	process of viewing
optic/o-	lenses; properties of light
opt/o-	eye; vision
-or	person or thing that produces or does
orbicul/o-	small circle
orbit/o-	orbit (eye socket)
orchi/o-	testis
orch/o-	testis
orex/o-	appetite
organ/o-	organ
or/o-	mouth
orth/o-	straight
-ory	having the function of
-ose	full of
-osing	a condition of doing
-osis	condition; abnormal condition; process
osm/o-	the sense of smell
osse/o-	bone
ossicul/o-	ossicle (little bone)
ossificat/o-	changing into bone
oste/o-	bone
ot/o-	ear
oure/o-	urine

Word Part	Definition(s) of Word Part
-ous	pertaining to
ovari/o-	ovary
ov/i-	ovum (egg)
ov/o-	ovum (egg)
ovul/o-	ovum (egg)
ox/i-	oxygen
ox/o-	oxygen
ox/y-	oxygen; quick

P

palat/o-	palate
palliat/o-	reduce the severity of
palpat/o-	touching; feeling
palpit/o-	to throb
pan-	all
pancreat/o-	pancreas
papill/o-	elevated structure
par-	beside
para-	beside; apart from; two parts of a pair; abnormal
parenchym/o-	parenchyma (functional cells of an organ)
-paresis	weakness
pareun/o-	sexual intercourse
pariet/o-	wall of a cavity
par/o-	birth
paroxysm/o-	sudden, sharp attack
part/o-	childbirth
-partum	childbirth
parturit/o-	to be in labor
patell/o-	patella (kneecap)
-path	disease; suffering
pathet/o-	suffering
path/o-	disease; suffering
-pathy	disease; suffering
pat/o-	to lie open
-pause	cessation
paus/o-	cessation
pect/o-	stiff
pector/o-	chest
pedicul/o-	lice
ped/o-	child
pelv/i-	pelvis (hip bone; renal pelvis)
pelv/o-	pelvis (hip bone; renal pelvis)
pendul/o-	hanging down

Word Part	Definition(s) of Word Part
-penia	condition of deficiency
pen/o-	penis
pepsin/o-	pepsin
peps/o-	digestion
peptid/o-	peptide (two amino acids)
pept/o-	digestion
per-	through; throughout
percuss/o-	tapping
perfor/o-	to have an opening
peri-	around
perine/o-	perineum
peripher/o-	outer aspects
peritone/o-	peritoneum
periton/o-	peritoneum
perone/o-	fibula (lower leg bone)
person/o-	person
petechi/o-	petechiae
-pexy	process of surgically fixing in place
phac/o-	lens (of the eye)
-phage	thing that eats
phag/o-	eating; swallowing
phak/o-	lens (of the eye)
phalang/o-	phalanx (finger or toe)
pharmaceutic/o-	medicine; drug
pharmac/o-	medicine; drug
pharyng/o-	pharynx (throat)
-pharynx	pharynx (throat)
phas/o-	speech
phe/o-	gray
-phil	attraction to; fondness for
-phile	person who is attracted to or fond of
phil/o-	attraction to; fondness for
phleb/o-	vein
phob/o-	fear or avoidance
phor/o-	to bear; to carry; range
phosph/o-	phosphorus
phot/o-	light
phren/o-	diaphragm; mind
phylact/o-	guarding or protecting
-phylaxis	condition of guarding or protecting
-phyma	tumor; growth
physic/o-	body
physi/o-	physical function

Word Part	Definition(s) of Word Part
-physis	state of growing
phys/o-	inflate or distend; grow
-phyte	growth
pigment/o-	pigment
pil/o-	hair
pituitar/o-	pituitary gland
pituit/o-	pituitary gland
placent/o-	placenta
plak/o-	plaque
-plasm	growth; formed substance
plasm/o-	plasma; formed substance
-plant	procedure to transfer or graft
plas/o-	growth; formation
plast/o-	growth; formation
-plasty	process of reshaping by surgery
-plegia	condition of paralysis
pleg/o-	paralysis
pleur/o-	pleura (lung membrane)
-plex	parts
-pnea	breathing
pne/o-	breathing
pneum/o-	lung; air
pneumon/o-	lung; air
pod/o-	foot
-poiesis	condition of formation
-poietin	a substance that forms
poikil/o-	irregular
polar/o-	two opposite poles
pol/o-	pole
poly-	many; much
polyp/o-	polyp
poplite/o-	back of the knee
por/o-	small openings; pores
port/o-	point of entry
post-	after; behind
poster/o-	back part
potent/o-	being capable of doing
pract/o-	medical practice
pre-	before; in front of
pregn/o-	being with child
presby/o-	old age
press/o-	pressure
preventat/o-	prevent
prevent/o-	prevent

Word Part	Definition(s) of Word Part
prim/i-	first
pro-	before
-probe	rodlike instrument
proct/o-	rectum and anus
product/o-	produce
project/o-	throw forward
pronat/o-	lying face down
prostat/o-	prostate gland
prosthet/o-	artificial part
protein/o-	protein
prote/o-	protein
proxim/o-	near the center or point of origin
prurit/o-	itching
psor/o-	itching
psych/o-	mind
-ptosis	state of prolapse or drooping; falling
-ptysis	abnormal condition of coughing up
puber/o-	growing up
pub/o-	pubis (hip bone)
pulmon/o-	lung
pulsat/o-	rhythmic throbbing
punct/o-	hole; perforation
pupill/o-	pupil (of the eye)
purul/o-	pus
pyel/o-	renal pelvis
pylor/o-	pylorus
py/o-	pus
pyret/o-	fever
pyr/o-	fire; burning

Q	
quadri-	four
quantitat/o-	quantity or amount

R	
radic/o-	all parts, including the root
radicul/o-	spinal nerve root
radi/o-	radius (forearm bone); x-rays; radiation
rap/o-	to seize and drag away
re-	again and again; backward; unable to
react/o-	reverse movement
recept/o-	receive
recess/o-	to move back
rect/o-	rectum

Word Part	Definition(s) of Word Part
recuper/o-	recover
reduct/o-	to bring back; decrease
refract/o-	bend or deflect
regurgitat/o-	flow backward
relax/o-	relax
remiss/o-	send back
ren/o-	kidney
repress/o-	press back
resect/o-	to cut out and remove
resist/o-	withstand the effect of
resuscit/o-	revive or raise up again
retard/o-	to slow down or delay
retent/o-	keep; hold back
reticul/o-	small network
retin/o-	retina (of the eye)
retro-	behind; backward
rex/o-	appetite
rhabd/o-	rod shaped
rheumat/o-	watery discharge
rhin/o-	nose
rhiz/o-	spinal nerve root
rhythm/o-	rhythm
rhytid/o-	wrinkle
rib/o-	ribonucleic acid
roentgen/o-	x-rays; radiation
rotat/o-	rotate
-rrhage	excessive flow or discharge
rrhag/o-	excessive flow or discharge
-rrhaphy	procedure of suturing
-rrhea	flow; discharge
rrhe/o-	flow; discharge
rrhythm/o-	rhythm
-rubin	red substance
rub/o-	red
rug/o-	ruga (fold)

S

sacchar/o-	sugar
sacr/o-	sacrum
sagitt/o-	going from front to back
saliv/o-	saliva
salping/o-	fallopian tube
-salpinx	fallopian tube
saphen/o-	standing

Word Part	Definition(s) of Word Part
sarc/o-	connective tissue
satur/o-	filled up
scal/o-	series of graduated steps
scaph/o-	boat shaped
scapul/o-	scapula (shoulder blade)
schiz/o-	split
scient/o-	science; knowledge
scint/i-	point of light
scintill/o-	point of light
scler/o-	hard; sclera (white of the eye)
scoli/o-	curved; crooked
-scope	instrument used to examine
scop/o-	examine with an instrument
-scopy	process of using an instrument to examine
scot/o-	darkness
script/o-	write
scrot/o-	a bag; scrotum
sebace/o-	sebum (oil)
seb/o-	sebum (oil)
secret/o-	produce; secrete
sect/o-	to cut
sedat/o-	to calm agitation
semi-	half; partly
semin/i-	spermatozoon; sperm
semin/o-	spermatozoon; sperm
sen/o-	old age
sensitiv/o-	affected by; sensitive to
sensit/o-	affected by; sensitive to
sens/o-	sensation
sensor/i-	sensory
septic/o-	infection
sept/o-	septum (dividing wall)
ser/o-	serum of the blood; serumlike fluid
sex/o-	sex
sial/o-	saliva; salivary gland
sigmoid/o-	sigmoid colon
sin/o-	hollow cavity; channel
sinus/o-	sinus
-sis	condition; abnormal condition
skelet/o-	skeleton
soci/o-	human beings; community
somat/o-	body
-some	a body
somn/o-	sleep

Word Part	Definition(s) of Word Part
som/o-	a body
son/o-	sound
sorb/o-	to suck up
-spasm	sudden, involuntary muscle contraction
spasm/o-	spasm
spasmod/o-	spasm
spast/o-	spasm
spermat/o-	spermatozoon; sperm
sperm/o-	spermatozoon; sperm
sphen/o-	wedge shape
sphenoid/o-	sphenoid bone or sinus
-sphere	sphere or ball
spher/o-	sphere or ball
sphincter/o-	sphincter
sphygm/o-	pulse
spin/o-	spine; backbone
spir/o-	breathe; a coil
splen/o-	spleen
spondyl/o-	vertebra
squam/o-	scalelike cell
stal/o-	contraction
-stalsis	process of contraction
staped/o-	stapes (stirrup-shaped bone)
-stasis	condition of standing still; staying in one place
stas/o-	standing still; staying in one place
stat/o-	standing still; staying in one place
steat/o-	fat
sten/o-	narrowness; constriction
stere/o-	three dimensions
stern/o-	sternum (breast bone)
-steroid	steroid
steroid/o-	steroid
-sterol	lipid-containing compound
steth/o-	chest
sthen/o-	strength
stigmat/o-	point; mark
stimul/o-	exciting; strengthening
stomat/o-	mouth
stom/o-	surgically created opening or mouth
-stomy	surgically created opening
strangul/o-	to constrict
strept/o-	curved
stress/o-	disturbing stimulus
styl/o-	stake

Word Part	Definition(s) of Word Part
sub-	below; underneath; less than
sucr/o-	sugar (cane sugar)
suct/o-	to suck
sudor/i-	sweat
su/i-	self
super-	above; beyond
superfici/o-	on or near the surface
super/o-	above
supinat/o-	lying on the back
supposit/o-	placed beneath
suppress/o-	press down
suppur/o-	pus formation
supra-	above
surg/o-	operative procedure
suspens/o-	hanging
sym-	together; with
symptomat/o-	collection of symptoms
syn-	together
syncop/o-	fainting
synovi/o-	synovium (membrane)
synov/o-	synovium (membrane)
system/o-	the body as a whole
-systole	contracting
systol/o-	contracting

T

tachy-	fast
tact/o-	touch
tampon/o-	stop up
tard/o-	late; slow
tars/o-	ankle
tax/o-	coordination
techn/o-	technical skill
tele/o-	distance
tempor/o-	temple (side of the head)
tendin/o-	tendon
tendon/o-	tendon
ten/o-	tendon
tens/o-	pressure; tension
terat/o-	bizarre form
termin/o-	end; boundary
testicul/o-	testis; testicle
tetr/a-	four
thalam/o-	thalamus

Word Part	Definition(s) of Word Part
thanat/o-	death
thec/o-	sheath or layers of membranes
theli/o-	cellular layer
therapeut/o-	treatment
therap/o-	treatment
-therapy	treatment
therm/o-	heat
thorac/o-	thorax (chest)
-thorax	thorax (chest)
thromb/o-	thrombus (blood clot)
thym/o-	thymus; rage
thyr/o-	shield-shaped structure (thyroid gland)
thyroid/o-	thyroid gland
tibi/o-	tibia (shin bone)
-tic	pertaining to
till/o-	to pull out
-tion	a process; being or having
toc/o-	labor and childbirth
toler/o-	to become accustomed to
-tome	instrument used to cut; an area with distinct edges
tom/o-	cut; slice; layer
-tomy	process of cutting or making an incision
ton/o-	pressure; tone
tonsill/o-	tonsil
-tope	place; position
topic/o-	a specific area
-tor	person or thing that produces or does
tort/i-	twisted position
-tous	pertaining to
toxic/o-	poison; toxin
tox/o-	poison
trabecul/o-	trabecula (mesh)
trache/o-	trachea (windpipe)
trac/o-	visible path
tract/o-	pulling
tranquil/o-	calm
trans-	across; through
transit/o-	changing over from one thing to another
transplant/o-	move something to another place
traumat/o-	injury
tremul/o-	shaking
-tresia	opening or hole
tri-	three
trich/o-	hair

Word Part	Definition(s) of Word Part
trigemin/o-	threefold
triglycerid/o-	triglyceride
-tripsy	the process of crushing
-triptor	thing that crushes
trochanter/o-	trochanter
trochle/o-	structure shaped like a pulley
-tron	instrument
troph/o-	development
-trophy	process of development
trop/o-	having an affinity for; stimulating; turning
tubercul/o-	nodule; tuberculosis
tuber/o-	nodule
tuberos/o-	knoblike projection
tub/o-	tube
tubul/o-	tube; small tube
turbin/o-	scroll-like structure; turbinate
tuss/o-	cough
-ty	quality or state
tympan/o-	tympanic membrane (eardrum)
-type	particular kind of; a model of

U

Word Part	Definition(s) of Word Part
-ual	pertaining to
-ula	small thing
-ular	pertaining to something small
ulcerat/o-	ulcer
-ule	small thing
uln/o-	ulna (forearm bone)
ultra-	beyond; higher
-um	a structure
umbilic/o-	umbilicus; navel
un-	not
ungu/o-	nail (fingernail; toenail)
uni-	single; not paired
-ure	system; result of
ureter/o-	ureter
urethr/o-	urethra
urin/o-	urine; urinary system
ur/o-	urine; urinary system
uter/o-	uterus (womb)
uve/o-	uvea (of the eye)

V

Word Part	Definition(s) of Word Part
vaccin/o-	giving a vaccine
vagin/o-	vagina

Word Part	Definition(s) of Word Part
vag/o-	vagus nerve
valv/o-	valve
valvul/o-	valve
varic/o-	varix; varicose vein
vascul/o-	blood vessel
vas/o-	blood vessel; vas deferens
vegetat/o-	growth
veget/o-	vegetable
venere/o-	sexual intercourse
ven/i-	vein
ven/o-	vein
ventilat/o-	movement of air
ventil/o-	movement of air
vent/o-	a coming
ventricul/o-	ventricle (lower heart chamber; chamber in the brain)
ventr/o-	front; abdomen
verd/o-	green
-verse	to travel; to turn
vers/o-	to travel; to turn
vertebr/o-	vertebra
vert/o-	to travel; to turn
vesic/o-	bladder; fluid-filled sac
vesicul/o-	bladder; fluid-filled sac
vestibul/o-	vestibule (entrance)
vest/o-	to dress
viril/o-	masculine
vir/o-	virus
viscer/o-	viscera (internal organs)
viscos/o-	thickness
vis/o-	sight; vision
vitre/o-	vitreous humor; transparent substance
voc/o-	voice
volunt/o-	done of one's own free will
vuls/o-	to tear away
vulv/o-	vulva

W–Z

xanth/o-	yellow
xen/o-	foreign
xer/o-	dry
xiph/o-	sword
-zoon	animal; living thing
zygomat/o-	zygoma (cheek bone)

PART B: DEFINITIONS AND MEDICAL WORD PARTS

Definition of Word Part	Word Part
A	
abdomen	**abdomin/o-**
	celi/o-
	lapar/o-
	ventr/o-
able to be	**-able**
able to conceive a child	**fertil/o-**
abnormal	**dys-**
	para-
abnormal condition	**-lysis**
	-osis
	-sis
abnormal condition of coughing up	**-ptysis**
abnormal condition of multiple masses or tumors	**-omatosis**
abnormal condition or process of slipping	**-olisthesis**
about	**circa-**
above	**epi-**
	hyper-
	super-
	super/o-
	supra-
absorb	**absorpt/o-**
accessory	**ancill/o-**
accessory connecting parts	**adnex/o-**
accumulation of fluid	**congest/o-**
acetabulum (hip socket)	**acetabul/o-**
acid (low pH)	**acid/o-**
acidic red dye (eosin)	**eosin/o-**
acromion	**acromi/o-**
across	**trans-**
action	**act/o-**
	-ade
	-ion
	-ment
activity	**erg/o-**
	-ergy
activity or manner of acting	**behav/o-**
adapt	**accommod/o-**
adorned	**cosmet/o-**
adrenal gland	**adrenal/o-**
	adren/o-

Definition of Word Part	Word Part
adult beginning	adolesc/o-
affected by	sensitiv/o-
	sensit/o-
affecting in a particular way	-ize
affects in a particular way, a thing that	-izer
after	meta-
	post-
again and again	re-
against	ant-
	anti-
	contra-
air	pneum/o-
	pneumon/o-
air movement	ventilat/o-
	ventil/o-
air sac (alveolus)	alveol/o-
albumin	albumin/o-
all	pan-
all parts, including the root	radic/o-
allergy	allerg/o-
almond shape	amygdal/o-
alveolus (air sac)	alveol/o-
amino acids of which there are two (peptide)	peptid/o-
amnion (fetal membrane)	amni/o-
amniotic fluid	-amnios
amount	quantitat/o-
aneurysm (dilation)	aneurysm/o-
angina	angin/o-
angle	goni/o-
animal	-zoon
ankle	tars/o-
anus	an/o-
anus and rectum	proct/o-
anvil-shaped bone (incus)	incud/o-
aorta	aort/o-
apart from	ana-
	para-
apex	apic/o-
appendix	appendic/o-
	append/o-
appetite	orex/o-
area between the posterior ribs and pelvis	lumb/o-
area of dead tissue	infarct/o-

Definition of Word Part	Word Part
area that is open	agor/a-
area that is small	macul/o-
area with distinct edges	-tome
arising from	gen/o-
arm	brachi/o-
armpit (axilla)	axill/o-
around	circum-
	peri-
arranged in a straight line	align/o-
arrangement	format/o-
arteriole	arteriol/o-
artery	arteri/o-
	arter/o-
artificial	factiti/o-
artificial part	prosthet/o-
asbestos	asbest/o-
ascites	ascit/o-
assistance	adjuv/o-
asthma	asthm/o-
atrium (upper heart chamber)	atri/o-
attached part that is small	appendicul/o-
attack that is sudden and sharp	paroxysm/o-
attraction to	-phil
	phil/o-
attractive	cosmet/o-
avoidance	phob/o-
away from	a-
	ab-
	apo-
	dis-
	ex-
	ex/o-
away from the center	dist/o-
away from the point of origin	dist/o-
axilla (armpit)	axill/o-
axis	axi/o-

B

back	dors/o-
back-laying position	supinat/o-
back of the head (occiput)	occipit/o-
back of the knee	poplite/o-
back part	poster/o-
backbone	spin/o-

Definition of Word Part	Word Part
backward	re-
	retro-
backward flow	regurgitat/o-
bacterium	bacteri/o-
bad	cac/o-
	mal-
bag	scrot/o-
ball	-sphere
	spher/o-
barrier that is blocking	obstruct/o-
base (high pH)	alkal/o-
base of a structure	bas/o-
base of an organ	basil/o-
basic (alkaline)	bas/o-
be controlled by	addict/o-
bear	fer/o-
	phor/o-
become accustomed to	toler/o-
before	ante-
	anter/o-
	pre-
	pro-
beginning	-arche
beginning of being an adult	adolesc/o-
behind	post-
	retro-
being capable of doing	potent/o-
being distinct	differentiat/o-
	different/o-
being or having	-ation
	-tion
being specialized	differentiat/o-
being with child	pregn/o-
belief that is false	delus/o-
below	hypo-
	infer/o-
	infra-
	sub-
bend	refract/o-
bending	flex/o-
beneath	infra-
bent	kyph/o-
beside	par-
	para-

Definition of Word Part	Word Part
besieged by thoughts	**obsess/o-**
between	**inter-**
between the posterior ribs and pelvis area	**lumb/o-**
beyond	**super-**
	ultra-
bile	**bil/i-**
	chol/e-
	chol/o-
bile duct	**cholangi/o-**
bile duct (common bile duct)	**choledoch/o-**
bilirubin	**bilirubin/o-**
bind	**ligat/o-**
birth	**nat/o-**
	par/o-
bizarre form	**terat/o-**
black	**melan/o-**
	melen/o-
bladder	**cyst/o-**
	vesic/o-
	vesicul/o-
block	**inhibit/o-**
	isch/o-
blocked by a barrier	**obstruct/o-**
blood	**hemat/o-**
	hem/o-
blood clot (thrombus)	**thromb/o-**
blood condition	**-emia**
blood flowing	**hemorrh/o-**
blood in the tissues	**ecchym/o-**
blood serum	**ser/o-**
blood vessel	**angi/o-**
	vascul/o-
	vas/o-
blue	**cyan/o-**
boat shaped	**scaph/o-**
body	**corpor/o-**
	physic/o-
	somat/o-
	-some
	som/o-
body as a whole	**system/o-**
body with a habitual condition	**hec/o-**
	hex/o-
bone	**osse/o-**
	oste/o-

Definition of Word Part	Word Part
bone growth area at the end of a long bone	epiphys/o-
bone making, changing	ossificat/o-
bone marrow	myel/o-
bone shaft	diaphys/o-
border	limb/o-
born	-nate
boundary	termin/o-
boundary between the earth and sky	horizont/o-
brain	encephal/o-
brain chamber (ventricle)	ventricul/o-
brain condition	-encephaly
brain's largest part (cerebrum)	cerebr/o-
brain's posterior part (cerebellum)	cerebell/o-
branching structure	dendr/o-
break down	ly/o-
	lys/o-
break down food	digest/o-
break into minute pieces	comminut/o-
break up	fract/o-
breaking down	catabol/o-
breaking down process	-lysis
breaking out	erupt/o-
breaks down substances, cell that	-clast
breast	mamm/a-
	mamm/o-
	mast/o-
breast bone (sternum)	stern/o-
breath	halit/o-
breathe	hal/o-
	spir/o-
breathe in	aspir/o-
breathing	-pnea
	pne/o-
bring	duc/o-
	duct/o-
bring back	reduct/o-
bring toward the center	affer/o-
bronchiole	bronchiol/o-
bronchus	bronchi/o-
	bronch/o-
bruising	contus/o-
build	construct/o-
building up	anabol/o-
bulblike	bulb/o-
bunion	bunion/o-

Definition of Word Part	Word Part
burning	caus/o-
	pyr/o-
bursa	burs/o-

C

calcaneus (heel bone)	calcane/o-
calcium	calc/i-
	calc/o-
calcium hardness	calcific/o-
calm	tranquil/o-
calming agitation	sedat/o-
calyx	calic/o-
	cali/o-
cancer	cancer/o-
	carcin/o-
	malign/o-
Candida (a yeast)	candid/o-
capillary	capill/o-
capsule (enveloping structure)	capsul/o-
carbohydrate	amyl/o-
carbon atoms	carb/o-
carbon dioxide	capn/o-
carbon monoxide	carbox/y-
caries (tooth decay)	cari/o-
carry	phor/o-
carrying	conduct/o-
cartilage	cartilagin/o-
	chondr/o-
cartilage that is crescent-shaped (meniscus)	menisc/o-
carving process	-mileusis
catheter	catheter/o-
cause of disease	eti/o-
cause specific for a disease	-ism
causing action	agon/o-
causing harm intentionally	malign/o-
cavity opening (foramen)	foramin/o-
cavity that is hollow	sin/o-
cavity wall	pariet/o-
cecum	cec/o-
cell	cellul/o-
	-cyte
	cyt/o-
cell that breaks down substances	-clast
cell that is immature	-blast

Definition of Word Part	*Word Part*
cell that is scalelike	**squam/o-**
cells that are the functional part of an organ (parenchyma)	**parenchym/o-**
cellular layer	**theli/o-**
center	**centr/o-**
cerebellum	**cerebell/o-**
cerebrum	**cerebr/o-**
cervix	**cervic/o-**
cessation	**-pause**
	paus/o-
change	**meta-**
	metabol/o-
	mutat/o-
changing into bone	**ossificat/o-**
changing over from one thing to another	**transit/o-**
channel	**sin/o-**
channel opening (foramen)	**foramin/o-**
cheek	**buccinat/o**
	bucc/o-
cheek bone (zygoma)	**zygomat/o-**
chemical	**chem/o-**
chemical element	**-ium**
chemical substance	**-ol**
	-one
chemical substance that is singular	**-nine**
chemically modified structure	**-ide**
chest (thorax)	**pector/o-**
	steth/o-
	thorac/o-
	-thorax
chewing	**masset/o-**
	mastic/o-
child	**ped/o-**
childbirth	**part/o-**
	-partum
	toc/o-
childbirth and pregnancy	**obstetr/o-**
chin	**ment/o-**
chloride	**chlor/o-**
cholesterol	**cholesterol/o-**
chorion (fetal membrane)	**chori/o-**
	chorion/o-
choroid	**choroid/o-**
ciliary body of the eye	**cycl/o-**
circle	**circul/o-**
	cycl/o-

Definition of Word Part	Word Part
circle that is small	orbicul/o-
circular route movement	circulat/o-
clavicle (collar bone)	clavicul/o-
	clav/o-
	cleid/o-
clear and shining	luc/o-
clear, glasslike substance	hyal/o-
close against	occlus/o-
close association	fratern/o-
clotting	coagul/o-
clumping	agglutin/o-
coal	anthrac/o-
coccyx (tail bone)	coccyg/o-
cochlea	cochle/o-
coil	helic/o-
	spir/o-
cold	cry/o-
collar bone (clavicle)	clavicul/o-
	clav/o-
	cleid/o-
collection of symptoms	symptomat/o-
colon	col/o-
	colon/o-
color	chrom/o-
colored part of the eye (iris)	ir/o-
	irid/o-
coming	vent/o-
coming together	converg/o-
common bile duct	choledoch/o-
communicate	express/o-
community	soci/o-
compacted feces	constip/o-
compel	compuls/o-
compensate	compens/o-
complete	dia-
completely through	dia-
composed of	-ate
	-ated
compound containing lipids	-sterol
comprehensive	glob/o-
conceive	concept/o-
conception ability	fertil/o-
conception to birth	gest/o-
	gestat/o-

Definition of Word Part	Word Part
condition	-ema
	-esis
	-ety
	-ia
	-ias
	-ion
	-ity
	-osis
	-sis
condition of being	-ency
condition of blood	-emia
condition of coughing up that is abnormal	-ptysis
condition of deficiency	-penia
condition of dilation	-ectasis
condition of doing	-osing
condition of fingers	-dactyly
condition of formation	-poiesis
condition of frenzy	-mania
condition of guarding	-phylaxis
condition of having	-ition
condition of inflammation	-isy
condition of movement	-kinesis
condition of multiple tumors that is abnormal	-omatosis
condition of paralysis	-plegia
condition of protecting	-phylaxis
condition of rapid relaxing and contracting	-clonus
condition of slipping that is abnormal	-olisthesis
condition of softening	-malacia
condition of speech	-lalia
condition of standing still	-stasis
condition of the body that is habitual	hec/o-
	hex/o-
condition of the brain	-encephaly
condition of the fingers or toes	-dactyly
condition of the intestine	-entery
condition of the neck	-collis
condition of vision	-opia
condition pertained to	-ated
condition that is abnormal	-lysis
	-osis
	-sis
condition that is painful	-algia
cone	con/o-
conjunctiva	conjunctiv/o-

Definition of Word Part	Word Part
connective tissue	sarc/o-
constipation that is severe	obstip/o-
constrict	strangul/o-
constriction	sten/o-
contracting	-systole
	systol/o-
contracting and relaxing condition that is rapid	-clonus
contraction	stal/o-
contraction, process of	-stalsis
contributing part	access/o-
contrived	factiti/o-
conveying	conduct/o-
coordination	tax/o-
cornea (of the eye)	corne/o-
	kerat/o-
cortex (outer region)	cortic/o-
cough	tuss/o-
coughing up that is an abnormal condition	-ptysis
counterbalance	compens/o-
cover	integu/o-
cranium (skull)	crani/o-
creating process	-ization
creation	gener/o-
crescent-shaped cartilage (meniscus)	menisc/o-
crooked	scoli/o-
crowding together	aggreg/o-
crushing, process of	-tripsy
crushing, thing that	-triptor
cul-de-sac	culd/o-
curved	scoli/o-
	strept/o-
cut	cis/o-
	sect/o-
	tom/o-
cut apart	dissect/o-
cut into	incis/o-
cut off	amputat/o-
	amput/o-
cut out	excis/o-
cut out and remove	resect/o-
cutting instrument	-tome
cutting process	-tomy
cycle	cycl/o-

Definition of Word Part	Word Part
D	
danger exposure	**compromis/o-**
darkness	**scot/o-**
dead tissue area	**infarct/o-**
death	**mort/o-**
	necr/o-
	thanat/o-
decrease	**reduct/o-**
deep unconsciousness	**comat/o-**
deficiency condition	**-penia**
deficient	**hypo-**
deflect	**refract/o-**
degree, increase in	**augment/o-**
delay	**retard/o-**
density	**densit/o-**
depressed area that is small	**fove/o-**
derived from one that is identical	**clon/o-**
destroy	**ablat/o-**
development	**troph/o-**
development process	**-trophy**
diabetes	**diabet/o-**
diaphragm	**diaphragmat/o-**
	phren/o-
diet	**dietet/o-**
	diet/o-
different	**different/o-**
difficult	**dys-**
digest	**digest/o-**
digestion	**peps/o-**
	pept/o-
digit (finger or toe)	**digit/o-**
dilate	**dilat/o-**
dilating	**diastol/o-**
dilation	**ectat/o-**
dilation condition	**-ectasis**
dimness	**ambly/o-**
direction of	**-ad**
discharge	**-rrhea**
	rrhe/o-
discharge that is excessive	**-rrhage**
	rrhag/o-
discharge that is watery	**rheumat/o-**

Definition of Word Part	Word Part
disease	morbid/o-
	morb/o-
	-path
	path/o-
	-pathy
disease cause	eti/o-
disease from a specific cause	-ism
disease within	infect/o-
disk	disk/o-
dissolve	ly/o-
	lys/o-
dissolved substance	-lyte
dissolving, process of	-lysis
distance	tele/o-
distend	phys/o-
distended	distent/o-
distinct edges of an area	-tome
disturbing stimulus	stress/o-
diverticulum	diverticul/o-
dividing wall (septum)	sept/o-
do away with	efface/o-
dog, resembling a	can/o-
doing	-ing
doing, capable of	potent/o-
doing, condition of	-osing
dominant part	centr/o-
done of one's own free will	volunt/o-
dorsum	dors/o-
dose	dos/i-
double	dipl/o-
down	cata-
drag away	rap/o-
drawn together	constrict/o-
dress	vest/o-
drive	compuls/o-
drooping state	-ptosis
droplets of fat suspended in a liquid	emulsific/o-
drug	chem/o-
	pharmaceutic/o-
	pharmac/o-
dry	xer/o-
dry up	desicc/o-
duct	-duct
	duct/o-

Definition of Word Part	Word Part
duodenum	duoden/o-
dura mater	dur/o-
dust	coni/o-

E

Definition of Word Part	Word Part
ear	aur/i-
	auricul/o-
	ot/o-
eardrum (tympanic membrane)	myring/o-
	tympan/o-
earth and sky boundary	horizont/o-
eating	phag/o-
eats, thing that	-phage
echo (sound wave)	ech/o-
edge	limb/o-
egg (ovum)	o/o-
	ov/o-
	ovul/o-
elbow	cubit/o-
electricity	electr/o-
electrolyte	mineral/o-
element, chemical	-ium
elevated structure	papill/o-
embolus	embol/o-
embryo	embryon/o-
embryonic	blast/o-
embryonic tissue	germin/o-
encircling structure	coron/o-
enclosed space	claustr/o-
end	termin/o-
end of a long bone, growth area at the	epiphys/o-
enlarged organ returns to normal size	involut/o-
enlargement	-megaly
entrance (vestibule)	vestibul/o-
entry point	port/o-
enveloping structure (capsule)	capsul/o-
enzyme	-ase
eosin (acidic red dye)	eosin/o-
eruption of teeth	dentit/o-
esophagus	esophag/o-
examine with an instrument	scop/o-
examining instrument	-scope
examining process using an instrument	-scopy
excessive	ana-

Definition of Word Part	Word Part
excessive discharge	-rrhage
	rrhag/o-
excessive flow	-rrhage
	rrhag/o-
excision done surgically	-ectomy
exciting	stimul/o-
expel	elimin/o-
expel suddenly	ejaculat/o-
expert	-ician
	-itian
exposed to danger	compromis/o-
external	ex/o-
extremity	acr/o-
eye	ocul/o-
	ophthalm/o-
	opt/o-
eye pupil	pupill/o-
eye socket (orbit)	orbit/o-
eyelid	blephar/o-

F	
face	faci/o-
face down	pronat/o-
fainting	syncop/o-
falling	-ptosis
falling off	decidu/o-
fallopian tube	fallopi/o-
	salping/o-
	-salpinx
false belief	delus/o-
false perception	illus/o-
farthest from the opening (fundus)	fund/o-
	fundu/o-
fascia	fasci/o-
fast	tachy-
fat (lipid)	adip/o-
	lipid/o-
	lip/o-
	obes/o-
	steat/o-
fat droplets suspended in a liquid	emulsific/o-
fatty deposit	atheromat/o-
fatty substance that is soft	ather/o-
fear	anxi/o-
	phob/o-

Definition of Word Part	Word Part
feces	**copr/o-**
	fec/o-
feces compacted	**constip/o-**
feces, to pass	**chez/o-**
feeling	**esthes/o-**
	esthet/o-
	palpat/o-
female	**estr/a-**
	estr/o-
	gynec/o-
female external genitalia (vulva)	**episi/o-**
femur (thigh bone)	**femor/o-**
fetal membrane (chorion)	**chori/o-**
	chorion/o-
fetus	**fet/o-**
fever	**pyret/o-**
fiber	**fibr/o-**
fibers that hold together	**coll/a-**
fibrin	**fibrin/o-**
fibrous protein that is hard	**kerat/o-**
fibula	**fibul/o-**
	perone/o-
filled up	**satur/o-**
filter	**filtr/o-**
filtering	**filtrat/o-**
finger (digit)	**digit/o-**
finger (phalanx)	**phalang/o-**
fingers or toes, condition of the	**-dactyly**
fire	**pyr/o-**
first	**prim/i-**
flat area on the vertebra (lamina)	**lamin/o-**
flatus (gas)	**flatul/o-**
flexing	**elast/o-**
flow	**-flux**
	-rrhea
	rrhe/o-
flow backward	**regurgitat/o-**
flow that is excessive	**-rrhage**
	rrhag/o-
flowing of blood	**hemorrh/o-**
fluid	**hydr/o-**
fluid accumulation	**congest/o-**
fluid that is oozing	**exud/o-**
fluid that is serumlike	**ser/o-**

Definition of Word Part	Word Part
fluid-filled sac	cyst/o-
	vesic/o-
	vesicul/o-
fluid-filled vesicles	hydatidi/o-
fluorescence	fluor/o-
focus	nid/o-
folds (rugae)	rug/o-
follicle (small sac)	follicul/o-
fondness for	-phil
	phil/o-
food	aliment/o-
food breakdown	digest/o-
foods	dietet/o-
	diet/o-
foot	pod/o-
foramen (opening into a cavity or channel)	foramin/o-
forceful resistance	oppos/o-
forearm bone	uln/o-
foreign	xen/o-
forgetfulness	amnes/o-
form	concept/o-
form of	-form
form that is immature	embryon/o-
formation	plas/o-
	plast/o-
formation, condition of	-poiesis
formation of pus	suppur/o-
formed substance	-plasm
	plasm/o-
forward	ante-
four	quadri-
	tetr/a-
free will	volunt/o-
frenzy condition	-mania
friction producer	-frice
from conception to birth	gestat/o-
	gest/o-
front	front/o-
	ventr/o-
front part	anter/o-
front to back	sagitt/o-
fruit	fruct/o-
full of	-ose
fully perceived	appercept/o-
function of	-ory

Definition of Word Part	Word Part
functional cells of an organ (parenchyma)	**parenchym/o-**
fundus (part farthest from the opening)	**fund/o-**
	fundu/o-
fungus	**fung/o-**
	myc/o-
fuse together, procedure to	**-desis**
fused together	**ankyl/o-**

G	
gall	**bil/i-**
	chol/e-
	chol/o-
gallbladder	**cholecyst/o-**
ganglion	**ganglion/o-**
gangrene	**gangren/o-**
gene	**-gene**
	gene/o-
genetic inheritance	**heredit/o-**
	hered/o-
genitalia	**genit/o-**
genitalia (vulva) that is external in a female	**episi/o-**
giant	**gigant/o-**
give ability	**habilitat/o-**
give as a gift	**donat/o-**
giving a vaccine	**vaccin/o-**
giving help	**adjuv/o-**
gland	**aden/o-**
	glandul/o-
glans penis	**balan/o-**
glasslike substance that is clear	**hyal/o-**
globe shaped	**glob/o-**
	globul/o-
glomerulus	**glomerul/o-**
glottis (of the larynx)	**glott/o-**
glucose (sugar)	**gluc/o-**
	glyc/o-
	glycos/o-
glycerol (sugar alcohol)	**glycer/o-**
go into	**invas/o-**
go out from the center	**effer/o-**
going	**-grade**
going from front to back	**sagitt/o-**
going toward	**-ly**
gonads (ovaries and testes)	**gonad/o-**

Definition of Word Part	Word Part
good	eu-
graft procedure	-plant
granule	granul/o-
gray	phe/o-
green	verd/o-
grind the teeth	brux/o-
groin	inguin/o-
group or set	gemin/o-
grow	phys/o-
growing state	-physis
growing up	puber/o-
growth	-phyma
	-phyte
	-plasm
	plas/o-
	plast/o-
	vegetat/o-
growth area at the end of a long bone	epiphys/o-
guarding	phylact/o-
guarding condition	-phylaxis
gums	gingiv/o-

H

habitual condition of the body	hec/o-
	hex/o-
hair	pil/o-
	trich/o-
hairlike structure	capill/o-
	cili/o-
hairy	hirsut/o-
half	semi-
half of one	hemi-
hand	chir/o-
	manu/o-
hang onto	depend/o-
hanging	suspens/o-
hanging down	pendul/o-
hard	scler/o-
hard, fibrous protein	kerat/o-
hard from calcium	calcific/o-
harm that is intentionally caused	malign/o-
have an influence on	affect/o-
have an opening	perfor/o-
having	-ation
	-tion

Definition of Word Part	Word Part
having an affinity for	**trop/o-**
having the form of	**-form**
having the function of	**-ory**
having the quality of	**-ility**
having the same angle	**conform/o-**
having the same scale	**conform/o-**
head	**cephal/o-**
	-cephalus
	-ceps
health	**hygien/o-**
hearing	**acous/o-**
	-acusis
hearing, sense of	**acus/o-**
	audi/o-
	audit/o-
heart	**card/i-**
	cardi/o-
heat	**calor/o-**
	therm/o-
held together by fibers	**coll/a-**
hemoglobin	**hemoglobin/o-**
hemorrhoid	**hemorrhoid/o-**
hernia	**-cele**
	herni/o-
hidden	**crypt/o-**
high pH (base)	**alkal/o-**
higher	**ultra-**
highest point	**acr/o-**
hilum (indentation in an organ)	**hil/o-**
hip bone	**pelv/i-**
	pelv/o-
hold back	**inhibit/o-**
	retent/o-
hold together	**contin/o-**
hold together, fibers that	**coll/a-**
holds things together, substance that	**-glia**
	gli/o-
hole	**punct/o-**
	-tresia
hollow cavity	**sin/o-**
hollow space	**cavit/o-**
	cav/o-
hormone	**hormon/o-**
human beings	**soci/o-**
humerus	**humer/o-**
humpbacked	**kyph/o-**

Definition of Word Part	Word Part
I	
identical group derived from one	clon/o-
ileum (third part of small intestine)	ile/o-
ilium (hip bone)	ili/o-
imagined perception	hallucin/o-
immature	blast/o-
immature cell	-blast
immature form	embryon/o-
immune response	-immune
	immun/o-
impart	communic/o-
implant tissue	-graft
imprison	incarcer/o-
in	em-
	en-
	in-
in front of	pre-
in one place	loc/o-
in the direction of	-ad
inadequate	defici/o-
	mal-
incision-making process	-tomy
incomplete	atel/o-
increase	exacerb/o-
increase in degree	augment/o-
increase in size	augment/o-
incus (anvil-shaped bone)	incud/o-
indentation in an organ (hilum)	hil/o-
independent	autonom/o-
individual	idi/o-
infection	septic/o-
inflammation, condition of	-isy
inflammation of	-itis
inflate	phys/o-
influence on	affect/o-
inheritance that is genetic	heredit/o-
	hered/o-
injury	traumat/o-
inner region (medulla)	medull/o-
innermost	endo-
insert	inject/o-
inserting process	-ization
inside	intern/o-

Definition of Word Part	Word Part
instrument	-tron
instrument that is rodlike	-probe
instrument used to cut	-tome
instrument used to examine	-scope
instrument used to measure	-meter
instrument used to record	-graph
insulin	insulin/o-
intentionally causing harm	malign/o-
intercourse, sexual	coit/o-
	pareun/o-
	venere/o-
internal organs (viscera)	viscer/o-
intestinal condition	-entery
intestine	enter/o-
	intestin/o-
introduce	insert/o-
involuntary, muscle contraction that is sudden and	-spasm
inward	en-
	es/o-
iodine	iodin/o-
	iod/o-
iris	irid/o-
	ir/o-
iron	ferrit/o-
	ferr/o-
irregular	poikil/o-
ischium (hip bone)	ischi/o-
island	insul/o-
itching	prurit/o-
	psor/o-

J	
jarring that is violent	concuss/o-
jaundice	icter/o-
jejunum	jejun/o-
joined together	conjug/o-
joint	arthr/o-
	articul/o-
joint socket	glen/o-
jugular (throat)	jugul/o-

K	
keep	retent/o-
keep back	isch/o-

Definition of Word Part	Word Part
kernel, to remove the	enucle/o-
ketones	ket/o-
	keton/o-
kidney	nephr/o-
	ren/o-
killing	cid/o-
kind that is particular	-type
kneecap (patella)	patell/o-
knob of tissue (node)	nod/o-
knobby mass that is small	nodul/o-
knoblike projection	tuberos/o-
knowledge	gnos/o-
	-ics
	scient/o-

	L
labium	labi/o-
labor and childbirth	toc/o-
labor, to be in	parturit/o-
labyrinth	labyrinth/o-
lacking	defici/o-
lacrimal sac	dacry/o-
lamina	lamin/o-
large	macr/o-
	meg/a-
	megal/o-
larynx (voice box)	laryng/o-
late	tard/o-
lattice structure	cancell/o-
layer	tom/o-
layers of membranes	thec/o-
lead to	ag/o-
leading in	induct/o-
leaf	foli/o-
left	lev/o-
leg	-cnemius
lens (of the eye)	lenticul/o-
	lent/o-
	phac/o-
	phak/o-
lenses	optic/o-
less than	sub-
lessening	mi/o-
lice	pedicul/o-

Definition of Word Part	Word Part
lie open	**pat/o-**
life	**bi/o-**
ligament	**ligament/o-**
light	**phot/o-**
light point	**scint/i-**
	scintill/o-
light properties	**optic/o-**
like a bulb	**bulb/o-**
limb	**appendicul/o-**
limping pain	**claudicat/o-**
lining membrane	**ependym/o-**
lip	**cheil/o-**
	labi/o-
lipid (fat)	**lipid/o-**
	lip/o-
lipid-containing compound	**-sterol**
listening	**auscult/o-**
little bone (ossicle)	**ossicul/o-**
little granule	**chondri/o-**
little thing	**-elle**
liver	**hepat/o-**
living organisms	**bi/o-**
living thing	**-zoon**
living tissue	**bi/o-**
lobe of an organ	**lob/o-**
looking at	**inspect/o-**
lower back	**lumb/o-**
lower jaw (mandible)	**mandibul/o-**
lower part of the body	**caud/o-**
lumen (opening)	**lumin/o-**
lung	**pneum/o-**
	pneumon/o-
	pulmon/o-
lung membrane (pleura)	**pleur/o-**
lying face down	**pronat/o-**
lying on the back	**supinat/o-**
lymph	**lymph/o-**
lymphatic system	**lymph/o-**
lymphatic vessel	**angi/o-**

M

magnet	**magnet/o-**
make stable	**fixat/o-**
make still	**fixat/o-**

Definition of Word Part	Word Part
make thin	emaci/o-
making, process of	-ization
making urine	micturi/o-
male	andr/o-
malleolus	malleol/o-
malleus (hammer-shaped bone)	malle/o-
man	hom/i-
mandible (lower jaw)	mandibul/o-
manner of acting	behav/o-
manner of activity	behav/o-
many	mult/i-
	poly-
mark	stigmat/o-
marrow of the bone	myel/o-
masculine	viril/o-
mass	-oma
	om/o-
	onc/o-
mass that is fatty	atheromat/o-
mastoid process	mast/o-
	mastoid/o-
mature	matur/o-
maxilla (upper jaw)	maxill/o-
measured quantity	-dose
measurement	metr/o-
measuring instrument	-meter
measuring process	-metry
mediastinum	mediastin/o-
medical practice	pract/o-
medical treatment	iatr/o-
	-iatry
medicine	clinic/o-
	medic/o-
	pharmaceutic/o-
	pharmac/o-
medulla (inner region)	medull/o-
membrane layers	thec/o-
membrane that lines	ependym/o-
meninges	meningi/o-
	mening/o-
meniscus	menisc/o-
mesentery	mesenter/o-
mesh (trabecula)	trabecul/o-

Definition of Word Part	Word Part
middle	medi/o-
	mesi/o-
	mes/o-
	mid-
milk	galact/o-
	lact/i-
	lact/o-
millionth, one	micr/o-
mind	ment/o-
	phren/o-
	psych/o-
mind, state of	affect/o-
mineral	mineral/o-
miterlike structure (tall hat with 2 points)	mitr/o-
mixing	-crasia
model of	-type
month	men/o-
monthly discharge of blood	menstru/o-
mood	affect/o-
moon	lun/o-
more than normal	hyper-
mouth	or/o-
	stomat/o-
mouth, surgically created	stom/o-
move	duc/o-
	duct/o-
move back	recess/o-
move something to another place	transplant/o-
movement	cin/e-
	dynam/o-
	-kine
	kines/o-
	kin/o-
	mot/o-
movement, condition of	-kinesis
movement in a circular route	circulat/o-
movement of air	ventil/o-
	ventilat/o-
movement, thing that produces	-motor
moving	emot/o-
much	poly-
mucous membrane	mucos/o-
mucus	muc/o-
mucus-like substance	myx/o-
multiple masses, abnormal condition of	-omatosis

Definition of Word Part	Word Part
multiple tumors, abnormal condition of	-omatosis
muscle	muscul/o-
	my/o-
	myos/o-
muscle contraction that is sudden and involuntary	-spasm
muscle fiber	fibrill/o-
myelin	myelin/o-
	myel/o-

N

nail	onych/o-
	ungu/o-
nape of the neck	nuch/o-
narrowed	constrict/o-
narrowness	sten/o-
nausea	nause/o-
navel	omphal/o-
	umbilic/o-
near	myop/o-
near the center or point of origin	proxim/o-
near the surface	superfici/o-
neck	cervic/o-
	nuch/o-
neck, condition of the	-collis
neck, nape of the	nuch/o-
needle	acu/o-
nephron	nephr/o-
nerve	nerv/o-
	neur/o-
nerve fiber	fibrill/o-
nerve root, spinal	radicul/o-
	rhiz/o-
nest	nid/o-
network that is small	reticul/o-
new	ne/o-
night	noct/o-
nipple, small area surrounding	areol/o-
node (knob of tissue)	nod/o-
nodule	tubercul/o-
	tuber/o-
none	null/i-
normal	eu-
	norm/o-

Definition of Word Part	Word Part
nose	**nas/o-**
	rhin/o-
not	**an-**
	im-
	in-
	non-
	un-
not paired	**uni-**
not taking part	**neutr/o-**
nourishment	**aliment/o-**
	nutri/o-
	nutriti/o-
nucleolus	**kary/o-**
	nucleol/o-
nucleus (of a cell or an atom)	**nucle/o-**
nucleus, removal of the	**enucle/o-**

O

obliterate	**efface/o-**
occiput (back of the head)	**occipit/o-**
occluding plug (embolus)	**embol/o-**
oil (sebum)	**sebace/o-**
	seb/o-
old age	**ger/o-**
	presby/o-
	sen/o-
omentum	**oment/o-**
one	**mon/o-**
one half	**hemi-**
one millionth	**micr/o-**
one tenth	**dec/i-**
one who performs	**-eon**
one who specializes in	**-ist**
oozing fluid	**exud/o-**
open area or space	**agor/a-**
opening	**lumin/o-**
	perfor/o-
	-tresia
opening into a cavity (foramen)	**foramin/o-**
opening into a channel (foramen)	**foramin/o-**
opening, surgically created	**stom/o-**
	-stomy
opening that is small	**por/o-**
operative procedure	**surg/o-**
opportunity taken advantage of	**opportun/o-**

Definition of Word Part	*Word Part*
oppose	**antagon/o-**
opposite poles	**polar/o-**
orbit	**orbit/o-**
organ	**organ/o-**
organ, base of an	**basil/o-**
organ, indentation (hilum) in an	**hil/o-**
organ, lobe of an	**lob/o-**
organs that are internal (viscera)	**viscer/o-**
origin	**-id**
ossicle	**ossicul/o-**
other	**all/o-**
	heter/o-
out	**e-**
	ec-
	ex-
out from the center	**effer/o-**
outer aspects	**peripher/o-**
outer region (cortex)	**cortic/o-**
outermost	**ecto-**
outside	**ecto-**
	ectop/o-
	extern/o-
	extrins/o-
outside of	**extra-**
outward	**ec-**
	ex/o-
ovaries and testes (gonads)	**gonad/o-**
ovary	**oophor/o-**
	ovari/o-
ovum (egg)	**o/o-**
	ov/o-
	ovul/o-
ovum (seed)	**gon/o-**
own free will, done of one's	**volunt/o-**
oxygen	**ox/i-**
	ox/o-
	ox/y-

P	
pain	**alg/o-**
	dyn/o-
	odyn/o-
pain causing limping	**claudicat/o-**
pain, sensation of	**alges/o-**

Definition of Word Part	Word Part
painful	**dys-**
painful condition	**-algia**
pair, two parts of a	**para-**
palate	**palat/o-**
pancreas	**pancreat/o-**
paralysis	**pleg/o-**
paralysis condition	**-plegia**
parenchyma (functional cells of an organ)	**parenchym/o-**
part farthest from the opening (fundus)	**fund/o-**
	fundu/o-
particles suspended in a solution	**emulsific/o-**
particular kind of	**-type**
partly	**semi-**
parts	**-plex**
pass stool	**chez/o-**
patella (kneecap)	**patell/o-**
pelvis (hip bone; renal pelvis)	**pelv/i-**
	pelv/o-
penis	**pen/o-**
people	**dem/o-**
pepsin	**pepsin/o-**
peptide (two amino acids)	**peptid/o-**
perceived fully	**appercept/o-**
perception that is false	**illus/o-**
perception that is imagined	**hallucin/o-**
perforation	**punct/o-**
perform a procedure	**operat/o-**
performs, one who	**-eon**
perineum	**perine/o-**
peritoneum	**peritone/o-**
	periton/o-
person	**person/o-**
person that does or produces	**-ator**
	-er
	-or
	-tor
person who is attracted to or fond of	**-phile**
person who is the object of an action	**-ee**
pertaining to	**-ac**
	-al
	-alis
	-an
	-ant
	-ar

Definition of Word Part	Word Part
pertaining to (continued)	-aris
	-ary
	-ate
	-atic
	-ative
	-atory
	-eal
	-ed
	-ent
	-etic
	-iac
	-ial
	-ian
	-ic
	-ical
	-ile
	-ine
	-ior
	-ious
	-istic
	-ive
	-ous
	-tic
	-tous
	-ual
pertaining to a condition	-ated
pertaining to a person	-arian
pertaining to a process	-iatic
pertaining to a process or state	-iatic
pertaining to a single chemical substance	-nine
pertaining to a state	-iatic
pertaining to a substance	-ine
pertaining to a substance in the blood	-emic
pertaining to blood	-emic
pertaining to something small	-ular
pertains to, thing that	-ite
petechiae	petechi/o-
pH that is high (base)	alkal/o-
pH that is low (acid)	acid/o-
phalanx (finger or toe)	phalang/o-
pharynx (throat)	pharyng/o-
	-pharynx
phosphorus	phosph/o-
physical function	physi/o-

Definition of Word Part	Word Part
physician	iatr/o-
	medic/o-
picture	-gram
pigment	pigment/o-
pituitary gland	hypophys/o-
	pituitar/o-
	pituit/o-
place	locat/o-
	-tope
placed beneath	supposit/o-
placed within	implant/o-
placenta	placent/o-
plant a seed	insemin/o-
plaque	plak/o-
plasma	plasm/o-
platelike structure	-elasma
pleasure	hedon/o-
pleura (lung membrane)	pleur/o-
plug that occludes (embolus)	embol/o-
point	cusp/o-
	stigmat/o-
point of activity	foc/o-
point of entry	port/o-
point of light	scint/i-
	scintill/o-
poison	toxic/o-
	tox/o-
pole	pol/o-
poles that are opposite	polar/o-
polyp	polyp/o-
poor	cac/o-
population	dem/o-
pores	por/o-
position	-tope
potassium	kal/i-
pouring	fus/o-
pouring out	effus/o-
power	dynam/o-
practice	-ics
pregnancy	-gravida
pregnancy and childbirth	obstetr/o-
prematurely stopped	abort/o-
present at birth	congenit/o-
press back	repress/o-

Definition of Word Part	Word Part
press down	**depress/o-**
	suppress/o-
press together	**compress/o-**
pressed together	**coarct/o-**
pressure	**press/o-**
	tens/o-
	ton/o-
prevent	**preventat/o-**
	prevent/o-
procedure of fusing together	**-desis**
procedure of suturing	**-rrhaphy**
procedure, operative	**surg/o-**
procedure, perform a	**operat/o-**
procedure to fuse together	**-desis**
procedure to graft	**-plant**
procedure to puncture	**-centesis**
procedure to transfer	**-plant**
process	**-ade**
	-ation
	-ism
	-osis
	-tion
process of	**-ery**
	-iasis
process of breaking down	**-lysis**
process of carving	**-mileusis**
process of contraction	**-stalsis**
process of creating	**-ization**
process of crushing	**-tripsy**
process of cutting	**-tomy**
process of development	**-trophy**
process of examination using an instrument	**-scopy**
process of inserting	**-ization**
process of making	**-ization**
process of making an incision	**-tomy**
process of measuring	**-metry**
process of recording	**-graphy**
process of reshaping by surgery	**-plasty**
process of slipping	**-olisthesis**
process of surgically fixing in place	**-pexy**
process of using an instrument to examine	**-scopy**
process of viewing	**-opsy**
process of working	**-ergy**

Definition of Word Part	Word Part
process, pertaining to a	-iatic
process related to the specialty of	-istry
produce	product/o-
	secret/o-
produced by	gen/o-
producer	-gen
produces friction	-frice
produces movement	-motor
produces, that which	-gen
production	gener/o-
professional who is skilled	-ician
	-itian
projection	cusp/o-
projection that is knoblike	tuberos/o-
prolapsed state	-ptosis
properties of light	optic/o-
prostate gland	prostat/o-
protecting	phylact/o-
protecting condition	-phylaxis
protein	protein/o-
	prote/o-
provoke	exacerb/o-
pubis (hip bone)	pub/o-
pull out	till/o-
pull together	contract/o-
pulley-shaped structure	trochle/o-
pulling	tract/o-
pulse	sphygm/o-
puncture, procedure to	-centesis
pupil (of the eye)	cor/o-
	pupill/o-
pus	purul/o-
	py/o-
pus formation	suppur/o-
put in	inject/o-
	insert/o-
pylorus	pylor/o-

Q

quality	-ty
quality of having	-ility
quantity	quantitat/o-
quantity that is measured	-dose
quick	ox/y-

Definition of Word Part	Word Part
R	
radiation	radi/o-
	roentgen/o-
radius (forearm bone)	radi/o-
rage	thym/o-
raise up again	resuscit/o-
range	phor/o-
rapid contracting and relaxing	clon/o-
rapid contracting and relaxing, condition of	-clonus
rays of the sun	actin/o-
receive	recept/o-
receive within	intussuscep/o-
record	-gram
	graph/o-
recording instrument	-graph
recording process	-graphy
recover	recuper/o-
rectum	rect/o-
rectum and anus	proct/o-
red	erythr/o-
	rub/o-
red dye that is acidic (eosin)	eosin/o-
red substance	-rubin
redness	erythemat/o-
redness and warmth	inflammat/o-
reduce the severity of	palliat/o-
relationship	fratern/o-
relax	relax/o-
relaxing and contracting condition that is rapid	-clonus
remove	elimin/o-
remove the kernel	enucle/o-
remove the nucleus	enucle/o-
removing from the body	excret/o-
renal pelvis	pyel/o-
resembling	-id
	-oid
resembling a dog	can/o-
reshaping by surgery, process of	-plasty
resistance that is forceful	oppos/o-
response, immune	-immune
	immun/o-
result of	-ure
retina (of the eye)	retin/o-

Definition of Word Part	Word Part
reversal of	de-
reverse movement	react/o-
revive	resuscit/o-,
rhythm	rhythm/o-
	rrhythm/o-
rhythmic throbbing	pulsat/o-
rib	cost/o-
ribonucleic acid	rib/o-
right	dextr/o-
rod shaped	rhabd/o-
rodlike instrument	-probe
root, all other parts including the	radic/o-
rotate	rotat/o-
rugae (folds)	rug/o-
running	-drome

S

sac that is fluid filled	cyst/o-
	vesic/o-
	vesicul/o-
sacrum	sacr/o-
saliva	saliv/o-
	sial/o-
salivary gland	sial/o-
same	home/o-
same angle	conform/o-
same scale	conform/o-
sausage	botul/o-
scalelike cell	squam/o-
scanty	olig/o-
scapula (shoulder blade)	scapul/o-
science	scient/o-
sclera (white of the eye)	scler/o-
scrape off	abras/o-
scroll-like structure	turbin/o-
scrotum	scrot/o-
search out	explorat/o-
sebum (oil)	sebace/o-
	seb/o-
secrete	crin/o-
	secret/o-
secretes, a thing that	-crine
seed (ovum or spermatozoon)	gon/o-
seed, plant a	insemin/o-

Definition of Word Part	Word Part
seize and drag away	rap/o-
seizure	convuls/o-
	eclamps/o-
	epilept/o-
	ict/o-
	-lepsy
self	aut/o-
	su/i-
self-governing	autonom/o-
semisolid cyst	cyst/o-
send	mitt/o-
send back	remiss/o-
send out	emiss/o-
sensation	esthes/o-
	esthet/o-
	sens/o-
sensation of pain	alges/o-
sense of hearing	acus/o-
	audi/o-
	audit/o-
sense of smell	olfact/o-
	osm/o-
sense of taste	gustat/o-
sensitive to	sensitiv/o-
	sensit/o-
sensory	sensor/i-
separate	analy/o-
	ly/o-
separation of	-crit
septum (dividing wall)	sept/o-
series of graduated steps	scal/o-
serum of the blood	ser/o-
serumlike fluid	ser/o-
servant	ancill/o-
set	gemin/o-
severe constipation	obstip/o-
severity, reduce the	palliat/o-
sex	sex/o-
sexual intercourse	coit/o-
	pareun/o-
	venere/o-
shaft of a bone	diaphys/o-
shaking	tremul/o-

Definition of Word Part	Word Part
shaking that is violent	concuss/o-
shape	morph/o-
shaped like a globe	glob/o-
	globul/o-
shaped like a wedge	sphen/o-
sharp attack that is sudden	paroxysm/o-
sharpness	acu/o-
sheath	thec/o-
shield-shaped structure (thyroid gland)	thyr/o-
shin bone (tibia)	tibi/o-
shining and clear	luc/o-
short	brachy-
shoulder blade (scapula)	scapul/o-
showing	exhibit/o-
side	later/o-
sieve	ethm/o-
sight	vis/o-
sigmoid colon	sigmoid/o-
single	mon/o-
	uni-
single chemical substance	-nine
sinus	sinus/o-
size, increase in	augment/o-
skeleton	skelet/o-
skilled professional	-ician
	-itian
skin	cutane/o-
	cut/i-
	derm/a-
	-derma
	dermat/o-
	derm/o-
	integument/o-
skin, to take out	excori/o-
skull (cranium)	crani/o-
sleep	carot/o-
	hypn/o-
	narc/o-
	somn/o-
slice	tom/o-
slipping, process of	-olisthesis
slow	brady-
	tard/o-

Definition of Word Part	Word Part
slow down	**retard/o-**
small	**micr/o-**
small area	**macul/o-**
small area around the nipple	**areol/o-**
small attached part	**appendicul/o-**
small circle	**orbicul/o-**
small, depressed area	**fove/o-**
small, knobby mass	**nodul/o-**
small network	**reticul/o-**
small openings	**por/o-**
small sac (follicle)	**follicul/o-**
small structure hanging from a larger structure	**append/o-**
small thing	**-cle**
	-ole
	-ula
	-ule
small tube	**tubul/o-**
smell, the sense of	**olfact/o-**
	osm/o-
smooth	**lei/o-**
snake	**ophidi/o-**
socket of a joint	**glen/o-**
soft, fatty substance	**ather/o-**
softening	**malac/o-**
softening, condition of	**-malacia**
sound	**acous/o-**
	son/o-
sound wave (echo)	**ech/o-**
source	**-id**
space	**agor/a-**
space that is enclosed	**claustr/o-**
space that is hollow	**cavit/o-**
	cav/o-
spaces within tissue	**interstiti/o-**
spark of electricity	**fulgur/o-**
spasm	**spasm/o-**
	spasmod/o-
	spast/o-
specialized or being distinct	**differentiat/o-**
speciality, process related to a	**-istry**
specific area	**topic/o-**
specific cause of a disease	**-ism**
speech	**phas/o-**

Definition of Word Part	Word Part
speech condition	-lalia
sperm	semin/i-
	semin/o-
	spermat/o-
	sperm/o-
spermatozoon	gon/o-
	semin/i-
	semin/o-
	spermat/o-
	sperm/o-
sphenoid bone	sphenoid/o-
sphere	-sphere
	spher/o-
spherical bacterium	cocc/o-
	-coccus
sphincter	sphincter/o-
spider, spider web	arachn/o-
spinal cord	myel/o-
spinal nerve root	radicul/o-
	rhiz/o-
spine	spin/o-
spleen	splen/o-
split	schiz/o-
splitting	fiss/o-
spot	macul/o-
stable, to make	fixat/o-
stake	styl/o-
stand up	erect/o-
standing	saphen/o-
standing still	stas/o-
	stat/o-
standing still, condition of	-stasis
stapes (stirrup-shaped bone)	staped/o-
starch	amyl/o-
starlike structure	astr/o-
state	-ety
	-ia
	-ity
	-ment
	-ty
state of	-ance
	-ancy
	-ence
	-iasis

Definition of Word Part	Word Part
state of drooping	-ptosis
state of growing	-physis
state of mind	affect/o-
state of prolapse	-ptosis
state, pertaining to a	-iatic
staying in one place	-stasis
	stas/o-
	stat/o-
steal	klept/o-
steps in a graduated series	scal/o-
sternum (breast bone)	stern/o-
steroid	-steroid
	steroid/o-
stick to	adhes/o-
sticking	agglutin/o-
stiff	ankyl/o-
	pect/o-
still, to make	fixat/o-
stimulating	trop/o-
stimulus that is disturbing	stress/o-
stirring up	emot/o-
stirrup-shaped bone (stapes)	staped/o-
stomach	gastr/o-
stone	calcul/o-
	lith/o-
	-lith
stool	copr/o-
	fec/o-
stool that is compacted	constip/o-
stop prematurely	abort/o-
stop up	tampon/o-
straight	orth/o-
straight line, arranged in a	align/o-
straightening	extens/o-
straining	filtrat/o-
strange	all/o-
strength	sthen/o-
strengthening	stimul/o-
stretched	distent/o-
stretching	elast/o-
structure	-body
	format/o-
	-ium
	-ix
	-on
	-um

Definition of Word Part	Word Part
structure like a miter (tall hat with 2 points)	mitr/o-
structure shaped like a pulley	trochle/o-
structure that branches	dendr/o-
structure that encircles	coron/o-
structure that is chemically modified	-ide
structure that is hairlike	capill/o-
	cili/o-
structure that is platelike	-elasma
structure that is scroll-like	turbin/o-
structure that is small and hanging from a larger structure	append/o-
structure that is starlike	astr/o-
structure that is threadlike	mit/o-
structure that is U-shaped	hy/o-
structure, the base of a	bas/o-
study of	log/o-
	-logy
stupor	carot/o-
	narc/o-
subsequent to	meta-
substance	-in
	-on
substance in the blood	-emia
substance that forms	-poietin
substance that holds things together	-glia
	gli/o-
substance that is a chemical	-ol
	-one
substance that is dissolved	-lyte
substance that is formed	-plasm
	plasm/o-
substance that is mucuslike	myx/o-
substance that is transparent	vitre/o-
substance that is watery	aque/o-
substance that is waxy	-cere
suck	suct/o-
suck in	aspir/o-
suck up	sorb/o-
sudden and involuntary muscle contraction	-spasm
sudden, sharp attack	paroxysm/o-
suddenly expel	ejaculat/o-
suffering	-path
	pathet/o-
	path/o-
	-pathy

Definition of Word Part	Word Part
sugar	sacchar/o-
sugar (cane sugar)	sucr/o-
sugar alcohol (glycerol)	glycer/o-
supplement	access/o-
supplemental part	access/o-
surface, on the	superfici/o-
surgery	operat/o-
surgical excision	-ectomy
surgically created mouth or opening	stom/o-
surgically fixing in place	-pexy
surrender to	addict/o-
suturing, procedure of	-rrhaphy
swallowing	degluti/o-
	phag/o-
swayback	lord/o-
sweat	hidr/o-
	sudor/i-
sweating	diaphore/o-
swelling	-edema
sword	xiph/o-
symptoms, collection of	symptomat/o-
synovium (membrane)	synovi/o-
	synov/o-
system	-ure
system composed of	-ature

T	
tail	caud/o-
tail bone (coccyx)	coccyg/o-
take away	ablat/o-
take in	absorpt/o-
take out skin	excori/o-
taking advantage of an opportunity	opportun/o-
tapping	percuss/o-
taste, sense of	gustat/o-
tear away	vuls/o-
tearing	lacer/o-
tears	dacry/o-
	lacrim/o-
technical skill	techn/o-
teeth eruption	dentit/o-
teeth grinding	brux/o-
teeth, without	edentul/o-
temple	tempor/o-

Definition of Word Part	Word Part
tendon	**tendin/o-**
	tendon/o-
	ten/o-
tension	**tens/o-**
testicle	**testicul/o-**
testing place	**laborat/o-**
testis	**-didymis**
	didym/o-
	gonad/o-
	orchi/o
	orch/o-
	testicul/o-
thalamus	**thalam/o-**
thickness	**viscos/o-**
thigh bone (femur)	**femor/o-**
thin	**man/o-**
thing	**-body**
	-ia
	-ie
	-il
thing that affects in a particular way	**-izer**
thing that crushes	**-triptor**
thing that does	**-ator**
	-er
	-or
thing that eats	**-phage**
thing that pertains to	**-ite**
thing that produces	**-ator**
	-er
	-or
thing that produces friction	**-frice**
thing that produces movement	**-motor**
thing that secretes	**-crine**
thinking	**cognit/o-**
thirst	**dips/o-**
thorax (chest)	**thorac/o-**
	-thorax
thoughts, besieged by	**obsess/o-**
threadlike structure	**mit/o-**
three	**tri-**
three dimensions	**stere/o-**
threefold	**trigemin/o-**
throat	**jugul/o-**
	pharyng/o-
	-pharynx

Definition of Word Part	Word Part
throb	palpit/o-
throbbing that is rhythmic	pulsat/o-
thrombus (blood clot)	thromb/o-
through	per-
	trans-
through completely	dia-
throughout	per-
throughout the body, widely scattered	dissemin/o-
throw forward	project/o-
thymus	thym/o-
thyroid gland	thy/o-
	thyroid/o-
tibia	tibi/o-
tie up	ligat/o-
time	chron/o-
tip (apex)	apic/o-
tissue	histi/o-
tissue implant	-graft
tissue knob (node)	nod/o-
tissue that is embryonic	germin/o-
tissue that is living	bi/o-
tissue transplant	-graft
tissue with blood in it	ecchym/o-
toe (digit)	digit/o-
toe (phalanx)	phalang/o-
toe, condition of the	-dactyly
together	converg/o-
	sym-
	syn-
together by crowding	aggreg/o-
together by fusion	ankyl/o-
together by joining	conjug/o-
tone	ton/o-
tongue	gloss/o-
	lingu/o-
tonsil	tonsill/o-
tooth	dent/i-
	dent/o-
	odont/o-
tooth decay (caries)	cari/o-
touch	tact/o-
touching	palpat/o-
toward	ad-
	-ad

Definition of Word Part	Word Part
toward the center	**affer/o-**
toxin	**toxic/o-**
trabecula	**trabecul/o-**
trachea (windpipe)	**trache/o-**
transfer procedure	**-plant**
transformation	**metabol/o-**
transition	**meta-**
transmit	**communic/o-**
transparent substance	**vitre/o-**
transplant tissue	**-graft**
travel	**-verse**
	vers/o-
	vert/o-
treatment	**therapeut/o-**
	therap/o-
	-therapy
treatment, medical	**iatr/o-**
	-iatry
triangle	**delt/o-**
triglyceride	**triglycerid/o-**
trochanter	**trochanter/o-**
tube	**-duct**
	duct/o-
	tub/o-
tuberculosis	**tubercul/o-**
tubular structures, uniting of two	**anastom/o-**
tumor	**kel/o-**
	-oma
	om/o-
	onc/o-
	-phyma
turbinate	**turbin/o-**
turn	**-verse**
	vers/o-
	vert/o-
turning	**trop/o-**
twins	**gemin/o-**
twisted position	**tort/i-**
two	**bi-**
	di-
	du/o-
two opposite poles	**polar/o-**
two parts of a pair	**para-**

Definition of Word Part	Word Part
tympanic membrane	myring/o-
	tympan/o-

U

ulcer	aphth/o-
	ulcerat/o-
ulna	uln/o-
umbilicus	omphal/o-
	umbilic/o-
unable to	re-
unconsciousness that is deep	comat/o-
underneath	sub-
unequal	anis/o-
unite two tubular structures	anastom/o-
unknown	idi/o-
upon	epi-
uppermost part	dors/o-
ureter	ureter/o-
urethra	urethr/o-
urinary system	urin/o-
	ur/o-
urinate in	enur/o-
urine	oure/o-
	urin/o-
	ur/o-
urine, making	micturi/o-
U-shaped structure	hy/o-
usual	norm/o-
uterus (womb)	hyster/o-
	metri/o-
	metr/o-
	uter/o-
uvea (of the eye)	uve/o-

V

vaccine, giving a	vaccin/o-
vagina	colp/o-
	vagin/o-
vagus nerve	vag/o-
valve	valv/o-
	valvul/o-
varicose vein	varic/o-
varix	varic/o-
vas deferens	vas/o-
vegetable	veget/o-

Definition of Word Part	Word Part
vein	**phleb/o-**
	ven/i-
	ven/o-
ventricle	**ventricul/o-**
vertebra	**spondyl/o-**
	vertebr/o-
vertebra, flat area (lamina) on the	**lamin/o-**
vesicles filled with fluid	**hydatidi/o-**
vestibule	**vestibul/o-**
viewing, process of	**-opsy**
violent shaking or jarring	**concuss/o-**
virus	**vir/o-**
viscera (internal organs)	**viscer/o-**
visible path	**trac/o-**
vision	**opt/o-**
	vis/o-
vision, condition of	**-opia**
vitreous humor	**vitre/o-**
voice	**voc/o-**
voice box (larynx)	**laryng/o-**
vomit	**emet/o-**
vomiting, condition of	**-emesis**
vulva	**episi/o-**
	vulv/o-

W

walking	**ambulat/o-**
wall of a cavity	**pariet/o-**
warmth and redness	**inflammat/o-**
water	**hydr/o-**
watery discharge	**rheumat/o-**
watery substance	**aque/o-**
waxy substance	**-cere**
weakened	**attenu/o-**
weakness	**-paresis**
wedge	**sphen/o-**
wedge shape	**sphen/o-**
wedged in	**impact/o-**
weight	**bar/o-**
well timed	**opportun/o-**
white	**albin/o-**
	leuk/o-
white of the eye (sclera)	**scler/o-**
whole body	**system/o-**
widely scattered throughout the body	**dissemin/o-**
widen	**dilat/o-**

Definition of Word Part	Word Part
widening	mydr/o-
windpipe (trachea)	trache/o-
with	con-
	sym-
withdrawal	apher/o-
within	en-
	endo-
	in-
	intra-
without	a-
	an-
	de-
without place or position	athet/o-
without teeth	edentul/o-
withstand the effect of	resist/o-
woman	gynec/o-
womb	hyster/o-
	metri/o-
	metr/o-
	uter/o-
word	lex/o-
	log/o-
word origin	etym/o-
work	erg/o-
work against	antagon/o-
working, process of	-ergy
workplace	laborat/o-
worry	anxi/o-
wrinkle	rhytid/o-
wrist	carp/o-
write	script/o-
X–Z	
x-ray	radi/o-
	roentgen/o-
yellow	cirrh/o-
	xanth/o-
youth	hebe/o-
zygoma (cheek bone)	zygomat/o-

Glossary of Medical Words and Phrases

Locate Medical Word and Phrase Definitions

Understanding the definition of a medical word or phrase is crucial to understanding medical language. Knowing word parts and their meanings is important, but sometimes you need a full definition to understand a medical word or phrase. This section provides that for you.

This section provides an alphabetical listing of the medical words and phrases found in *Medical Language,* the comprehensive textbook that is a companion to this reference guide. Some of the definitions provided in this section will not *exactly* match the definitions found in the textbook. Some editing was performed to allow for quick referencing, and some changes were made to match the body as a whole, instead of an individual body system.

Table Key		
word [ICD-9 *]	Definition of the word. [*see also:* other words located in this section that are related to this word]	cross-reference **
	Sx *** Symptoms	
	Dx *** Diagnosis	
	Tx *** Treatment	

* ICD-9 coding requires five digits. Only the first three digits are provided here because of the general application of the definitions. Further investigation and analysis is required in order to code accurately because of the need for the fourth and fifth digits, as indicated by an ".xx" following the first three digits. Some of the diseases in this section do not have an ICD-9 code listed with them, as additional information (such as the cause or location of the disease) is required before an accurate category code can be assigned. Some more recently named diseases are not listed or assigned codes in the current edition of ICD–9.

** The far right column in this table provides a cross-reference to other sections in this reference guide: **A** = Abbreviation Section, **F** = Figures Section, **L** = Laboratory Section, and **S** = Synonyms Section.

*** Selected diseases contain information on Sx (Symptoms), Dx (Diagnosis), and Tx (Treatment), some of which are further classified as to ♂ (male) and ♀ (female).

GLOSSARY OF MEDICAL WORDS AND PHRASES

0-9

24-hour creatinine clearance	Urine test that collects all urine for 24 hours to measure the total amount of creatinine "cleared" (excreted) by the kidneys. The result is compared to the level of creatinine in the blood to determine the level of kidney function. [see also: blood urea nitrogen, creatinine]	S

A

abdominal cavity	Cavity that is surrounded by the diaphragm superiorly, the abdominal wall anteriorly, and the spinal column posteriorly. [see also: laparoscopy]	
abdominopelvic cavity	Continuous cavity within the abdomen and pelvis that contains the abdominal cavity superiorly and the pelvic cavity inferiorly.	
abducens nerve	Cranial nerve VI, responsible for movement of the eyeball. [see also: convergence]	S
ABO blood group	Category that includes blood types A, B, AB, and O. Blood types are hereditary. Each blood type has antigens on its erythrocytes and antibodies against other blood types in the plasma. [see also: blood group, Rh blood group]	
above-the-knee amputation	An above-the-knee amputation is performed at the level of the femur. Most commonly performed on diabetic patients who have had a gangrenous infection. The progression of the diabetes and/or infection determines the level of the amputation, whether it is above the knee or below the knee. [see also: amputation, diabetes mellitus, gangrene, prosthesis]	A
abrasion	Sliding injury that mechanically removes the epidermal layer of the skin to reveal the dermis beneath. [see also: excoriation]	S
abruptio placentae [641.xx]	Complete or partial separation of the placenta from the uterine wall before the third stage of labor, resulting in uterine hemorrhage that threatens the life of the mother as well as the life of the fetus. [see also: dystocia]	
	Dx Vaginal bleeding in the last two trimesters of pregnancy; ultrasound to visualize the placenta.	
	Tx Depends on severity. Bedrest or possible delivery, either vaginally or by cesarean section.	
abscess	Localized, pus-containing pocket caused by a bacterial infection. [see also: incision and drainage]	
absorption	Process by which digested food nutrients move through villi of the small intestine into the blood.	
accessory nerve	Cranial nerve XI. Movement of the vocal cords and muscles of the neck and upper back. Two of its nerve branches also assist the vagus nerve. [see also: vagus nerve]	S
accommodation	Medical procedure to test the ability of the ciliary muscles of the eye to contract and flex the lens as demonstrated on near and distance visual acuity tests. [see also: cilia, lens, phorometry, presbyopia, visual acuity testing]	
acetylcholine	Neurotransmitter for the parasympathetic nervous system. It is released by the vagus nerve and slows the heart rate. [see also:	A

acetylcholine receptor antibodies, Alzheimer's disease, Botox injections, myasthenia gravis, Parkinson's disease, somatic nervous system, Tensilon test, thymectomy]

acetylcholine receptor antibodies
Blood test for myasthenia gravis. It detects antibodies that the body has formed against its own acetylcholine receptors. [*see also*: acetylcholine, myasthenia gravis]

acid phosphatase
Blood test for an enzyme found mostly in the prostate gland; it can help detect prostate cancer. There are also concentrated levels in semen, so the presence of acid phosphatase in the vagina indicates sexual intercourse and is sometimes used in rape investigations.

acne rosacea
[695.xx]
Chronic skin condition with redness of the face in middle-aged patients. The sebaceous glands secrete excessive amounts of sebum, causing papules and pustules. [*see also*: blepharitis, comedo, laser surgery, rhinophyma]

acne vulgaris
[706.xx]
During puberty, the sebaceous glands produce large amounts of sebum. Excess sebum builds up around the hair shaft, hardens, and blocks the follicle. [*see also*: comedo]

acoustic neuroma
[225.xx]
Benign tumor of the nerve cells of the auditory nerve. Depending on its location in the ear, it can cause symptoms of pain, dizziness, or hearing loss. [*see also*: brainstem auditory evoked response, conductive hearing loss, mixed hearing loss, sensorineural [hearing loss]   **S**

acquired immunodeficiency syndrome
[042.xx]
Infection caused by the retrovirus HIV. Once infected, it takes about three months for the body to develop enough antibodies against HIV to give a positive serology test. HIV uses helper T cells (CD4 lymphocytes) to reproduce, which in turn suppresses the normal immune response and leaves the patient immuno-compromised and defenseless against infection and cancer. [*see also*: human immunodeficiency virus, Kaposi's sarcoma, *Pneumocystis carinii* pneumonia]   **L S**

Sx Fever, night sweats, weight loss, fatigue.

Dx H&P. In order to diagnose AIDS, the patient must first be HIV+, second, have a CD4 count below 200 cells/mL of blood, and third, currently have one of the following: a wasting disease, an opportunistic infection, or cancer. Once a patient has all three, an AIDS diagnosis is confirmed.

Tx Medication. (The type of medications used to treat AIDS patients and those who are HIV positive varies depending on several different factors. Outside resources and medical professionals should be consulted.)

acrocyanosis
[443.xx]
Temporary bluish coloration of the skin of the head, hands, and feet; sometimes occurring after birth.   **S**

acromegaly
[253.xx]
Hypersecretion of growth hormone during adulthood. Because the growth plates at the ends of the long bones are already fused, the patient cannot grow taller. Growth hormone causes the facial features and jaw to become wider and enlarged. The hands and feet become wider. [*see also*: gigantism]   **L S**

activated clotting time
Blood test to monitor the effectiveness of the anticoagulant drug heparin when it is given in high dosages. [*see also*: partial thromboplastin time]   **A**

A = Abbreviations Section   **F** = Figures Section   **L** = Laboratory Section   **S** = Synonyms Section
Sx (Symptoms)   **Dx** (Diagnosis)   **Tx** (Treatment)

active immunity

The body's continuing immune response and defense against pathogens it has seen before. [*see also*: immunoglobulin G, passive immunity]

acute coronary syndrome [411.xx]

General category that includes acute ischemia of the myocardium with unstable angina pectoris. [*see also*: angina pectoris, myocardial infarction]   A

acute renal failure [584.xx]

Disease in which the kidney's urine production progressively decreases and may stop, due to trauma, severe blood loss, or overwhelming infection. It is accompanied by the sudden destruction of a large number of nephrons and their tubules. [*see also*: renal failure]   A

Dx   Lab tests for BUN, creatinine, and other metabolic functions of the kidney to determine how well, or poorly, the kidney is functioning. Monitoring of intake and output to establish fluid levels. [*see also*: anuria, blood urea nitrogen, creatinine, intake and output, oliguria]

Tx   Treat underlying cause with IV fluids, transfusions, medication. [*see also*: dialysis]

acute tubular necrosis [584.xx]

The sudden destruction of large numbers of nephrons and their tubules that occurs during acute renal failure. [*see also*: acute renal failure, anuria, dialysis, oliguria]   A L

Dx   Lab tests and a UA to determine kidney function. Other tests may be performed to rule out causes for acute renal failure. Monitoring of intake and output to establish fluid level. [*see also*: blood urea nitrogen, creatinine, intake and output]

Tx   Treat underlying cause with IV fluids, transfusions, medication.

adaptive device

A device that increases mobility or independence by helping the physically challenged patient to perform activities of daily living. Examples: a grasper to extend the reach, spoons that can be attached to the wrist, and pens with extra-large barrels.

Addison's disease [255.xx]

Hyposecretion of cortisol. This is an autoimmune disease in which the body produces antibodies that destroy the adrenal cortex. (It can also be caused by hyposecretion of adrenocorticotropic hormone from the anterior pituitary gland.) [*see also*: autoimmune diseases, cortisol]   S L

Dx   Blood and urine cortisol levels are measured before and after the administration of adrenocorticotropic hormone. [*see also*: ADH stimulation test]

Tx   Hormone replacement.

adductor

Muscle that produces adduction when it contracts.

ADH stimulation test

Urine test that measures the concentration of urine to evaluate the function of the posterior pituitary gland. Water is withheld for 12 hours and a urine specimen is obtained. ADH (vasopressin) is given, the patient drinks water, and another urine specimen is obtained. In a patient with diabetes insipidus, the second urine specimen will be more concentrated because of the ADH. [*see also*: Addison's disease, diabetes insipidus]   S

adhesions [568.xx]

Abnormal fibrous bands of tissue that form after surgery. They connect the intestines to each other or to another organ in the abdominopelvic cavity. They can bind so tightly that peristalsis and intestinal function are affected. [*see also*: endometriosis]

Dx	H&P. Barium swallow, CT scan, or endoscopic procedure to visualize the abdominal cavity and its contents. [*see also*: barium swallow, culdoscopy]	
Tx	Depending on severity of symptoms, the adhesions may be left alone or excised. Surgery isn't always a first option because surgery may be the cause of subsequent adhesions. Medications are provided to treat the symptoms associated with the adhesions. [*see also*: bowel resection and anastomosis]	

adipose tissue — Fatty tissue in the subcutaneous layer of the skin. It contains lipocytes. [*see also*: lipocyte, lipoma, liposuction]   **S**

adrenal cortex — Outermost part of the adrenal gland. It produces and secretes three groups of hormones that are related to or control salt, sugar, and sex. Salt: Mineralocorticoids (aldosterone). Sugar: Glucocorticoids (cortisol). Sex: Some androgens (male hormones).

adrenal glands — Endocrine glands on top of the kidneys. Each adrenal gland contains two parts: the adrenal cortex and the adrenal medulla. Each part secretes different hormones. [*see also*: adrenal cortex, adrenal medulla]   **S**

adrenal medulla — Innermost part of the adrenal gland. It produces and secretes the hormones epinephrine and norepinephrine. [*see also*: pheochromocytoma, vanillylmandelic acid]

adrenocorticotropic hormone — Hormone secreted by the anterior pituitary gland. It stimulates the adrenal cortex to secrete all three of its hormones (aldosterone, cortisol, androgens). [*see also*: Cushing's, hyperaldosteronism]   **A** **S**

adrenogenital syndrome [255.xx] — Hypersecretion of androgens. Caused by an adenoma in the adrenal gland. In boys, it causes precocious puberty. In girls, it causes the clitorus and labia to enlarge and resemble a penis and scrotum. In adult females, it causes virilism with masculine facial features and body build, hirsutism, and amenorrhea. [*see also*: amenorrhea, androgens, hirsutism]

Dx	Lab tests to determine hormone blood levels; karyotyping is performed to determine gender.
Tx	Steroid therapy and hormone replacement is considered. Surgery to remove the adenoma. Gender assignment surgery may be discussed as an option.

adult respiratory distress syndrome [518.xx] — Precipitated by a severe infection, burns that affect the entire body, or a direct injury to the lung tissue (aspiration of vomit or inhalation of chemical fumes). The alveoli are damaged because of lack of blood flow, are unable to make surfactant, and collapse with each breath. [*see also*: aspiration pneumonia, Legionnaire's disease, pneumonia, septicemia, severe acute respiratory syndrome, tuberculosis]   **A**

Dx	H&P. ABGs and PFTs to determine lung function, chest x-ray to visualize the lungs. Lab tests including a CBC and a C&S. [*see also*: pulmonary function tests]
Tx	Oxygen therapy along with mechanical ventilation to support respiratory function. Medications and other treatments based on the underlying cause, if known. [*see also*: endotracheal intubation, oxygen therapy]

affect — Outward display on the face of the inward emotions and thoughts. [*see also*: schizophrenia]

A = Abbreviations Section   F = Figures Section   L = Laboratory Section   S = Synonyms Section
Sx (Symptoms)   Dx (Diagnosis)   Tx (Treatment)

afferent nerves	Nerves that carry sensory nerve impulses to the brain or spinal cord from the body. [*see also*: efferent nerves]
aggregation	Process of platelets sticking to a damaged area in the blood vessel wall and forming clumps.
agranulocyte	Category of leukocytes with nearly invisible granules in the cytoplasm. Includes lymphocytes and monocytes.
albinism [270.xx]	White-to-light pink skin coloration. Genetic mutation associated with melanocytes that do not produce melanin. There is a lack of pigment in the skin, hair, and iris of the eyes. **S**
albumin	Most abundant plasma protein. [*see also*: albuminuria, metabolic panel, nephrotic syndrome, plasma proteins, plasmapheresis] **L**
albuminuria [791.xx]	Presence of albumin in the urine, which is not normally there. The albumin molecules are too large to pass through the pores in the glomerulus. But if the membrane is damaged by kidney disease or infection, albumin passes through and is excreted in the urine. An important first sign of kidney disease. It is also present in pregnant women who are developing preeclampsia. [*see also*: glomerulonephritis, nephrotic syndrome, preeclampsia, renal failure] **S**
aldosterone	Most abundant and biologically active of the mineralocorticoid hormones secreted by the adrenal cortex. It regulates the balance of electrolytes, keeping sodium (and water) in the blood while excreting potassium in the urine. [*see also*: hyperaldosteronism, hypoaldosteronism, renin]
allergen	Cells from plants or animals (foods, pollens, molds, animal dander), as well as dust, chemicals, and drugs that cause an allergic response in a hypersensitive person. [*see also*: allergic reaction, conjunctivitis, contact dermatitis, hypersensitivity, local reaction, radioallergosorbent test, scratch test, systemic reaction]
allergic reaction [995.xx]	Response to an allergen in a hypersensitive person. An allergic reaction is based on the release of histamine. [*see also*: anaphylactic shock, gluten enteropathy, immunoglobulin E, pruritus, urticaria] **S**
allergic rhinitis [477.xx]	Allergy symptoms in the nose. In response to an inhaled antigen, the immune response releases histamine, producing nasal stuffiness, sneezing, rhinorrhea, hypertrophy of the turbinates with red, edematous, and boggy mucous membranes, and postnasal drip. [*see also*: hay fever]
allograft	Uses a graft taken from a living donor or a cadaver donor. [*see also*: autograft, bone graft, bone marrow donation, graft-versus-host disease, skin grafting, xenograft] **S**
alopecia [704.xx]	Acute or chronic loss of scalp hair. [*see also*: radiation therapy] **S**
alpha fetoprotein	Amniotic Fluid: Used to diagnose a congenital neural tube defect, such as a meningocele or meningomyelocele. The fetal liver makes alpha fetoprotein, which is normally present in small amounts. However, increased levels indicate that alpha fetoprotein is leaking into the amniotic fluid from a neural tube defect. [*see also*: amniocentesis, meningocele] **A**
	Blood Test: Not normally present in adults, elevated levels are seen with cancer of the liver, testes, and ovaries. The higher the level, the more advanced the cancer. AFP can also be elevated in noncancerous conditions such as cirrhosis and hepatitis.
alveolus	Hollow sphere of cells in the lungs where oxygen and carbon dioxide are exchanged. [*see also*: atelectasis, surfactant] **F**

A = Abbreviations Section   **F** = Figures Section   **L** = Laboratory Section   **S** = Synonyms Section
Sx (Symptoms)   **Dx** (Diagnosis)   **Tx** (Treatment)

Alzheimer's disease [331.xx]	A hereditary dementia that is known to run in families with inherited mutations on chromosomes 1, 14, and 21. At autopsy, the neurons show characteristic neurofibrillary tangles that distort the cells. There are also microscopic senile plaques. The brain also has decreased levels of the neurotransmitter acetylcholine. [*see also*: dementia, positron emission tomography scan, presenile dementia]	
amblyopia [368.xx]	To prevent double vision, the brain ignores the visual image from an eye with strabismus (the most common cause) or an eye in which the vision is unfocused or cloudy. May continue even after the strabismus or other defect is surgically corrected. [*see also*: convergence, esotropia, exotropia, strabismus]	S
amenorrhea	Absence of monthly menstrual periods. (This is normal before puberty, during pregnancy, and after menopause.) Caused by a hormone imbalance, thyroid disease, or tumors of the uterus or ovaries. [*see also*: androgenital syndrome, Cushing's syndrome]	S
amnesia	Partial or total loss of recent or long-term memory due to trauma or disease of the hippocampus. [*see also*: anterograde amnesia, global amnesia, retrograde amnesia]	S
amniocentesis	Amniotic fluid test. With ultrasound guidance, a needle is inserted through the abdominal wall and into the uterus to withdraw amniotic fluid. The test is done between 15 to 18 weeks' gestation. [*see also*: alpha fetoprotein, chorionic villus sampling, chromosome studies, lecithin/sphingomyelin ratio, sickle cell anemia]	
amnion	Part of the zygote that becomes the amniotic membrane and holds amniotic fluid. [*see also*: amniotic fluid]	S
amniotic fluid	Fluid produced by the amnion. It surrounds and cushions the developing embryo and fetus. [*see also*: amnion, oligohydramnios, polyhydramnios]	
amniotomy	Medical procedure in which a hook is inserted into the cervix to rupture the amniotic sac and induce labor. [*see also*: induction of labor]	S
amputation	Removal of all or part of an extremity, either from a surgical procedure or through trauma. A muscle flap is wrapped over the end of the bone to provide a cushion and support a prosthesis. [*see also*: above-the-knee amputation, below-the-knee amputation, prosthesis]	
amygdaloid body	Almond-shaped area within each temporal lobe. It interprets facial expressions and new social situations to identify danger. It integrates with long-term memory and is particularly active in the emotions of fear, anger, and rage. [*see also*: limbic system]	
amylase	Digestive enzyme from the pancreas and in saliva. It breaks down carbohydrates and starch in the duodenum into simple sugars and food fibers.	
anacusis	Total deafness. [*see also*: conductive hearing loss, conversion disorder, mixed hearing loss, sensorineural hearing loss]	S
anaphylactic shock	Severe, systemic allergic reaction characterized by bronchoconstriction, hypotension, and shock. [*see also*: allergic reaction]	S
anaplasia	Condition in which normal cells that are mature and differentiated become cancerous cells that are undifferentiated in appearance and behavior.	S

A = Abbreviations Section   **F** = Figures Section   **L** = Laboratory Section   **S** = Synonyms Section
Sx (Symptoms)   **Dx** (Diagnosis)   **Tx** (Treatment)

anatomical position	Standard position of the body for the purpose of studying it. The body is erect, head up, hands by the side with palms facing forward, and the legs are straight with toes pointing forward.
anatomy	The study of the structure of the human body and its parts.
androgens	Category that includes naturally occurring male hormones like testosterone from the testes, other androgens from the adrenal cortex, as well as manufactured male hormones used in drugs. In females, androgens are secreted by cells around the follicles in the ovary and play a role in female sexual drive. [*see also*: adrenogenital syndrome, Cushing's syndrome, gynecomastia]
anemia	The number of erythrocytes in the blood is decreased because too few erythrocytes are produced, erythrocytes have been destroyed, or erythrocytes have been lost. Anemias can be classified by their cause or by the size, shape, and appearance of the erythrocytes. [*see also*: aplastic anemia, iron deficiency anemia, folic acid anemia, pernicious anemia, and sickle cell anemia]

L

anencephaly [655.xx]	Rare congenital condition in which some or all of the cranium and cerebrum are missing in a newborn. The infant breathes because the respiratory center in the medulla oblongata is intact, but only survives a few hours or days. [*see also*: cerebrum]

S

anesthesia	Condition in which sensation of any type has been completely lost. Unconsciousness is accompanied by an inability to perceive any sensation, which is the basis for the use of drugs that induce general anesthesia. [*see also*: epidural, pain management]

S

aneurysm [442.xx]	Area of dilation and weakness in the wall of an artery. This can be congenital or where arteriosclerosis has damaged the artery. With each heartbeat, the weakened artery wall balloons outward. Aneurysms can rupture without warning. [*see also*: arteriosclerosis, diabetic retinopathy, dissecting aneurysm]
	Dx Angiogram or Doppler ultrasound to visualize the aneurysm. [*see also*: angiography, aortography, arteriography]
	Tx Surgical graft to repair the aneurysm, medications to control underlying causes. [*see also*: aneurysmectomy]
aneurysmectomy	Surgical procedure to remove an aneurysm and repair the defect in the artery wall. [*see also*: aneurysm, dissecting aneurysm]

angina pectoris [413.xx]	Mild-to-severe chest pain caused by ischemia of the myocardium. Atherosclerosis blocks the flow of oxygenated blood through the coronary arteries to the myocardium. Men may feel a crushing, pressure-like sensation in the chest, with pain extending up into the neck or down the left arm, often accompanied by extreme sweating and a sense of doom. Women often experience angina as indigestion. Angina pectoris can occur during exercise or while resting and is a warning sign of an impending myocardial infarction. [*see also*: acute coronary syndrome, arteriosclerosis, atherosclerosis, cardiac enzymes, diaphoresis, stress test]

L
S

angiogenesis	Process by which a cancerous tumor causes blood vessels in the surrounding tissues to grow into the tumor and provide it with nutrients.
angiography	Uses an x-ray beam and iodinated contrast dye injected into an artery or vein to create an image of the blood vessel. [*see also*: aortography, arteriography, coronary angiography, digital subtraction angiography, rotational angiography, venography]

anhidrosis [705.xx]	Congenital absence of the sweat glands and inability to tolerate heat.	S
anisocoria [379.xx]	Unequal sizes of the pupils. Caused by glaucoma, head trauma, stroke, or a tumor that damages the cranial nerve that causes the iris to dilate or constrict. [see also: miosis, mydriasis, pupillary response]	
anisocytosis [790.xx]	Erythrocytes that are either too large or too small. [see also: anemia, poikilocytosis, thalassemia]	
ankylosing spondylitis [720.xx]	Chronic inflammation of the vertebrae that leads to fibrosis, restriction of movement of the vertebrae, and stiffening of the spine. [see also: spondylolisthesis]	S
anorexia [783.xx]	Decreased appetite because of disease or the gastrointestinal side effects of a drug. [see also: anorexia nervosa]	L
anorexia nervosa [307.xx]	Extreme, chronic fear of being fat and an obsession with becoming thinner. The patient is driven to decrease food intake to the point of starvation. Patients deny being too thin, deny abnormal eating habits, and try to keep these a secret from family and friends by making excuses for not eating and wearing clothes that conceal their extreme weight loss. [see also: bulimia]	L

Dx H&P. Body weight loss of 15% or more. Physical exam and psychological exam.

Tx Nutritional support. If needed, psychological or psychiatric intervention may be warranted. [see also: cognitive-behavioral therapy, psychotherapy]

anosmia [781.xx]	Loss of the sense of smell. Most often caused by head trauma.	S
anovulation [628.xx]	Failure of the ovaries to release a mature ovum at the time of ovulation, although the menstrual cycle and flow are normal. This results in infertility. A normal condition prior to menarche and during menopause. [see also: dysfunctional uterine bleeding, ovulation]	
anoxia	Complete lack of oxygen in the arterial blood and body tissues. Caused by a lack of oxygen in the inhaled air or by an obstruction that prevents oxygen from reaching the lungs. [see also: cyanosis, hypoxemia, pulse oximetry]	
antagonism	Process in which two hormones exert opposite effects.	
anteflexion	Normal position of the uterus in which the superior portion is tipped anteriorly on top of the bladder.	
antepartum	From the mother's standpoint, the period of time from conception until labor and delivery. [see also: postpartum]	
anterior	Pertaining to the front of the body, the front part of an organ, or the front of a structure. Opposite of posterior. [see also: coronal plane, oblique]	S
anterior chamber	Small area between the cornea and the surface of the iris. Aqueous humor circulates through it. [see also: hyphema, slit-lamp examination, trabecular meshwork]	
anterior pituitary gland	Part of the pituitary gland that secretes thyroid-stimulating hormone (TSH), follicle-stimulating hormone (FSH), luteinizing hormone (LH), prolactin, adrenocorticotropic hormone (ACTH), and growth hormone (GH). [see also: dwarfism, hypopituitarism, panhypopituitarism, pituitary gland]	S

A = Abbreviations Section   **F** = Figures Section   **L** = Laboratory Section   **S** = Synonyms Section
Sx (Symptoms)   **Dx** (Diagnosis)   **Tx** (Treatment)

anthracosis [500.xx]	The constant exposure to coal dust in the air causes pulmonary fibrosis in which the alveoli lose their elasticity. [*see also*: pneumoconiosis]	S
antibodies	Produced by a B cell that becomes a plasma cell. There are five classes of antibodies (also known as immunoglobulins): IgA, IgD, IgE, IgG, and IgM. [*see also*: autoimmune diseases]	S
antidiuretic hormone	Hormone produced by the hypothalamus but stored in and released by the posterior pituitary gland. It stimulates the kidneys to move water back into the blood to increase the volume of the blood. [*see also*: ADH stimulation test, diabetes insipidus, syndrome of inappropriate antidiuretic hormone]	A
antigen	A protein marker on the cell membrane of an erythrocyte that indicates the blood type. Also, a protein marker on the cell wall of pathogens (bacteria, viruses, and so forth) and cancerous cells that the body recognizes as foreign.	S
antisperm antibody test	Cervical mucus test that detects antibodies against sperm in the woman's cervical mucus. Some antibodies attack the tail of the spermatozoon so that it cannot swim; others prevent the spermatozoon from penetrating cervical mucus. Men produce antibodies to their own spermatozoa when the spermatozoa must be absorbed by the body after a vasectomy. These antibodies remain even after reversal of the vasectomy. [*see also*: hormone testing, semen analysis, vasovasostomy]	
antithyroglobulin antibodies	Blood test that detects antibodies against thyroglobulin (precursor hormone to T_3 and T_4) in the thyroid gland. A positive test result indicates Hashimoto's thyroiditis. [*see also*: Hashimoto's thyroiditis, hyperthyroidism, hypothyroidism, rheumatoid arthritis, systemic lupus erythematosus]	
antrum	Transition between the body of the stomach and the narrowing channel of the pylorus.	
anuria [788.xx]	Absence of urine production by the kidney. The underlying cause is acute or chronic renal failure. [*see also*: acute renal failure, chronic renal failure, dialysis]	
anus	External opening of the rectum. The external anal sphincter is under voluntary control. The perianal area is around the anus. [*see also*: hemorrhoids]	F
anxiety disorder [300.xx]	Dwelling on issues that involve "What if …" and predicting or fearing that the worst thing will happen to self, family, or friends. [*see also*: panic disorder]	
	Dx Symptoms are not due to another mental disorder and all medical conditions have been ruled out. For a six-month period, the patient has had more days filled with anxiety than days without it, and the patient has three out of the six criteria listed in the DSM-IV.	
	Tx If needed, psychological or psychiatric intervention may be warranted. [*see also*: cognitive-behavioral therapy, hypnosis, psychotherapy]	
aorta	Largest artery in the body. It receives blood from the left ventricle of the heart. Parts of the aorta include the ascending aorta, the aortic arch, the thoracic aorta, and the abdominal aorta. [*see also*: aneurysm, aortography, coarctation of the aorta, ductus arteriosus]	F

aortic valve	Heart valve located between the left ventricle and the aorta. [*see also*: rheumatic heart disease]
aortography	Radiologic procedure in which radiopaque contrast dye is used to outline the aorta to look for stenosis or an aortic aneurysm. [*see also*: aneurysm, angiography, arteriography, coronary angiography, dissecting aneurysm, rotational angiography, venography]
Apgar score	Medical procedure that assigns a score to a newborn at one and five minutes after birth. Points (0–2) are given for heart rate, respiratory rate, muscle tone, response to stimulation, and skin color.
aphakia [379.xx]	Condition in which the lens of the eye has been surgically removed. In most patients, an artificial intraocular lens is put into the eye during the cataract surgery. Some cataract patients are not good candidates for an artificial intraocular lens. Their cataract is removed, but they wear special cataract eyeglasses, and they remain aphakic. [*see also*: cataract, cataract extraction, extracapsular cataract extraction, phacoemulsification]
aphasia	Loss of the ability to communicate verbally or in writing because of injury to the areas of the brain that deal with language and the interpretation of sounds and symbols. [*see also*: cerebrovascular accident, expressive aphasia, global aphasia, receptive aphasia] **S**
apheresis	Medical procedure that separates out one specific type of blood cell. The rest of the blood is returned to the donor. The collected cells are then given as a transfusion to a patient. [*see also*: plasmapheresis, stem cell transplantation]
aphthous stomatitis [528.xx]	Canker sores; they present as small ulcers of the oral mucosa. [*see also*: stomatitis] **S**
aplastic anemia [284.xx]	Failure of the bone marrow to produce erythrocytes because it has been damaged by disease, cancer, radiation, or chemotherapy drugs.The total number of erythrocytes is decreased, even though individual erythrocytes are normal in size and color. [*see also*: anemia, pancytopenia, radiation therapy] **L** **S**
apnea	Brief or prolonged absence of spontaneous respirations. [*see also*: neonatal apnea, polysomnography, sleep apnea]
aponeurosis	Flat, wide, white sheet of fibrous connective tissue that attaches a muscle to a bone or other structure. Primarily located in the abdominal region, dorsal lumbar region, and palmar region. [*see also*: transverse rectus abdominis muscle flap]
apoptosis	Programmed cell death in which the p53 gene directs the cell to shut down when its DNA is too damaged to be repaired.
appendicitis [540.xx–543.xx]	Inflammation and infection of the appendix. **L** **S**
	Dx H&P. Rebound tenderness in the LLQ, CBC to determine the number and presence of WBCs. Depending on the presentation of symptoms, a barium enema may be performed to see if they can visualize the appendix and the extent of its growth; an endoscopy may be performed for direct visualization. [*see also*: barium enema]
	Tx Surgery. Depending on the severity, either laparoscopically or through an open incision.
appendix	Long, thin pouch on the exterior wall of the cecum. It does not play a role in digestion. It contains lymphatic tissue and is active in the body's immune response. [*see also*: appendicitis, cecum] **F**

aqueous humor	Clear, watery fluid produced by the ciliary body. It circulates through the posterior and anterior chambers and takes nutrients and oxygen to the cornea and lens. [*see also*: glaucoma]
arachnoid	Thin, middle layer of the meninges. [*see also*: meninges, subarachnoid space]
areola	Pigmented area around the nipple of the breast. [*see also*: Tanner staging]
arrhythmia [427.xx]	Any type of irregularity in the rate or rhythm of the heart. **S** Arrhythmias include bradycardia, dysrhythmia, tachycardia, heart block, flutter, and fibrillation. [*see also*: automatic implantable cardiac defibrillator, cardioversion, electrocardiography, electrophysiology study, Holter monitor, radiofrequency catheter ablation, stress test] [*see also the following rhythms*: bradycardia, fibrillation, flutter, heart block, left bundle branch block, premature contraction, right bundle branch block, sick sinus syndrome, tachycardia]
arterial blood gases	Blood test to measure the partial pressure (P) of the gases oxygen **A** (PO_2) and carbon dioxide (PCO_2) in arterial blood. The pH, how **L** acid or alkaline the blood is, is also measured. The more carbon dioxide, the more acidic the blood and the lower the pH. [*see also*: deoxygenated, hypercapnea, hypoxemia, oxygen therapy]
arteriography	Radiologic procedure in which radiopaque iodinated contrast dye is injected into an artery to create an image that shows blockage, narrowed areas, or aneurysms. [*see also*: angiography, aortography, coronary angiography, digital subtraction angiography, rotational angiography]
arteriole	Smallest branch of an artery.
arteriosclerosis [440.xx]	Progressive degenerative changes that produce a narrowed, **L** hardened artery. The process begins with a small tear in the endothelium that is caused by chronic hypertension. Then LDLs in the blood deposit cholesterol and form an atheromatous plaque inside the artery, which can enlarge, making the lumen of the artery narrower and narrower. [*see also*: aneurysm, atherosclerosis, coronary artery disease, diabetic nephropathy, peripheral artery disease]
arteriovenous malformation	Abnormality in which arteries connect directly to veins (rather **A** than to capillaries), forming a twisted nest of blood vessels that can rupture and cause a stroke. Most commonly found in the brain. [*see also*: cerebrovascular accident]
	Dx Angiography to visualize the vessels. Sometimes a CT scan or MRI may be performed to assist in locating the vessel prior to performing the angiography.
	Tx Medications for general symptoms. Surgical intervention or irradiation therapy to correct the problem.
artery	Blood vessel that carries blood away from the heart. All arteries **F** carry oxygen-rich blood, except the pulmonary arteries that carry oxygen-poor blood to the lungs for oxygenation.
arthralgia [719.xx]	Pain in the joint from an injury, inflammation, or an infection from various causes. [*see also*: arthrography, avascular necrosis]
arthrocentesis	Surgical procedure to remove an accumulation of fluid in a joint by using a needle or trocar inserted into the joint space. [*see also*: bursitis, gout, hemarthrosis]

arthrodesis	Surgical procedure to fuse the bones in a degenerated, unstable joint. Used mostly in the extremities and when joint replacement isn't an option. Used to restore stability and for relief of severe pain. With the advancements in joint replacement, this procedure is being used less and less. [*see also*: bone graft, joint replacement surgery]
arthrography	Contrast dye is injected into the joint. It outlines the bones, capsule, and soft tissue structures of the joint. In magnetic resonance imaging, a noniodinated contrast dye medium is used and an MRI scan creates the image of the joint. [*see also*: arthralgia, degenerative joint disease, magnetic resonance imaging, torn meniscus]
arthropathy	Disease of a joint from any cause. [*see also*: avascular necrosis, bursitis, degenerative joint disease, gout, rheumatoid arthritis, temporomandibular joint syndrome]
arthroscopy	Surgical procedure that uses an arthroscope inserted into the joint to visualize the inside of the joint and its structures. Various instruments can be inserted through the arthroscope to scrape or cut damaged cartilage and smooth sharp bone edges. [*see also*: bursitis, degenerative joint disease, hemarthrosis, torn meniscus]
articular cartilage	Cartilage that covers the bone ends in a synovial joint. [*see also*: cartilage transplantation, torn meniscus, synovial joint]
articulation	A joint where two bones come together and join or articulate. [*see also*: joint] **S**
asbestosis [501.xx]	Constant exposure to inhaled particles of asbestos, causing pulmonary fibrosis in which the alveoli lose their elasticity. [*see also*: pneumoconiosis]
ascites [789.xx]	Accumulation of ascitic fluid in the abdominopelvic cavity, usually from an underlying disease. [*see also*: nephrotic syndrome, portal hypertension] **S**
aspiration pneumonia [507.xx]	Pneumonia caused by foreign matter, such as vomit, that is inhaled into the lungs. [*see also*: meconium aspiration, pneumonia, sudden infant death syndrome]
assisted delivery	Procedure in which obstetrical forceps or a vacuum extractor is used to facilitate delivery of the head of the fetus. [*see also*: dystocia]
asthma [493.xx]	Sudden onset of hyperreactivity of the bronchi and bronchioles with bronchospasm (contraction of the smooth muscle). Inflammation and swelling severely narrow the lumens. Attacks recur intermittently and are triggered by exposure to dust, mold, cigarette smoke, inhaled chemicals, exercise, cold air, or emotional stress. [*see also*: status asthmaticus] **L** **S**
	Dx H&P. Auscultation of the lungs. ABGs to determine lung function.
	Tx Medication and oxygen therapy to support episodes and long-term treatments. Depending on severity, mechanical ventilation may be required. [*see also*: endotracheal intubation]
astigmatism [367.xx]	Surface of the cornea is curved more steeply on one side of the eye than on the other, so there is no single point of focus. The patient's vision is blurry both near and at a distance. [*see also*: cornea, phacoemulsification, phorometry]

A = Abbreviations Section   **F** = Figures Section   **L** = Laboratory Section   **S** = Synonyms Section
Sx (Symptoms)   **Dx** (Diagnosis)   **Tx** (Treatment)

astrocyte	Star-shaped cell that provides structural support for neurons, connects them to capillaries, and forms the blood–brain barrier. [*see also*: neuroglia]	S
asystole	Complete absence of a heartbeat. [*see also*: automatic external defibrillator, cardiopulmonary resuscitation, conduction system, defibrillator, electrocardiography, systole]	S
ataxia [781.xx]	Incoordination of the muscles during movement, particularly the gait. Caused by diseases of the brain or spinal cord, cerebral palsy, or an adverse reaction to a drug. [*see also*: bradykinesia, cerebral palsy, dyskinesia, hyperkinesia]	S
atelectasis [518.xx]	Incomplete expansion or collapse of part or all of a lung due to mucus, tumor, trauma, or a foreign body that blocks the bronchus. [*see also*: adult respiratory distress syndrome, pneumoconiosis, pyothorax, ventilation-perfusion scan]	S
atherosclerosis [440.xx]	When atheromatous plaques are formed inside an artery, collagen fibers form underneath the plaque, and the artery wall becomes hard and nonelastic. [*see also*: angina pectoris, arteriosclerosis, bruit, coronary artery disease]	
atrial septal defect [745.xx]	Permanent hole in the interatrial septum of the fetal heart, caused by a congenital defect that is present at birth.	A
atrial tachycardia [427.xx]	Arrhythmia in which there is a fast but regular rhythm (up to 200 beats/minute). It occurs when an ectopic group of cells somewhere in the atrium produces an electrical impulse that overrides the SA node rhythm. [*see also*: cardioversion, dysrhythmia, radiofrequency catheter ablation, tachycardia]	
atrioventricular node	Small knot of tissue located between the right atrium and right ventricle. The AV node is part of the conduction system of the heart and receives electrical impulses from the SA node. [*see also*: conduction system]	A F
atrium	Upper chamber of the heart. There are two atria. [*see also*: foramen ovale]	F
atrophy	Loss of muscle bulk in one or more muscles. It can be caused by malnutrition or can occur in any part of the body that is paralyzed where the muscles receive no electrical impulses from the nerves. [*see also*: flaccid paralysis, muscle biopsy, muscular dystrophy, spastic paralysis]	S
attention-deficit hyperactivity disorder [314.xx]	Distractability, short attention span, inability to follow directions, restlessness, hyperactivity, emotional lability, and impulsiveness. It may be caused by mild brain damage at birth, genetic factors, or other abnormalities. It is five times more common in boys than in girls. Most children outgrow the symptoms by late childhood.	A S
	Dx The diagnosis of ADHD remains controversial. DMS-IV and medical professionals should be consulted. The patient will exhibit hyperactivity, impulsiveness, and inability to focus, but these are only a small part of a definitive diagnosis.	
	Tx If needed, psychological or psychiatric intervention may be warranted. [*see also*: psychotherapy]	
audiometry	Hearing test that measures hearing acuity and documents hearing loss. The patient puts on headphones that are connected to an audiometer that produces a series of pure tones, each at a different frequency and varying in intensity. The patient presses a button to signal when the sound is heard. Used to assist in determining whether a patient needs a hearing aid. [*see also*: brainstem	

	auditory evoked response, cochlear implant, conductive hearing loss, Ménière's disease, presbyacusis, Rinne and Weber hearing tests, sensorineural hearing loss, tympanometry]
auditory cortex	Area of the temporal lobe of the brain where nerve impulses from the auditory nerve are interpreted for the sense of hearing. [see also: auditory nerve, brainstem auditory evoked response, temporal lobe]
auditory nerve	Cranial nerve VIII that conducts nerve impulses from the semicircular canals and the cochlea to the brain, to maintain balance and for the sense of hearing. [see also: acoustic neuroma, auditory cortex, cochlea, semicircular canals, sensorineural hearing loss, vertigo] S
augmentation mammaplasty	Surgical procedure to enlarge the size of a small breast by inserting a breast prosthesis or implant under the skin or chest muscles. [see also: mammaplasty, reconstructive mammaplasty, reduction mammaplasty] S
aura	Before the onset of a seizure, some epileptics experience a visual, olfactory, sensory, or auditory sign that warns them of an impending seizure. [see also: epilepsy, seizure]
auscultation	Medical procedure that uses a stethoscope to listen to sounds within the body, such as breath sounds, heart sounds, and bowel sounds.
autism [299.xx]	Inability to communicate or form significant relationships with others, and a lack of interest in doing so. Patients may be of normal intelligence or may be mentally retarded. Speech may not develop or may be abnormal, with echolalia. Patients avoid physical contact and eye contact, but are fascinated by certain objects. There are ritualistic, repetitive behaviors.
	Dx H&P. Emphasis on a neurological exam to demonstrate deficiencies. CT scan and MRI to view structural problems within the brain.
	Tx Treatment depends on the patient and the severity. An educational program specifically designed for the patient's deficits. Some patients will need around-the-clock care.
autograft	Uses a graft taken from another part of the patient's body. [see also: allograft, bone grafting, graft-versus-host disease, skin grafting, xenograft] S
autoimmune disease	Disease in which the body makes antibodies against its own tissues. Specific tissues are attacked, causing pain and loss of function. [see also: antibodies, Addison's disease, choroiditis, Cushing's syndrome, diabetes mellitus type 1, Graves' disease, Hashimoto's thyroiditis, iritis, multiple sclerosis, myasthenia gravis, polymyositis, psoriasis, rheumatic heart disease, rheumatoid arthritis, scleroderma, systemic lupus erythematosus, thymoma, uveitis, vitiligo] L S
automatic external defibrillator	A portable computerized device kept on emergency response vehicles and in public places like airports. It analyzes the patient's heart rhythm and delivers an electrical shock to stimulate a heart in cardiac arrest. An AED is designed to be used by nonmedical persons. [see also: asystole, defibrillator] S
automatic implantable cardiac defibrillator	An implanted device under the skin of the chest. It has leads (wires) that go to the heart, sense its rhythm, and the defibrillator delivers an electrical shock, if needed. [see also: defibrillator, dysrhythmia] A

A = Abbreviations Section   **F** = Figures Section   **L** = Laboratory Section   **S** = Synonyms Section
Sx (Symptoms)   **Dx** (Diagnosis)   **Tx** (Treatment)

autonomic nervous system

Division of the nervous system that carries nerve impulses to the heart, involuntary smooth muscles, and glands. It includes the parasympathetic nervous system and the sympathetic nervous system. [*see also*: parasympathetic nervous system, sympathetic nervous system]

avascular necrosis [733.xx]

Death of cells in the epiphysis of a long bone, often the femur. **S** Caused by an injury, fracture, or dislocation that damages nearby blood vessels or by a blood clot that interrupts the blood supply to the bone. [*see also*: arthralgia, epiphysis, joint replacement surgery]

aversion therapy

The patient thinks about a desired, but destructive, behavior and the thought is coupled with a mild electrical shock or noxious smell, such as ammonia. This is a form of conditioning that creates an aversion to that behavior. Used to treat drug and cigarette addiction and sexual identity issues.

avoidant personality [301.xx]

Avoidance of social contact because of excessive shyness and extreme fear and sensitivity to criticism or rejection.

avulsion

An injury that causes the muscle to tear away from the tendon **S** or the tendon to tear away from the bone.

axon

Part of the neuron that is a single, elongated branch at the opposite end from the dendrites. It conducts the electrical impulse and releases neurotransmitters into the synapse. Large axons are covered by an insulating layer of myelin. [*see also*: myelin, oligodendroglia, Schwann cell, white matter]

B

B cell

Type of lymphocyte that matures in the red bone marrow. B cells are activated by macrophages and become plasma cells that make antibodies. B cells also activate helper T cells. [*see also*: antibodies, immunoglobulin D, interleukin, leukocyte, lymphocyte, macrophage, multiple myeloma, spleen, T cell, vaccination]

Babinski's sign

Neurologic test in which the lateral sole of the foot is stroked **S** from heel to toes. A normal test (or negative Babinski) shows downward curling of the toes. An abnormal test (or positive Babinski) shows upward extension of the great toe and lateral fanning of the other toes and indicates injury to the parietal lobe of the brain or to the spinal nerves. [*see also*: central nervous system, parietal lobe, reflex]

bacterial vaginosis [616.xx]

Bacterial infection of the vagina due to *Gardnerella vaginalis*. There is a white or grayish vaginal discharge that has a fishy odor. [*see also*: vaginitis]

bacteriuria [599.xx]

Presence of bacteria in the urine. Normally, urine is sterile. The presence of bacteria indicates a urinary tract infection. [*see also*: cystitis, epididymitis, nonspecific urethritis, orchitis, prostatitis, pyelonephritis, sexually transmitted disease, urinary tract infection]

balanitis [607.xx]

Inflammation and infection of the glans penis caused by bacteria, viruses, yeasts, or fungi. Often associated with phimosis and inadequate hygiene of the prepuce. [*see also*: circumcision, phimosis]

band

Immature neutrophil in the blood. It has a nucleus shaped like a **F** curved band. [*see also*: neutrophil]

barium

Radiopaque contrast dye made of small, chalky particles **A** suspended in a liquid. Used for radiologic procedures of the digestive tract. [*see also*: barium enema, barium swallow]

barium enema	Radiologic procedure that uses a liquid radiopaque contrast dye (barium), introduced through the rectum, that outlines and coats the walls of the rectum and colon. An x-ray is then taken. [*see also:* appendicitis, Crohn's disease, diverticulitis, double contrast enema, inflammatory bowel disease, polyps]	A S
barium swallow	Radiologic procedure that uses a liquid radiopaque contrast dye (barium) that is swallowed. Barium coats and outlines the walls of the esophagus, stomach, and duodenum. Fluoroscopy is used to follow the barium through the small intestine. Individual x-rays are taken at specific times throughout the procedure. Used to identify ulcers, tumors, or obstruction. [*see also:* adhesions, bulimia, gastroesophageal reflux disease, hiatal hernia]	S
basal cell carcinoma [173.xx]	Arises from the basal layer of the epidermis. It is the most common type of skin cancer. It most often appears as a raised, pearly bump. A slow-growing cancer that does not metastasize to other parts of the body. [*see also:* Moh's surgery, premalignant skin lesions]	
basophil	Least numerous of the leukocytes. It is classified as a granulocyte because granules in its cytoplasm stain dark blue to purple with basic dye. It releases histamine and heparin at the site of tissue damage. [*see also:* complement proteins, complete blood count, histamine, immunoglobulin E]	A F L
Beck Depression Inventory	Screening tool that assesses the degree of depression. This is a self-assessment filled out by the patient, and each item offers four answers that show progressively more depressed emotions. [*see also:* bipolar disorder, dysthymia, major depression, premenstrual dysphoric disorder, postpartum depression, seasonal affective disorder]	A
Bell's palsy [351.xx]	Usually caused by a viral infection. Inflammation of cranial nerve VII causes weakness, drooping, or actual paralysis of one side of the face. [*see also:* blepharoptosis, facial nerve]	
	Dx H&P. Diagnostic tests to rule out other causes of paralysis.	
	Tx Medications to treat the pain and other symptoms. Physical therapy and speech therapy to strengthen the muscles.	
below-the-knee amputation	A below-the-knee amputation is performed at the level of the tibia and fibula. Most commonly performed on diabetic patients who have had a gangrenous infection. The progression of the diabetes and/or infection determines the level of the amputation, whether it is above the knee or below the knee. [*see also:* amputation, diabetes mellitus, gangrene, prosthesis]	S
Bence Jones protein	Urine test used to monitor the course of multiple myeloma. The cancerous plasma cells produce this abnormal immunoglobulin that can be detected in the urine. [*see also:* multiple myeloma]	
benign prostatic hypertrophy [600.xx]	Benign, gradual enlargement of the prostate gland that compresses the urethra and causes the bladder to retain urine. [*see also:* acid phosphatase, digital rectal examination, hydronephrosis, prostate gland, transurethral resection of the prostate]	A S
bile	Yellow-green, bitter fluid produced by the liver and stored in the gallbladder. It is released into the duodenum to digest the fat in foods. [*see also:* bile ducts, cholecystokinin, cholelithiasis, emulsification, gallbladder, lipase, liver]	
bile ducts	Bile produced by the liver flows into the right and left hepatic ducts. Bile leaves the gallbladder through the cystic duct, which	S F

A = Abbreviations Section   F = Figures Section   L = Laboratory Section   S = Synonyms Section
Sx (Symptoms)   Dx (Diagnosis)   Tx (Treatment)

joins the hepatic duct to form the common bile duct. All of these ducts form a treelike structure known as the biliary tree. [*see also*: bile, cholangiography, cholangitis, choledocholithiasis, choledocholithotomy, gallbladder, tumor marker (CA 19-9)]

biopsy

Surgical procedure to remove tissue for the purpose of diagnosis. **A** The biopsy specimen is sent to the pathology department for examination and diagnosis. [*see also*: bronchoscopy, *Campylobacter*-like organism test, core needle biopsy, endoscopic sinus surgery, excisional biopsy, fine-needle biopsy, frozen section, incisional biopsy, interventional radiology, punch biopsy, shave biopsy, stereotactic biopsy and neurosurgery, vacuum-assisted biopsy]

bladder

Expandable reservoir for storing urine. [*see also*: cystectomy, cystitis, cystometry, cystoscopy, interstitial cystitis, KUB x-ray, neurogenic bladder, radiation cystitis, stone basketing, trigone, vesicocele, vesicovaginal fistula]

bladder neck suspension

Surgical procedure to correct stress incontinence. A supportive sling of muscle tissue or synthetic material is inserted around the base of the bladder and the urethra, elevating them to a normal position. [*see also*: incontinence]

blepharitis [373.xx]

Inflammation or infection of the eyelid with redness, crusts, and scales at the bases of the eyelashes. Acute blepharitis is caused by allergy or infection. Chronic blepharitis is caused by acne rosacea, seborrheic dermatitis, or an infection from microscopic mites that live in the sebaceous glands and eyelash follicles. [*see also*: acne rosacea, chalazion, eczema, sebaceous glands, stye]

blepharoplasty

Plastic surgery procedure for the removal of fat and drooping or sagging skin from around the eyelids. [*see also*: blepharoptosis, orbicularis oculi muscle, rhytidectomy]

blepharoptosis [374.xx]

Drooping of the upper eyelid from excessive fat or sagging of the tissues due to age. Can also be from a disease that affects the muscles or nerves. [*see also*: Bell's palsy, blepharoplasty, cerebrovascular accident, myasthenia gravis, oculomotor nerve, orbicularis oculi muscle, rhytidectomy, trigeminal nerve]

blindness [369.xx]

Condition of complete or partial loss of vision. Caused by trauma, eye diseases, or defects in the structure of the eye, optic nerve, or visual cortex in the brain. [*see also*: color blindness, conversion disorder, glaucoma, legally blind, night blindness, retinitis pigmentosa, sexually transmitted disease]

blister

Repetitive rubbing injury that mechanically separates the epidermis **S** from the dermis and releases tissue fluid. A blister is a fluid-filled sac with a thin, transparent covering of epidermis.

blood

Type of connective tissue that contains plasma and blood cells. The blood transports oxygen, carbon dioxide, nutrients, and waste products of metabolism. [*see also*: ABO blood group, anemia, apheresis, blood dyscrasia, blood type, circulatory system, clotting factors, dialysis, erythrocyte, hemorrhage, hemostasis, immune response, leukocyte, oxyhemoglobin, phlebotomy, plasma, polycythemia vera, Rh blood group, stem cell, thrombocyte]

blood chemistries

Blood test used to determine the levels of various chemicals in the blood. [*see also*: metabolic panel, phlebotomy]

blood donation

Medical procedure in which a unit of whole blood is collected from a donor for transfusion. The unit is labeled as to blood type and is stored as whole blood, or it is divided into its component parts (erythrocytes, platelets, plasma) to meet the needs of a specific patient. [*see also*: blood transfusion, type and crossmatch, p24 antigen test]

blood dyscrasia	Any disease condition involving blood cells. [*see also*: hemophilia, leukemia, sickle cell anemia, thrombocytopenia]
blood smear	Blood test done manually to examine the characteristics of erythrocytes and leukocytes under the microscope when an abnormal automated CBC suggests leukemia, anemia, etc. [*see also*: complete blood count, leukemia]
blood transfusion	Whole blood, blood cellular products, or plasma given by intravenous transfusion. [*see also*: apheresis, blood donation, erythropoietin, hemolytic reaction, hemophilia, p24 antigen test, type and crossmatch]
blood type	Blood test that determines the blood type (A, B, AB, or O) and Rh factor (positive or negative) of the patient's blood. [*see also*: ABO blood group, Rh blood group, type and crossmatch]
blood urea nitrogen	Blood test that measures the amount of urea in the blood. Used to monitor kidney function and the progression of kidney disease or to watch for signs of nephrotoxicity. [*see also*: creatinine, kidney, metabolic panel, urea] **A L**
blood vessels	Channels through which the blood circulates throughout the body. These include arteries, capillaries, and veins. [*see also*: angiogenesis, angiography, arteriovenous malformation, artery, capillary, ductus arteriosus, endothelium, hemangioma, hemodialysis, vein] **S**
body dysmorphic disorder [300.xx]	Overconcern with minor defects in the appearance of the body, particularly the face, with the demand for frequent plastic surgery. [*see also*: dermatoplasty, rhinoplasty, rhytidectomy]
boil	A localized abscess around a hair follicle that causes the skin to be elevated, painful, and red. Also known as a furuncle. [*see also*: carbuncle, folliculitis, incision and drainage, pilonidal sinus] **S**
bone density test	Radiologic procedure that measures the bone mineral density to determine if demineralization from osteoporosis has occurred. The heel or wrist bone can be tested, but the hip and spine bones give more accurate results. [*see also*: densitometry, osteoporosis, vertebra]
bone grafting	Surgical procedure that uses whole bone or bone chips to repair fractures with extensive bone loss or defects due to bone cancer. Bone can be taken from the patient's own body or from a donor.
bone marrow aspiration	Procedure to remove red bone marrow from the posterior iliac crest of the hip bone to diagnose leukemia or lymphoma. [*see also*: bone marrow donation, bone marrow testing, bone marrow transplantation, leukemia]
bone marrow donation	Procedure to harvest bone marrow from a healthy donor to give to a patient who needs a bone marrow transplantation. [*see also*: allograft, bone marrow aspiration, bone marrow testing, bone marrow transplantation, leukemia]
bone marrow testing	Cytology test of the red bone marrow to examine all the stages of cell development (stem cell to mature cell). Used to help diagnose leukemia or lymphoma and monitor its progression. [*see also*: bone marrow donation, bone marrow transplantation, leukemia, lymphoma]
bone marrow transplantation	Red marrow is harvested by aspirating it from the hip bone of a matched donor. The patient is treated with high-dose chemo- **A**

therapy drugs or radiation to destroy all cancerous cells (this also destroys all the cells in the red marrow). The donor marrow is then filtered and given to the patient intravenously. The donated bone marrow cells travel through the blood to the bones, where they implant. After two to four weeks, the patient's marrow begins to produce normal blood cells. [*see also*: bone marrow donation, bone marrow testing, leukemia, stem cell transplantation]

bone scintigraphy
Nuclear medicine procedure in which phosphate compounds are tagged with a radioactive tracer, injected intravenously, and taken up into the bone. A gamma scintillation camera detects gamma rays from the radioactive tracer. Areas of increased uptake, "hot spots," indicate increased bone metabolism due to arthritis, fracture, osteomyelitis, cancerous tumors of the bone, or areas of bony metastasis. [*see also*: degenerative joint disease, fracture, rheumatoid arthritis, osteomyelitis]

borderline personality
[301.xx]
Inability to sustain a stable relationship. Patients fear abandonment and panic when they are alone, rushing into intense but self-destructive relationships. They tend to see things in black and white—all good or all bad with no middle ground. They are hypersensitive, with strong emotions that can easily change. They have poor tolerance to stress and often overreact.

Botox injection
Medical procedure in which the drug Botox is injected into the muscles that cause deep skin wrinkles on the face. The drug inhibits the release of acetylcholine and keeps these muscles from contracting. This treatment is effective for several months. [*see also*: rhytidectomy]

bowel resection and anastomosis
Surgical procedure to remove a section of diseased intestine and rejoin the intestine. The cut ends are then sutured together, or the end of one segment is sutured to the side of the other. [*see also*: adhesions, inflammatory bowel disease, volvulus]

Bowman's capsule
Sphere-shaped structure that surrounds the glomerulus and collects filtrate. [*see also*: glomerulus, nephron]   S

brace
Orthopedic device that supports a body part with weak muscles. It keeps it in anatomical alignment and may permit some movement depending on the type of brace applied. [*see also*: orthosis]

brachytherapy
Category that includes internal, interstitial, and intracavitary radiotherapy in which a radioactive substance is placed in, or a short distance from, the tumor.

bradycardia
[427.xx]
Arrhythmia in which the heart beats too slowly. [*see also*: dysrhythmia, hypothyroidism]

bradykinesia
[332.xx]
Abnormally slow muscle movements or a decrease in the number of spontaneous muscle movements. Usually associated with Parkinson's disease. [*see also*: ataxia, Huntington's chorea, hyperkinesis, Parkinson's disease]

bradypnea
Abnormally slow rate of breathing. May be caused by a chemical imbalance or neurological damage that affects the respiratory center of the brain.

brain
Largest organ of the nervous system. It is part of the central nervous system and is located in the cranial cavity. [*see also*: anencephaly, brainstem, cerebrum, cerebellum, frontal lobe, occipital lobe, parietal lobe, temporal lobe]   F

brain death
[997.xx]
A condition in which there is irreversible loss of all brain function, as confirmed by an electroencephalography (EEG) that is flat,

showing no brain wave activity of any kind for 30 minutes.
[*see also*: coma, electroencephalography]

brainstem

Most inferior part of the brain that joins with the spinal cord. It is composed of the midbrain, pons, and medulla oblongata.

brainstem auditory evoked response

Analyzes the brain's response to sounds. The patient listens as an audiometer produces a series of clicks. An EEG is performed at the same time. A lesion or tumor in the auditory cortex of the brain or on the auditory nerve will produce an abnormal brainstem auditory evoked response. [*see also*: acoustic neuroma, auditory cortex, auditory nerve]   A S

Braxton Hicks contractions
[644.xx]

Irregular uterine contractions during the last trimester. These strengthen the uterine muscle in preparation for labor. [*see also*: premature labor]   S

BRCA1 or **BRCA2 gene**

Blood test for the BRCA1 or BRCA2 gene, a genetic mutation that significantly increases the risk of breast cancer. The BRCA1 gene also increases the risk of ovarian cancer. [*see also*: receptor assays]

breast self-examination

Systematic palpation of all areas of the breast and under the arm to detect lumps, masses, or enlarged lymph nodes. A BSE should be done monthly to detect early signs of breast cancer.   A

breech birth
[652.xx]

Birth position in which the presenting part of the fetus is the buttocks, buttocks and the feet, or just the feet. [*see also*: dystocia]

brittle diabetic

One who is being treated for diabetes mellitus but has difficulty controlling blood glucose levels, with frequent swings from hyperglycemia to hypoglycemia. [*see also*: diabetes mellitus, glycosylated hemoglobin]

broad ligament

Double layer of peritoneum that supports and suspends the uterus, fallopian tubes, and ovaries within the pelvic cavity. [*see also*: peritoneum, uterine prolapse, uterine suspension]

bronchiectasis
[494.xx]

Chronic, permanent enlargement and loss of elasticity of the bronchi and bronchioles. [*see also*: pneumoconiosis]

   Dx   H&P. CT scan and bronchoscopy to visualize (and remove mucus from) the lungs. [*see also*: bronchoscopy]

   Tx   Medication to treat the symptoms, oxygen therapy to improve lung function, possible surgery.

bronchiole

Small tubular air passageway that branches off the bronchus. It carries inhaled and exhaled air to and from the alveoli. [*see also*: bronchitis]   F

bronchitis
[466.xx; 491.xx]

Acute or chronic inflammation or infection of the bronchi. Inflammation due to pollution or smoking; infections are caused by bacteria or viruses. [*see also*: chronic bronchitis]

   Dx   H&P. X-ray to visualize the chest, pulmonary function tests to determine lung performance.

   Tx   Medications to treat the underlying symptoms. Oxygen therapy, if necessary, to improve blood oxygen levels. Relieve any underlying causes, such as smoking.

bronchoscopy

Surgical procedure that uses a flexible, lighted scope inserted through the mouth to examine the trachea and bronchi. Attachments on the scope can be used to remove foreign bodies, suction thick mucus, or perform a biopsy.

bronchus

Tubular air passageway that branches off the trachea to the right or left and enters each lung. It carries inhaled and exhaled air to and from the bronchiole. [*see also*: bronchiole, bronchitis, cilia]   F

A = Abbreviations Section   **F** = Figures Section   **L** = Laboratory Section   **S** = Synonyms Section
Sx (Symptoms)   **Dx** (Diagnosis)   **Tx** (Treatment)

bruise	Blunt trauma that causes bleeding in the muscle but does not break the skin. [*see also*: ecchymosis]	
bruit	A harsh, rushing sound made by blood passing through an artery narrowed and roughened by atherosclerosis. The bruit can be heard when a stethoscope is placed over the artery. [*see also*: carotid artery, cerebrovascular accident]	
bulbourethral glands	Small, bulblike glands below the prostate that secrete mucus into the urethra during ejaculation.	F S
bulimia [307.xx]	Patients gorge themselves on excessive amounts of food (binge eating) and then, for fear of gaining weight, they rid (purge) themselves of food by using laxatives or by self-induced vomiting. Long-term vomiting wears away tooth enamel, causes inflammation and ulcers in the esophagus and can lead to death. [*see also*: anorexia nervosa, barium swallow, polyphagia]	S

Dx H&P. Lab chemistries to show loss of electrolytes due to purging. Psychological exam.

Tx Psychological and/or psychiatric intervention, including medications; nutritional support. [*see also*: cognitive-behavioral therapy]

bundle branches	Parallel fiber bundles of the conduction system of the heart that begin at the bundle of His and travel down the interventricular septum. At the apex of the heart, the right bundle branch turns to the right ventricle and the left bundle branch turns to the left ventricle. Then, each bundle divides into the Purkinje fibers. [*see also*: conduction system]	F
bundle of His	Section of the conduction system of the heart after the AV node. It splits into the right and left bundle branches. [*see also*: conduction system]	F S
bunionectomy	Surgical procedure to remove the prominent part of a metatarsal bone that is causing a bunion.	
burns [940.xx–949.xx]	Heat (fire, hot objects, steam, boiling water), electrical current (lightning, electrical outlets or cords), chemicals, or radiation or x-rays (sunshine or prescribed radiation therapy) can cause a burn injury to the superficial or deep tissues. [*see also*: first-degree burn, second-degree burn, third-degree burn]	L

Dx H&P. Other diagnostic procedures vary depending on the degree and cause of the burn.

Tx The degree of burn will dictate the appropriate treatment.

bursa	Fluid-filled sac that decreases friction where a tendon rubs against a bone near a synovial joint. It contains synovial fluid. [*see also*: bursitis, synovial joint]	
bursitis [726.xx–727.xx]	Inflammation of the bursal sac because of repetitive muscular activity or pressure on the bone underneath the bursa. Most often occurs in the shoulders and knees. [*see also*: bursa]	S

Dx H&P. X-ray of the bursa and underlying bone.

Tx Medication for symptoms, surgical aspiration of the joint, laboratory analysis of joint fluid. [*see also*: arthocentesis, joint replacement surgery]

C

calcitonin	Hormone secreted by the thyroid gland. Along with parathyroid hormone, it regulates the amount of calcium in the blood. If the calcium level is too high, calcitonin moves calcium from the blood	S

	and deposits it in the bones. [see also: calcium, thyroid gland, parathyroid gland]	
calcium	Blood test that measures the level of calcium. Most commonly used to evaluate the function of the parathyroid gland. [see also: calcitonin, metabolic panel, parathyroid gland, osteoporosis]	A L
callus [700.xx]	Repetitive rubbing injury that causes the epidermis to gradually thicken into a wide, elevated pad. A corn is a callus with a hard central area with a pointed tip that causes pain and inflammation of deeper skin tissues.	S
calix	Ducts at the tip of each renal pyramid. The minor calices take urine to the major calices. Calyx is an alternate spelling.	F
Campylobacter-like organism test	Rapid screening test to detect the presence of the bacterium *Helicobacter pylori*. A biopsy of gastric mucosa is placed in contact with the substance urea. If *H. pylori* bacteria are present, they will metabolize the urea to ammonia, and ammonia changes the color of the test pad. *Campylobacter* was reclassified to the genus *Helicobacter*. [see also: peptic ulcer disease]	A
cancer	General word for any type of cancerous cell or tumor. There are four broad categories of cancer: carcinoma, sarcoma, leukemia, and embryonal cell carcinoma. The way in which the cancer is treated depends on the type and extent of the cancer.	L S
candidiasis [112.xx]	Yeast infection due to *Candida albicans*. Usually occurs after taking an antibiotic drug for a bacterial infection and is seen in immunocompromised patients. [see also: thrush, vaginal candidiasis]	
capillary	Smallest blood vessel in the body. It connects the arterioles to the venules. The exchange of oxygen and carbon dioxide takes place in the capillaries. [see also: petechiae]	
capsulotomy	Surgical procedure that is only done after a cataract extraction when the remaining posterior lens capsule becomes cloudy or wrinkled. A laser is used to make an opening in the capsule to restore normal vision. [see also: cataract extraction]	
carbon dioxide	Exhaled gas that is a waste product of cellular metabolism. [see also: arterial blood gases, cyanosis, deoxygenated, hypercapnia]	A
carboxyhemoglobin	Blood test to measure the level of carbon monoxide, a byproduct of fires or engines that burn fuel. In unventilated spaces, carbon monoxide from smoke or car exhaust builds up, combining with hemoglobin in the blood to form carboxyhemoglobin. This prevents the hemoglobin from carrying oxygen or carbon dioxide molecules. Carboxyhemoglobin blood levels above 50% are fatal.	A
carbuncle [680.xx]	Composed of large furuncles with connecting channels through the subcutaneous tissue or to the skin surface. [see also: boil]	
carcinoembryonic antigen	Blood test that detects a protein normally present in an embryo, but not in adults. Elevated levels of CEA are seen with several different cancers. The higher the level, the more advanced the cancer is. CEA can also be elevated in patients with noncancerous diseases of the colon or liver and in patients who smoke.	
carcinogen	Environmental substance that can contribute to the development of cancer. [see also: cancer]	
carcinoid syndrome [259.xx]	A set of symptoms caused by the release of the hormone serotonin from a carcinoid tumor, a slow-growing cancerous tumor that seldom metastasizes. Occurring mainly in the digestive tract, it does not exhibit all of the characteristics of cancer.	

A = Abbreviations Section **F** = Figures Section **L** = Laboratory Section **S** = Synonyms Section
Sx (Symptoms) **Dx** (Diagnosis) **Tx** (Treatment)

	Dx	H&P. Lab tests and UA to determine hormone levels and metabolic effects on the body. A CT scan, MRI, or endoscopy with biopsy may be performed to visualize the tumor.
	Tx	Depending on location: Medication, surgery, radiation therapy, or chemotherapy.

carcinoid tumor Slow-growing cancerous tumor that seldom metastasizes. It does not exhibit all of the characteristics of cancer. It occurs mainly in the digestive tract. [*see also*: carcinoid syndrome]

carcinoma Cancer of epithelial cells in the skin and mucous membranes of organs. Carcinomas grow more slowly than sarcomas, but they occur more frequently. Carcinomas usually metastasize via the lymphatic system. [*see also*: basal cell carcinoma, metastasis] A

carcinomatosis General word for a condition in which cancerous tumors are present in multiple sites in the body. [*see also*: metastasis] S

cardia Small area where the esophagus enters the stomach. It is the part of the stomach that is nearest the heart. [*see also*: cardiac sphincter, gastroesophageal reflux disease, heartburn]

cardiac catheterization Diagnostic procedure performed to evaluate the arteries that supply the heart muscle with blood. A catheter is inserted into the femoral or brachial artery and threaded to the left atrium. Then radiopaque contrast dye is injected to outline the coronary arteries and show narrow or blocked areas. If blockages of the coronary arteries are present, an angioplasty may be performed at that time. [*see also*: coronary artery disease, myocardial infarction]

cardiac cycle One contraction of the heart and the rest period that follows. [*see also*: asystole, conduction system, diastole, dysrhythmia, murmur, systole]

cardiac enzymes Blood test to measure the levels of enzymes that are released into the blood when myocardial cells die. They include CK-MB and LDH. Cardiac enzymes are measured every few hours for several days. [*see also*: angina pectoris, creatine phosphokinase MB bands, lactate dehydrogenase, myocardial infarction, troponin] L

cardiac sphincter Muscular ring in the esophagus that keeps food in the stomach from going back into the esophagus. [*see also*: cardia, gastro-esophageal reflux disease, heartburn] S

cardiac tamponade [423.xx] When fluid, either from the pericardium or another source, presses on the heart and prevents it from beating. [*see also*: parietal pericardium, pericarditis]

	Dx	H&P. Presence of Beck's triad: hypotension, jugular vein distention, muffled heart sounds. Chest x-ray to visualize the heart outline, an EKG to determine heart function, and an echocardiogram to visualize the heart function. [*see also*: echocardiography]
	Tx	Medications; surgery to remove the fluid or insert a permanent drain. [*see also*: pericardiocentesis]

Cardiolite stress test Nuclear medicine procedure that combines a cardiac exercise stress test with intravenous injections of radioactive tracers of thallium-201 and technetium-99m. The radioactive tracers collect in those parts of the myocardium that have the best perfusion. The artery must be about 70% blocked before any abnormality is evident on the image. (When technetium-99m is joined to a synthetic molecule—sestamibi—the radioactive tracer combination is known as Cardiolite.) [*see also*: stress test] S

cardiomegaly [429.xx]	Enlargement of the heart, usually due to congestive heart failure. [*see also*: cardiomyopathy, congestive heart failure]	**S**

> **Dx** H&P. EKG to determine heart function, echocardiogram to visualize heart function and thickness of heart chambers. [*see also*: echocardiography, electrocardiography, radionuclide ventriculography]
>
> **Tx** Medication to improve heart function, possible surgery to remove excess muscle. An AICD may be considered.

cardiomyopathy
[425.xx]

Any disease condition of the heart muscle that includes heart enlargement and heart failure. [*see also*: cardiomegaly, congestive heart failure, cor pulmonale, dilated cardiomyopathy, echocardiography, idiopathic cardiomyopathy, radionuclide ventriculography]

cardiopulmonary bypass   **L**

Technique used during open-heart surgery in which the patient's blood is rerouted through a cannula in the femoral vein to a heart-lung machine. There, the blood is oxygenated, carbon dioxide and waste products are removed, and the blood is pumped back into the body via a cannula in the femoral artery. Cardiopulmonary bypass takes over the functions of the heart and lungs during the surgery. [*see also*: coronary artery bypass graft]

cardiopulmonary resuscitation   **A**

Medical procedure to ventilate the lungs and artificially circulate the blood if the patient has stopped breathing and the heart has stopped beating. Air is forced into the lungs by mouth or Ambu bag, while the chest is compressed to manually pump blood through the heart. [*see also*: asystole]

cardiovascular system

Body system that includes the heart, arteries, veins, and capillaries. It circulates the blood throughout the body.

cardioversion

Medical procedure to treat life-threatening arrhythmias or some abnormal rhythms. An electrical shock is sent to the heart in hopes of overriding the current electrical cycle. Sometimes, a low-voltage shock is synchronized with the EKG to occur at a specific moment during the cardiac cycle. [*see also*: cardiac cycle, de-fibrillator, dysrhythmia, fibrillation, flutter]

carotid artery   **F**

Major artery that carries blood to the face, head, and brain. If this artery is compressed, the lack of blood to the brain will cause a person to become unconscious. [*see also*: bruit, carotid duplex scan]

carotid duplex scan

Radiologic procedure that uses ultrasound to produce a two-dimensional image to visualize areas of stenosis and plaque in the carotid arteries. [*see also*: carotid artery, carotid endarterectomy, cerebrovascular accident]

carotid endarterectomy

Surgical procedure to remove plaque from the carotid artery. This opens up the lumen of the artery, restores blood flow to the brain, and decreases the possibility of a stroke. [*see also*: carotid artery, cerebrovascular accident]

carpal tunnel syndrome [354.xx]   **A**

Chronic condition with tingling in the hand because of inflammation and swelling of the tendons that go through the carpal tunnel of the wrist bones to reach the hand. The swelling compresses the median nerve. Caused by repetitive motions of the hand and wrist. [*see also*: cumulative trauma disorder]

> **Dx** H&P. Phalen's maneuver, Tinel's sign to demonstrate nerve compression. An MRI might be performed to visualize the internal structures of the wrist. Also, an EMG may provide

	information on nerve function. [see also: electromyelography, nerve conduction study, paresthesia]
Tx	Depends on severity: Medications to treat underlying symptoms, braces/splints to rest the affected area, physical or occupational therapy to strengthen the muscles, surgery to correct deficits and relieve pressure.

cartilage transplantation	Surgical procedure that is an alternative to a total knee replacement. Used to treat middle-aged adults (as opposed to elderly) with degenerative joint disease of the knee who have an active lifestyle. [see also: articular cartilage, joint replacement surgery]
caruncle	Red, triangular tissue at the medial corner of the eye.
cast	Medical procedure in which a cast of plaster or fiberglass is applied around a fractured bone and adjacent areas to immobilize the fracture in a fixed position to facilitate healing. [see also: fracture, orthosis]
cataract [366.xx]	Clouding of the lens. Protein molecules in the lens begin to clump together. Caused by aging, sun exposure, eye trauma, smoking, and some medications. Vision becomes dull and blurry, with faded colors and a yellowish tint around lights. [see also: aphakia, cataract extraction, lens]
cataract extraction	Surgical procedure to remove a lens affected by a cataract. Preoperatively, a laser is used to measure the length of the eye and the curvature of the cornea so that a customized intraocular lens can be created that corrects the patient's vision. [see also: aphakia, capsulotomy, extracapsular cataract extraction, phacoemulsification]
cauda equina	Group of nerve roots that begin where the spinal cord ends and continue inferiorly within the spinal cavity. They look like the individual hairs in the tail of a horse. [see also: spinal cord] **S**
caudad	Toward the tail bone, feet, or lower part of the body. Opposite of cephalad. [see also: cephalad] **S**
causalgia [354.xx–355.xx]	Severe, burning pain along a nerve and its branches. [see also: complex regional pain syndrome, neuralgia, pain management, paresthesia, radiculopathy, sciatica]
cavity	Hollow space surrounded by bones or muscles and containing organs and structures. [see also the following cavities: abdominal, abdominopelvic, cranial, nasal, oral, pelvic, spinal, and thoracic]
CD4 count	Measures the number of CD4 cells (helper T cells). Used to monitor the progression of the HIV virus and its response to antiretroviral drugs. The CD4:CD8 ratio is also monitored. [see also: acquired immune deficiency syndrome, human immunodeficiency virus, T cell]
cecum	First part of the large intestine. A short, pouchlike area. The appendix is attached to the cecum's external wall. [see also: appendix] **F**
celiac trunk	Part of the abdominal aorta from which arteries arise to take blood to the stomach, small intestine, liver, gallbladder, and pancreas.
cell membrane	Permeable barrier that surrounds a cell and holds in the cytoplasm. It allows water and nutrients to enter and waste products to leave the cell.

A = Abbreviations Section   **F** = Figures Section   **L** = Laboratory Section   **S** = Synonyms Section
Sx (Symptoms)   **Dx** (Diagnosis)   **Tx** (Treatment)

cellulitis [682.xx]	Spreading inflammation and infection of the connective tissues of the skin and muscle. The infecting bacteria produce enzymes that dissolve cells and allow the infection to spread between the tissue layers.
central nervous system	Division of the nervous system that includes the brain and the spinal cord. [*see also*: Babinski's sign] **A**
cephalad	Toward the head of the body. Opposite of caudad. [*see also*: caudad] **S**
cephalalgia [784.xx]	Pain in the head that is commonly known as a headache. [*see also*: hypoglycemia, migraine headache, motion sickness, myelography, pheochromocytoma, scotoma, sinusitis] **S**
cephalic presentation	Position of the fetus in which the head is the presenting part that is first to go through the birth canal. Vertex presentation is a type of cephalic presentation in which the top of the head is the presenting part. [*see also*: dystocia]
cephalopelvic disproportion [653.xx]	The size of the fetal head exceeds the size of the opening in the mother's pelvic bones. [*see also*: cesarean section, dilation, failure to progress, pelvimetry] **A**
cerclage	Surgical procedure to place a purse-string suture around the cervix to prevent it from dilating prematurely. The suture is removed prior to delivery. [*see also*: incompetent cervix] **S**
cerebellum	Small, rounded structure that is the most posterior part of the brain. It monitors muscle tone and position and coordinates new muscle movements. [*see also*: cerebral cortex] **F**
cerebral angiography	Radiologic procedure in which a radiopaque contrast dye is injected into the carotid arteries and an x-ray is taken to visualize the arterial circulation in the brain. [*see also*: aneurysm, angiography, cerebrovascular accident]
cerebral contusion [851.xx]	A traumatic injury to the brain or spinal cord. There is no loss of consciousness, but there is bruising with some bleeding in the tissues. [*see also*: concussion]
cerebral cortex	The outermost surface of the cerebrum and cerebellum. It consists of gray matter. [*see also*: cerebrum, cerebellum, gray matter]
cerebral palsy [343.xx]	Cerebral palsy is caused by a lack of oxygen to parts of the baby's brain during birth. The extent of involvement varies, but can include spastic muscles and lack of coordination in walking, eating, and talking. There can be muscle paralysis, seizures, and mental retardation. [*see also*: assisted delivery, ataxia] **A**
cerebrospinal fluid	Clear, colorless fluid that circulates through the subarachnoid space, around the brain, through the ventricles, and the spinal cavity. It cushions and protects the brain and contains glucose and other nutrients. It is produced by the ependymal cells that line the ventricles and spinal canal. [*see also*: cerebrospinal fluid examination, ependymal cell, hydrocephalus, otorrhea, subarachnoid space]
cerebrospinal fluid examination	Laboratory test that examines the CSF for clarity, color, cells, proteins, and other substances. Normal CSF is clear and colorless. Red blood cells indicate bleeding in the brain from a stroke or trauma. White blood cells indicate an infection, such as meningitis or encephalitis. Elevated protein levels indicate infection or the presence of a tumor. The presence of oligoclonal bands points to multiple sclerosis. Myelin-basic protein is elevated in multiple

A = Abbreviations Section   **F** = Figures Section   **L** = Laboratory Section   **S** = Synonyms Section
Sx (Symptoms)   **Dx** (Diagnosis)   **Tx** (Treatment)

sclerosis and amyotrophic lateral sclerosis. [*see also*: Creutzfeldt-Jakob disease, encephalitis, hydrocephalus, Lou Gehrig's disease, lumbar puncture, meningitis, multiple sclerosis]

cerebrovascular accident [435.xx–436.xx]
Disruption or blockage of blood flow to the brain, usually caused by an embolus or thrombus, which causes tissue death and an area of necrosis known as an infarct. [*see also*: embolus, thrombus, transient ischemic attack]   A L S

> **Dx** H&P. Sudden onset of neurological deficiencies. CT, MRI, or angiogram to visualize possible reasons. [*see also*: blepharoptosis, bruit, carotid duplex scan, cerebral angiography, scotoma]
>
> **Tx** Medical emergency treatment with medications to dissolve the clot and thin the blood. Depending on the extent of the injury, the patient may have to undergo extensive rehabilitation. [*see also*: carotid endarterectomy]

cerebrum
The largest and most visible part of the brain. Its surface contains gyri and sulci and it is divided into two hemispheres. [*see also*: anencephaly, corpus callosum, electroencephalography, fissure, hemisphere]   F

cerumen
Sticky wax that traps dirt in the external auditory canal. [*see also*: cerumen impaction, external auditory canal]   S

cerumen impaction [380.xx]
Cerumen, epithelial cells, and hair form a mass that occludes the external auditory canal. Occurs most commonly in the elderly because of dryness of the skin, thick cerumen, and growth of hair in the external auditory canal. [*see also*: cerumen impaction, external auditory canal]

cervical dysplasia [622.xx]
Abnormal growth of squamous cells that make up the epithelium of the cervix. Seen on abnormal Pap smears. Severe dysplasia is a precancerous or cancerous condition. [*see also*: genital warts, Papanicolaou smear]

cervical vertebrae
Vertebrae C1 through C7 in the cervical spine. C1 is also known as the atlas; C2 is known as the axis.   F

cervix
Narrow, most inferior part of the uterus. It contains the cervical canal. Part of the cervix hangs down into the vagina. The cervical os is the small central opening in the cervix. [*see also*: cerclage, cervical dysplasia, dilation and curettage, dyspareunia, genital warts, incompetent cervix, internal genitalia, Papanicolaou smear, pelvic inflammatory disease]   F

cesarean section
Surgical procedure to deliver a fetus because of cephalopelvic disproportion, failure to progress during labor, the mother being past the due date, or health problems in the mother or fetus. The fetus is delivered through an incision in the abdominal wall and uterus. [*see also*: dystocia, Nägele's rule, pelvimetry]   A

chalazion [373.xx]
A semisolid, chronically inflamed and granular lump on the edge of the eyelid in a sebaceous gland. Also known as a meibomian cyst. [*see also*: blepharitis, stye]   S

cheilitis [528.xx]
Inflammation and cracking of the lips and corners of the mouth due to infection, allergies, or nutritional deficiency.

cheiloplasty
Surgical procedure to repair the lip, usually because of a laceration.

chemical peel
Uses a chemical to remove the epidermis. Alphahydroxy acid (glycolic acid) provides the mildest chemical peel. Stronger chemical peels using trichloroacetic acid and phenol are usually

---

A = Abbreviations Section   **F** = Figures Section   **L** = Laboratory Section   **S** = Synonyms Section
Sx (Symptoms)   **Dx** (Diagnosis)   **Tx** (Treatment)

	done in surgery. [see also: dermabrasion, exfoliation, laser skin resurfacing]
chest tube insertion	Surgical procedure that uses a clear plastic tube inserted between the ribs into the thoracic cavity to remove air or blood due to trauma or infection. The tube is connected to suction through a measuring container. Used to treat a pneumothorax, pyothorax, or hemothorax. [see also: hemothorax, pneumothorax]
Chlamydia [099.xx]	A sexually transmitted disease caused by *Chlamydia trachomatis*, a gram-negative coccus bacterium. It is the most commonly transmitted STD. [see also: sexually transmitted disease]

	Sx	♂ : May have no symptoms or may have painful urination with burning and itching. Thin, watery discharge from the urethra. [see also: epididymitis] ♀ : Frequently have no symptoms or slight vaginal discharge.	S
	Dx	Smear of discharge from urethra or cervix.	
	Tx	Oral antibiotic drugs.	

chloasma [374.xx]	Melanocyte-stimulating hormone can become active during pregnancy and cause dark, hyperpigmented areas on the face. [see also: linea nigra]	S
cholangiography	Radiologic procedure that uses a contrast dye to outline the bile ducts. An x-ray is taken to identify stones in the gallbladder and biliary ducts or thickening of the gallbladder wall. [see also: bile ducts, cholangitis, cholecystitis, choledocholithiasis, cholelithiasis, endoscopic retrograde cholangiopancreatography, gallbladder, hydroxyiminodiacetic acid scan, intravenous cholangiography, percutaneous transhepatic cholangiography]	
cholangitis [576.xx]	Acute or chronic inflammation of the bile ducts because of cirrhosis or gallstones. [see also: bile ducts, cholangiography, cholelithiasis, cirrhosis]	
cholecystectomy	Surgical procedure to remove the gallbladder. This is done as a minimally invasive laparoscopic cholecystectomy that utilizes an endoscope inserted through a small incision in the abdomen. [see also: gallbladder]	
cholecystitis [574.xx]	Acute or chronic inflammation of the gallbladder usually caused by gallstones. [see also: bile]	

	Dx	H&P. Ultrasound, cholangiography, CT scan, or MRI to visualize the anatomy. Lab tests will be performed to ascertain digestive and metabolic functions. [see also: cholangiography]
	Tx	Depends on symptoms. Medications to alleviate symptoms; surgery or lithotripsy to remove stones. [see also: bile, extracorporeal shock wave lithotripsy]

cholecystokinin	Hormone released by the duodenum when it receives food from the stomach. Cholecystokinin causes the gallbladder to release bile and the pancreas to release its digestive enzymes. [see also: bile, cholelithiasis]	
choledocholithiasis [574.xx]	Occurs when a gallstone becomes lodged in the common bile duct. [see also: bile ducts, cholangiography]	L
choledo- cholithotomy	Surgical procedure to make an incision in the common bile duct to remove a gallstone. [see also: bile ducts, cholelithiasis]	
cholelithiasis [574.xx]	One or more gallstones in the gallbladder. When the bile is too concentrated, it forms a thick sediment (sludge) that begins to	S

A = Abbreviations Section   F = Figures Section   L = Laboratory Section   S = Synonyms Section
Sx (Symptoms)   Dx (Diagnosis)   Tx (Treatment)

	form small crystals that gradually grow into gallstones. [*see also*: bile, cholangiography]
cholesteatoma [385.xx]	Benign, slow-growing mass in the middle ear composed of cholesterol deposits and epithelial cells. It can eventually destroy the bones of the middle ear and extend into the mastoid air cells. The underlying cause is usually chronic otitis media. [*see also*: ossicles, otitis media]
chondroma [213.xx]	Benign tumor of the cartilage.
chondromalacia patellae [717.xx]	Abnormal softening of the patella because of thinning and uneven wear. The thigh muscle pulls the patella in a crooked path that wears away the underside of the bone. [*see also*: osteomalacia] **S**
chordae tendineae	Ropelike strands that support the tricuspid and mitral valves and keep their leaflets tightly closed when the ventricles are contracting. [*see also*: endocarditis, endocardium, mitral valve prolapse, murmur, valve] **F**
chordee [752.xx]	Downward curvature of the penis during erection. Caused by a constricting, cordlike band of tissue along the underside of the penis. Congenital abnormality often associated with hypospadias. [*see also*: dyspareunia, hypospadias] **S**
chorion	Cellular area in a zygote that penetrates the endometrium of the uterus to bring nutrients and oxygen to the embryo. It later develops into the placenta. [*see also*: human chorionic gonadotropin, placenta] **S**
chorionic villus sampling	Genetic test of the chorionic villi from the placenta. A needle is inserted through the abdomen, or a catheter is inserted through the cervix, to aspirate tissue. This test is performed when a fetal genetic defect is suspected. It can be performed at 12 weeks, which is earlier than an amniocentesis, but it cannot detect neural tube defects in the fetus. [*see also*: amniocentesis]
choroid	Spongy membrane of blood vessels that begins at the iris and continues around the eye. In the posterior cavity, it is the middle layer between the sclera and the retina. [*see also*: choroiditis, retinal detachment, retinopexy, uveal tract] **F**
choroiditis [363.xx]	Inflammation or infection of the choroid membrane. Can be caused by infection in the eye or another part of the body, an allergy, trauma, or an autoimmune disease. [*see also*: autoimmune disease, choroid]
chromosome	Paired, rodlike structures within the nucleus. Each cell contains 46 chromosomes (23 pairs). [*see also*: Alzheimer's disease, chromosome studies, DNA, Down syndrome, gene, karyotype, nucleus]
chromosome studies	Test on fetal skin cells to determine the sex of the fetus and identify genetic abnormalities, such as Down syndrome. [*see also*: amniocentesis, chromosome, Down syndrome]
chronic bronchitis [491.xx]	Chronic inflammation or infection of the bronchi. Inflammation is due to pollution or smoking; infections are caused by bacteria or viruses. Chronic bronchitis is one of the component parts of chronic obstructive pulmonary disease. [*see also*: bronchitis, chronic obstructive pulmonary disease, pneumonia]
chronic obstructive pulmonary disease [496.xx]	Combination of conditions including chronic bronchitis and emphysema, caused by chronic exposure to pollution or smoking. [*see also*: chronic bronchitis, emphysema] **A** **L**

A = Abbreviations Section   **F** = Figures Section   **L** = Laboratory Section   **S** = Synonyms Section
Sx (Symptoms)   **Dx** (Diagnosis)   **Tx** (Treatment)

	Dx H&P. CT scan and chest x-ray to visualize the lungs. A pulmonary function test may be performed to determine lung function and capacity.
	Tx Directed toward halting destruction of the lungs. Medications, oxygen therapy to optimize blood oxygen levels. In some patients, surgery may be warranted to remove damaged lung tissue to optimize the functional lung tissue still left.
chronic renal failure [585.xx]	Disease in which the kidney's urine production progressively decreases and then stops altogether. Begins with renal insufficiency, followed by gradual worsening with progressive damage to the kidneys from diabetes mellitus, hypertension, or glomerulonephritis. [*see also*: renal failure] **A**
	Dx Urinary output remains low regardless of the amount of fluid taken in. Elevated laboratory levels of creatinine and other metabolic functions. [*see also*: anuria, blood urea nitrogen, creatinine, oliguria]
	Tx Depends on severity. Medications to treat symptoms. Dialysis to remove waste products from the blood. If severe enough, a kidney transplant may be considered. [*see also*: dialysis]
chyme	Food mixed with digestive enzymes in the stomach and small intestine. [*see also*: amylase, lipase, peptidase, protease]
cicatrix	Fibrous tissue composed of collagen that replaces injured skin tissue as the injury heals. Also known as a scar. **S**
cilia	Small hairs that flow or beat in waves to propel articles or things toward a desired position, whether it is outside the body or into an organ or area.
ciliary body	Extension of the choroid layer. It lies posterior to the iris. It has muscles that change the shape of the lens. It also produces aqueous humor. [*see also*: aqueous humor] **F**
circulatory system	Circular route that the blood takes as it moves through the body. Circulation is the process of moving the blood through this system.
circumcision	Surgical procedure to remove the prepuce (foreskin). This can be done to correct a tight prepuce and allow better hygiene of the glans penis. The foreskin is often removed because of social customs or religious requirements. [*see also*: balanitis, phimosis]
cirrhosis [571.xx]	Chronic, progressive inflammation and finally irreversible degeneration of liver tissue, characterized by nodules and scarring. Most likely cause is alcoholism, but can be due to other pathology. [*see also*: alpha fetoprotein, carcinoembryonic antigen, cholangitis, hepatomegaly, human chorionic gonadotropin, jaundice] **L**
cleft palate [749.xx]	Congenital deformity in which the maxilla fails to join before birth. The resulting cleft in the bone and skin can be unilateral or bilateral. The cleft can also extend into the soft palate. [*see also*: palate, philtrum]
clitoris	Organ of sexual response in the female that enlarges and becomes engorged with blood. It is part of the female external genitalia. [*see also*: genitalia] **F**
closed fracture [829.xx]	Any type of fracture in which the bone does not break through the overlying skin. [*see also*: fracture]

A = Abbreviations Section   **F** = Figures Section   **L** = Laboratory Section   **S** = Synonyms Section
Sx (Symptoms)   **Dx** (Diagnosis)   **Tx** (Treatment)

closed reduction	Medical procedure in which manual manipulation of a displaced fracture is performed so that the bone ends go back into normal alignment without the need for surgery. [see also: fracture]
closed-angle glaucoma [365.xx]	Increased intraocular pressure because aqueous humor cannot circulate freely. The angle where the edges of the iris and cornea touch is too small and blocks the aqueous humor. Causes severe pain, blurred vision, and photophobia. [see also: glaucoma, gonioscopy]
clotting factors	A series of 12 protein factors that are released either from platelets or injured tissue or are produced by the liver. They activate each other in a series of steps that eventually form fibrin strands that trap erythrocytes and form a blood clot. [see also: disseminated intravascular coagulation, hemophilia]
clubbing [781.xx]	Abnormally curved fingernails and stunted growth of the fingers associated with a chronic lack of oxygen. [see also: cystic fibrosis, hypoxia, tetralogy of Fallot]
coagulation	The formation of a blood clot by platelets and the clotting factors. S [see also: disseminated intravascular coagulation]
coagulopathy [286.xx]	Any disease that affects the ability of the blood to clot normally.
coarctation of the aorta [747.xx]	The aorta is abnormally narrow at the aortic arch so that its two sides are pressed together, restricting blood flow. [see also: tetralogy of Fallot]
	Dx H&P. Echocardiography, angiography to visualize the vessel. [see also: echocardiography]
	Tx Surgical resection of the vessel, angioplasty and/or stent placement to open the vessel.
cochlea	Structure of the inner ear associated with the sense of hearing. F It relays information to the brain via the cochlear branch of the auditory nerve. [see also: auditory nerve, Ménière's disease]
cochlear implant	Surgical procedure to implant a small, battery-powered implant beneath the skin behind the ear. Wires are placed from the implant through the round window and into the cochlea of the inner ear. When the implant "hears" a sound, it sends an electrical impulse to stimulate the cochlear nerve. [see also: audiometry]
cognitive-behavioral therapy	Therapy based on the premise that beliefs and attitudes A (not people or events) cause undesirable or destructive emotions, and thought patterns and behaviors are learned and can be unlearned. Patients are taught to use guided imagery and self-counseling to produce desirable emotions and behavior. Used to treat anxiety, panic attacks, phobias, depression, eating disorders, and other behaviors.
cold sores [054.xx]	Skin infection caused by the herpes virus with vesicles that S rupture, releasing clear fluid that forms crusts. Occurring on the lips, these lesions tend to recur during illness and stress. After the initial infection, the virus remains dormant in the skin until triggers of stress, sunlight, illness, or menstruation cause it to erupt again. [see also: herpes, Tzanck test]
colic [789.xx]	Common disorder in babies. Symptoms include crampy S abdominal pain that occurs soon after eating.
collagen	Firm, white protein connective tissue fibers throughout the dermis. [see also: scleroderma]
collagen injection	Medical procedure in which a solution of the protein collagen is injected into wrinkles or acne scars. This plumps the skin and decreases the depth of the wrinkle or scar.

A = Abbreviations Section   F = Figures Section   L = Laboratory Section   S = Synonyms Section
Sx (Symptoms)   Dx (Diagnosis)   Tx (Treatment)

collecting duct	Common passageway that collects fluid from many nephrons. The final step of reabsorption takes place there, and the remaining fluid is known as urine.
Colles' fracture [813.xx]	Distal radius is broken by falling onto an outstretched hand. [see also: fracture]
colon	The longest part of the large intestine. It has four parts: the ascending colon, the transverse colon, the descending colon, and the S-shaped sigmoid colon. [see also: carcinoembryonic antigen, colostomy, diverticulitis, Crohn's disease, indium-111, irritable bowel syndrome, OncoScint scan, polyps, ulcerative colitis]
color blindness [368.xx]	Genetic condition in which the cones in the retina, particularly green or red ones, are absent or do not contain enough visual pigment to respond to the light from colored objects. [see also: blindness, color blindness testing, cones, retinitis pigmentosa]
color blindness testing	A visual exam used to determine if a patient has a defect in one of the three types of color receptors in the eye: blue, green, or red. The most common type is red and green color blindness. Each successive color plate requires a higher discrimination of color perception. Color plates with numbers are used to test adults, while color plates with circles, squares, or animals are used to test children. [see also: color blindness]
color flow duplex ultrasonography	Radiologic procedure that combines a two-dimensional ultrasound image with Doppler ultrasonography that color codes images of the blood according to their velocity and direction. It shows turbulence and variation in velocity by variations in brightness. This test is the "gold standard" for evaluating tortuous varicose veins and diagnosing deep venous thrombosis. [see also: Doppler ultrasonography, echocardiography, varicose veins]
colostomy	Surgical procedure to remove the diseased part of the colon and create a new opening in the abdominal wall where feces can leave the body. The colon is brought out through the abdominal wall, and the edges of the wall of the colon are rolled to make a mouth that is then sutured to the abdominal wall. The patient wears a plastic disposable pouch that adheres to the abdominal wall to collect feces. [see also: colon]
colostrum	First milk from the breasts. It is rich in nutrients and contains maternal antibodies to give the newborn passive immunity to common diseases. [see also: lactation, immunoglobulin A, passive immunity]
colporrhaphy	Surgical procedure to suture a weakness in the vaginal wall. This procedure is done to correct a cystocele or a rectocele. [see also: rectocele, vesicocele]
colposcopy	Medical procedure that uses a magnifying, lighted scope to visually examine the vagina and cervix. [see also: dystocia, Papanicolaou smear]
coma	Deep state of unconsciousness and unresponsiveness caused by trauma to or disease in the brain, metabolic imbalance with accumulation of waste products, or a deficiency of sugar in the blood. [see also: brain death, concussion, diabetic ketoacidosis, eclampsia, Glasgow Coma Scale, hypoglycemia, shaken baby syndrome]
comedo [706.xx]	During puberty, the sebaceous glands produce large amounts of sebum. The sebum turns black as its oil is oxidized from exposure to the air. [see also: acne rosacea, acne vulgaris, dermis, exocrine gland, sebaceous gland, seborrhea]

S

comminuted fracture [829.xx]	Fracture in which the bone is crushed into several pieces. [*see also*: cast, external fixation, fracture, open reduction and internal fixation]	
compartment syndrome [729.xx; 958.xx]	The enveloping fascia of a damaged muscle (usually in an extremity) acts like a compartment, holding in blood as it accumulates. The increased pressure causes cell death in the muscle and nerve damage. [*see also*: fasciotomy]	
complement proteins	Group of nine proteins in the plasma that are activated by the presence of bacteria, viruses, or parasites. They coat the pathogen and kill it by making holes in it. Complement proteins also cause basophils to release histamine in areas where the tissue has been injured. [*see also*: basophil, immune response, plasma proteins]	
complete blood count	Group of blood tests that are performed automatically by machine to determine the number, type, and characteristics of various cells in the blood. [*see also*: blood smear, basophil, eosinophil, lymphocyte, monocyte, neutrophil]	A L
complex partial seizures	Type of epilepsy in which there is some degree of impairment of consciousness. Involuntary contractions of one or several muscle groups. Obvious automatisms, such as lip smacking and patterns of muscle movement, can be present. [*see also*: epilepsy, seizure]	S
complex regional pain syndrome [337.xx; 354.xx]	Involves causalgia, with hyperesthesia, changes in skin color, warmth, and swelling. [*see also*: causalgia] **Dx** H&P. No specific diagnostic test exists; tests are conducted to rule out other disorders. **Tx** Medications to treat symptoms; surgery, implanted pumps to deliver pain medication, spinal cord stimulation to decrease the pain. [*see also*: pain management]	A
compound fracture [829.xx]	Any type of fracture in which the bone breaks through the overlying skin. [*see also*: fracture]	
compression fracture [829.xx]	Vertebrae are compressed together when a person falls onto the buttocks or when a vertebra collapses in on itself because of disease. [*see also*: fracture]	S
computerized axial tomography	Uses an x-ray beam that is controlled by a computer and moves around the body axis of a patient inside the CT scanner. Produces individual images as "slices," as well as a composite three-dimensional view. [*see also*: multidetector-row computerized tomography, spiral computerized tomography]	A
concussion [850.xx]	Traumatic injury to the brain that results in the immediate loss of consciousness for a brief or prolonged period of time. The patient must be watched closely for an enlarging hemorrhage in the brain. [*see also*: cerebral contusion, coma]	
condom catheter	Shaped like a condom (male contraceptive device), it fits snugly over the male penis. It collects the urine as it leaves the urethral meatus, directing it through a tube and into a collecting bag. [*see also*: Foley catheter, straight catheter, suprapubic catheter]	
conduct disorder [309.xx; 312.xx]	Persistent, aggressive behavior (fighting, arguing, provoking, annoying), defiance of and refusal to obey rules, disrespect for authority figures, with anger, stubbornness, and touchiness. More severe than oppositional defiant disorder in that patients physically and sexually assault others, destroy property, steal, set fires, or run away from home. [*see also*: oppositional defiant disorder, psychopath]	

conduction system	System that conveys the electrical impulse that makes the heart beat. It consists of the SA node, AV node, bundle of His, bundle branches, and Purkinje fibers. [*see also*: depolarization, dysrhythmia, ectopic sites, electrocardiography, electrophysiology study, depolarization]
conductive hearing loss [389.xx]	Progressive, permanent decline in the ability to hear sounds in one or both ears. A foreign body or infection in the external auditory canal, perforation of the tympanic membrane, fluid behind the tympanic membrane, or degeneration of the ossicles of the middle ear keep sound waves from reaching the inner ear. [*see also*: audiometry, mixed hearing loss, otosclerosis, sensorineural hearing loss]
cone	Light-sensitive cells in the retina that detect colored light. There are three types of cones, each of which responds to red, green, or blue light. [*see also*: color blindness, optic nerve, retina]
conformal radiotherapy	Uses a computer to map the location and create a three-dimensional image of a tumor. The external beam radiation is then matched to conform to the exact shape of the tumor to protect nearby vital organs. [*see also*: external beam radiotherapy]
congenital disease	Caused by an abnormality as the fetus develops or one that occurs during the birth process. Examples: Cleft lip and palate, cerebral palsy.
congenital dislocation of the hip [754.xx]	Displacement of the end of a bone from its normal position within a joint. Present at birth because the acetabulum is poorly formed or the ligaments are loose. **A**
congenital hypothyroidism [243.xx]	A deficiency of thyroid hormone production in an infant; if untreated, it causes mental retardation (cretinism). [*see also*: hypothyroidism]
congestive heart failure [428.xx]	Inability of the heart to pump sufficient amounts of blood. Caused by chronic coronary artery disease or hypertension. [*see also*: cardiomegaly, cardiomyopathy, coronary artery disease, cor pulmonale, hypertension, left-sided congestive heart failure, paroxysmal nocturnal dyspnea, pulmonary edema, right-sided congestive heart failure] **A** **L**
	Dx H&P. Laboratory studies, EKG, echocardiogram, x-ray. [*see also*: echocardiography, electrocardiography]
	Tx Lifestyle modification, fluid intake restrictions to reduce fluid accumulation, medications to treat symptoms. In severe cases, cardiac transplant surgery or the insertion of a left ventricular assist device (LVAD).
conization	Surgical procedure to remove a large, cone-shaped section of tissue that includes the cervical os and part of the cervical canal. Used to diagnosis a lesion or excise an abnormal area identified by a Pap smear. [*see also*: Papanicolaou smear]
conjunctiva	Delicate, transparent mucous membrane that covers the inside of the eyelids and the anterior surface of the eye. It produces clear, watery mucus. [*see also*: conjunctivitis, pink eye, scleral icterus] **F**
conjunctivitis [372.xx]	Inflamed, reddened, and swollen conjunctivae with dilated blood vessels on the sclerae. Caused by a foreign substance in the eye, a chemical splashed in the eye, allergens or pollution in the air, chlorinated water in swimming pools, mechanical irritation from **S**

eyelashes (entropion), or dryness due to a lack of tears. Also caused by a bacterial or viral infection. [*see also*: allergen, conjunctiva, pink eye]

constipation
[564.xx]
Failure to have regular, soft bowel movements. [*see also*: defecation, diverticulitis, hypothyroidism, obstipation]

contact dermatitis
[692.xx]
Topical reaction to physical contact with a substance that is an allergen or an irritant. The skin becomes inflamed and pruritic. Small vesicles may also appear. [*see also*: allergic reaction, dermatitis]   S

continuous ambulatory peritoneal dialysis
Medical procedure to remove waste products from the blood of patients in renal failure. A permanent catheter is inserted through the abdominal wall. Dialysate fluid flows through the catheter and remains in the abdominal cavity for several hours. During that time, the fluid pulls body wastes from the blood. Then the fluid is removed, carrying waste products with it. The patient is able to walk around between the three or four daily episodes of dialysis. [*see also*: continuous cycling peritoneal dialysis, dialysis, hemodialysis, peritoneal dialysis]   A

continuous cycling peritoneal dialysis
Medical procedure to remove waste products from the blood of patients in renal failure. A permanent catheter is inserted through the abdominal wall. Dialysate fluid flows through the catheter and remains in the abdominal cavity for several hours. During that time, the fluid pulls body wastes from the blood. Then the fluid is removed, carrying waste products with it. A machine inserts and removes dialysate fluid several times a night while the patient sleeps. [*see also*: continuous ambulatory peritoneal dialysis, dialysis, hemodialysis, peritoneal dialysis]   A

contraction
Shortening of the length of all muscle fibers in a group and of the muscle itself. Opposite of relaxation. [*see also*: epilepsy, muscle spasm, seizures]

contracture
[728.xx]
Inactivity or paralysis coupled with continuing nerve impulses causes an arm or leg to be progressively flexed and drawn into a position where it becomes nearly immovable. [*see also*: Dupuytren's contracture, fasciectomy, rehabilitation exercises]

contusion
[920.xx–924.xx]
An area of any size of hemorrhage under the skin. [*see also*: bruise, cerebral contusion, concussion, hemorrhage]   S

convergence
Medical procedure to test the ability of both eyes to turn medially. The physician holds up an index finger and moves it progressively closer to the patient's nose to test the function of the medial rectus muscles. The maximum convergence is called the near point. [*see also*: abducens nerve, amblyopia, esotropia, exotropia, gaze testing, oculomotor nerve, strabismus, trochlear nerve]

conversion disorder [300.xx]
Somatoform (neurologic, sensory, or motor) deficits that occur without any physical basis. There may be sudden blindness, deafness, paralysis, or the inability to speak. There is repression of overwhelming anxiety or internal conflict which then undergoes a conversion to physical symptoms. [*see also*: anacusis]

cor pulmonale
[415.xx]
A condition where there is lung disease and the right ventricle enlarges to pump harder. Cor is a Latin word that means heart. [*see also*: cardiomyopathy, congestive heart failure]   L

Dx   H&P. EKG, echocardiogram to determine heart function, x-ray to visualize the chest, ABGs to determine arterial blood oxygenation. [*see also*: echocardiography, electrocardiography, positron emission tomography scan]

A = Abbreviations Section   **F** = Figures Section   **L** = Laboratory Section   **S** = Synonyms Section
Sx (Symptoms)   **Dx** (Diagnosis)   **Tx** (Treatment)

	Tx Treat the underlying cause. Medications to treat the underlying symptoms and oxygen therapy to optimize the blood oxygen.	
core needle biopsy	A large-gauge needle is inserted into a tumor to obtain several long cores of tissue. [*see also:* biopsy]	
cornea	Transparent layer over the anterior part of the eye. It is a continuation of the white sclera. [*see also:* astigmatism, corneal abrasion, corneal transplant, phacoemulsification, slit-lamp examination]	F
corneal abrasion [918.xx]	Loss of the superficial layers of the cornea due to trauma or repetitive irritation, such as a foreign particle under a contact lens. Chronic bacterial infection in an abrasion causes a corneal ulcer, with sloughing off of necrotic tissue. [*see also:* cornea, fluorescein staining]	
corneal transplantation	Surgical procedure to replace a damaged or diseased cornea. The cornea is removed with a trephine, and then a donor cornea is sutured in place with zig-zag sutures. [*see also:* allograft, cornea]	
coronal plane	Plane that divides the body into front and back sections, anterior and posterior. [*see also:* midsagittal plane, oblique, projection, transverse plane]	S
coronal suture	Suture between the frontal bone and the parietal bones of the cranium.	F
coronary angiography	Radiologic procedure in which radiopaque contrast dye is injected into a coronary artery. A catheter is inserted into the femoral or brachial artery and threaded to the aorta. The radiopaque contrast dye outlines the coronary arteries and shows narrowing, stenosis, or blockage. [*see also:* angina pectoris, angiography, aortography, arteriography, coronary artery disease, myocardial infarction, rotational angiography, venography]	
coronary arteries	Arteries that bring blood to the myocardium. [*see also:* angina pectoris, arteriosclerosis, atherosclerosis, cardiac catheterization, coronary artery disease, myocardial infarction]	F
coronary artery bypass graft	Surgical procedure to bypass an occluded coronary artery and restore blood flow to the myocardium. A blood vessel (either the saphenous vein or the internal mammary artery) is used as the bypass graft. Oxygenated blood flows through the graft, past the blockage, and back into the coronary artery. [*see also:* cardiopulmonary bypass, coronary artery disease]	A
coronary artery disease [410.xx–414.xx; 429.xx]	Arteriosclerosis of the coronary arteries. They are filled with atheromatous plaque, and their narrowed lumens cannot carry enough oxygenated blood to the myocardium, resulting in angina pectoris. Severe arteriosclerosis (or a blood clot that forms on an atherosclerotic plaque) can completely block the lumen of a coronary artery, causing a myocardial infarction. [*see also:* angina pectoris, arteriosclerosis, atherosclerosis, congestive heart failure, myocardial infarction]	A
	Dx H&P. EKG to determine heart function, lab studies to determine cardiac function, angiography to visualize the vessel. [*see also:* cardiac catheterization, electrocardiography]	
	Tx Medications to treat the underlying symptoms. An angioplasty or stent placement to open the coronary artery. Depending on the severity and number of blocked arteries,	

coronary artery bypass graft surgery may be considered. [see also: coronary artery bypass graft, percutaneous transluminal coronary angioplasty]

corpus	The main part or body of an organ. Body or widest part of the uterus.
corpus callosum	Thick white band of nerves that connects the two hemispheres of the cerebrum and allows them to communicate and coordinate their activities. [see also: cerebrum]
corpus luteum	The remains of a ruptured ovarian follicle. The corpus luteum is filled with yellow fat and secretes estradiol and progesterone during the menstrual cycle. This continues after the ovum is fertilized until the placenta begins to secrete these hormones. Then the corpus luteum becomes white scar tissue. [see also: follicle, human chorionic gonadotropin, ischemic phase, luteinizing hormone, ovaries, placenta, progesterone, secretory phase]
cortex	Tissue layer of the kidney just beneath the renal capsule.
cortisol	Most abundant and biologically active of the glucocorticoid hormones secreted by the adrenal cortex. It increases the level of glucose in the blood, decreases the formation of proteins and new tissues, and has an anti-inflammatory effect. The adrenal cortex secretes cortisol when stimulated by adrenocorticotropic hormone from the anterior pituitary gland. [see also: Addison's disease, adrenal cortex, Cushing's syndrome]
	<u>Blood Test</u>: Measures the level of cortisol. Used to evaluate the function of the adrenal cortex and the anterior pituitary gland. A metabolite of cortisol, 17-hydroxycorticosteroids, can also be measured in the urine to measure indirectly the level of cortisol. [see also: adrenal cortex, anterior pituitary gland]
corticosteroid injection	Medical procedure in which a corticosteroid drug is given by intraarticular injection into one particular joint with degenerative joint disease to decrease inflammation and pain. [see also: degenerative joint disease]
costal cartilage	Smooth, firm, but flexible segments of connective tissue that join the ribs to the sternum. The area where the costal cartilage meets the rib is known as the costochondral joint.
cough	Protective mechanism to expel forcefully accidentally inhaled food, irritating particles (smoke, dust), or internally produced mucus. A cough may be nonproductive or productive of sputum. [see also: expectoration, intercostal muscles]
cranial cavity	Cavity in the head that is surrounded by the cranium and contains the brain, cranial nerves, and other structures.
cranial nerves	Twelve pairs of nerves that originate in the brain. They carry sensory nerve impulses to the brain and motor nerve impulses from the brain. Olfactory (I), optic (II), oculomotor (III), trochlear (IV), trigeminal (V), abducens (VI), facial (VII), vestibulocochlear (VIII), glossopharyngeal (IX), vagus (X), accessory (XI), hypoglossal (XII). [see also: medulla oblongata, pons, thalamus]
craniotomy	Surgical incision into the cranium to expose the brain tissue. A craniotomy is the first phase of any type of brain surgery (i.e., evacuation of a subdural hematoma or excising a brain tumor). [see also: subdural hematoma]
cranium	Bony structure of the head that contains the cranial cavity and the brain.
C-reactive protein	Blood test to measure the level of inflammation in the body. Inflammation from sites other than the cardiovascular system (such as inflammation of the gums or chronic urinary tract infections) can

F

S

F

A

A

produce inflammation of the walls of the blood vessels. This can lead to blood clot formation and a myocardial infarction. [*see also*: polymyositis, rheumatoid arthritis, systemic lupus erythematosus]

creatine kinase MB bands

Part of cardiac enzymes, a blood test to measure the levels of enzymes that are released into the blood when myocardial cells die. A specific form of creatine kinase, CK-MB is found exclusively in myocardial cells. The CK-MB level begins to rise 2–6 hours after a myocardial infarction. Cardiac enzymes are measured every few hours for several days. Also known as creatine phosphokinase (CPK). [*see also*: cardiac enzymes, myocardial infarction]

A
L

creatine phosphokinase MM bands

Blood test to measure the level of serum CPK-MM, an isoenzyme found in the muscles. High levels of CPK-MM are present in major trauma and various diseases, particularly muscular dystrophy, in which muscle tissue is being destroyed.

A

creatinine

Waste product from muscle contractions. It is removed from the blood by the kidneys.

Blood Test: Measures the amount of creatinine. Used to monitor kidney function and the progression of kidney disease. Creatinine is measured in conjunction with the BUN to give a comprehensive picture of kidney function. [*see also*: 24-hour creatinine clearance, blood urea nitrogen, metabolic panel, renal failure]

A
L

Creutzfeldt-Jakob disease [046.xx]

A fatal neurologic disorder caused by a prion contracted from eating meat from cows infected with mad cow disease (bovine spongiform encephalopathy), for which there is no known treatment or cure. [*see also*: cerebrospinal fluid examination]

S

Crohn's disease [555.xx]

A type of inflammatory bowel disease that affects the ileum and colon where there are areas of inflammation followed by areas of normal mucosa. [*see also*: colon, ileum, inflammatory bowel disease]

L
S

Dx H&P. Lab tests to determine metabolic functions and digestive problems. A barium x-ray, CT scan, or colonoscopy to visualize the intestines. [*see also*: barium enema, metabolic panel]

Tx Medications to treat the underlying symptoms. Dietary changes to reduce the frequency and severity of symptoms. Surgery may be indicated to remove an affected area of the intestine. [*see also*: bowel resection and anastomosis]

crowning

A large portion of the top of the fetal head is visible at the vaginal introitus just prior to birth. [*see also*: cephalic presentation, dystocia]

cryosurgery

Medical procedure in which liquid nitrogen is sprayed or painted onto a wart, mole, or lesion. The liquid nitrogen freezes and destroys the tissue. [*see also*: genital warts, verruca, solar keratoses]

cryptorchism [752.xx]

Failure of one or both of the testicles to descend through the inguinal canal into the scrotum. This causes a low sperm count and male infertility. Also known as cryptorchidism. [*see also*: infertility, inguinal canal, oligospermia, orchiopexy, testes]

S

culdoscopy

Surgical procedure in which an endoscope is inserted into the vagina and enters the pelvic cavity. This procedure is performed under local anesthesia and leaves no abdominal scars. Used to examine the cul-de-sac and the external surfaces of the uterus, fallopian tubes, and ovaries for signs of endometriosis or adhesions. [*see also*: adhesions, endometriosis]

A = Abbreviations Section   **F** = Figures Section   **L** = Laboratory Section   **S** = Synonyms Section
Sx (Symptoms)   **Dx** (Diagnosis)   **Tx** (Treatment)

culture and sensitivity	A specimen is placed in a Petri dish and cultured to diagnose the cause of an infection. Microorganisms present in the specimen may grow into colonies. The specific disease-causing pathogen is identified and then tested to determine its sensitivity to various drugs. Disks containing various drugs are placed in the culture dish. A drug that can kill that organism will have a ring of "no growth" around its disk. [see also: pathogen]	A
cumulative trauma disorder [354.xx]	Condition affecting the muscles, tendons, and sometimes the nerves as a result of trauma due to repetitious movements over an extended period of time. Includes tennis elbow, carpal tunnel syndrome, and other disorders. [see also: carpal tunnel syndrome, lateral epicondylitis, medial epicondylitis]	A S
curettage	Medical procedure that involves using a curet to scrape off the superficial part of a skin lesion. Curettage is often combined with electrodesiccation for complete removal of a lesion. [see also: dilation and curettage, electrodesiccation]	
Cushing's disease Cushing's syndrome [255.xx]	Excess cortisol breaks down too much glycogen and causes elevated levels of glucose in the blood. This results in weight gain, with deposits of fat in the face (moon face), upper back (buffalo hump), and abdomen. There is also a wasted appearance in the muscles of the extremities and weakness because of the lack of protein synthesis. Hypersecretion of adrenocorticotropic hormone from the pituitary gland causes the adrenal cortex to produce excess androgens, and this produces dark facial hair and amenorrhea in women. The difference between Cushing's disease and Cushing's syndrome is in the cause.	L
	Cushing's disease: Hypersecretion of adrenocorticotropic hormone by an adenoma in the anterior pituitary gland.	
	Cushing's syndrome: Hypersecretion of cortisol by an adenoma in the adrenal cortex. It can also occur in a patient who takes corticosteroid drugs on a long-term basis. [see also: adrenocorticotropic hormone, autoimmune diseases, cortisol]	
cuticle	Layer of dead skin that arises from the epidermis around the proximal end of the nail. It keeps microorganisms from entering the nail root. [see also: herpes whitlow, paronychia]	
cyanosis [728.xx]	Bluish-gray/purple discoloration of the skin and nails due to decreased oxygen and abnormally high levels of carbon dioxide in the blood. It can be seen around the mouth or in the nail beds. Can be caused by cardiac or respiratory disease. [see also: anoxia, deoxygenated, hypercapnia]	
cyclothymia [301.xx]	Chronic, mild bipolar disorder. In between mood swings, the patient is free from signs and symptoms for several months. [see also: bipolar disorder]	
cystectomy	Surgical procedure to remove the bladder because of bladder cancer. A radical cystectomy removes the bladder, surrounding tissues, and lymph nodes.	
cystic fibrosis [277.xx]	Inherited, eventually fatal disease caused by a recessive gene. CF affects all the exocrine cells that secrete mucus or enzymes, but the respiratory system is particularly affected.	A
	Dx H&P. Sweat test to show increased levels of chlorine and sodium in the sweat. Pulmonary function tests may be performed to determine lung capacity and function.	

A = Abbreviations Section   F = Figures Section   L = Laboratory Section   S = Synonyms Section
Sx (Symptoms)   Dx (Diagnosis)   Tx (Treatment)

Tx	Medications to treat the underlying symptoms. Oxygen therapy to optimize the blood oxygen levels, along with chest physiotherapy to break up secretions and clear the airway.
cystitis	Inflammation or infection of the bladder, commonly caused by a bacterial infection of the urethra that ascends into the bladder. [*see also*: bacteriuria, dysuria, hematuria, interstitial cystitis, nocturia, radiation cystitis, urinary tract infection]
cystometry	Diagnostic procedure that evaluates the function of the nerves to the bladder. A catheter is used to inflate the bladder with liquid or gas. A cystometer attached to the catheter measures the amount of liquid and the pressure in the bladder. The patient indicates when the first urge to urinate occurs. [*see also*: diabetes mellitus, incontinence, multiple sclerosis, neurogenic bladder, overactive bladder, spinal cord injury, urinary retention]
cystoscopy	Surgical procedure that uses a rigid or flexible scope inserted through the urethra in order to examine the bladder. A wide-angle lens and a light allow a full view of the bladder. A video attachment can be used to create a permanent visual record. [*see also*: retrograde pyelography, stone basketing] A
cytokines	Protein molecules released by damaged tissues. Cytokines call leukocytes to that area. [*see also*: histamine, leukocytes]
cytoplasm	Gel-like intracellular substance. Organelles are embedded in it.

D

dacryocystitis [375.xx]	Infection of the lacrimal sac by the bacterium that causes skin, nose, and ear infections. The lacrimal sac is tender and contains pus.
debridement	Medical or surgical procedure in which necrotic tissue is debrided (removed) from a burn, wound, or ulcer. Debridement is done to remove dead tissue that can become the source of infection, assess the extent or depth of a wound, and create a clean, raw surface that is ready to heal or receive a skin graft.
debulking	Surgical procedure to excise part of a bulky, unresectable tumor. This is done to reduce the size of the tumor and make the patient more comfortable or to leave a smaller tumor that can be treated with chemotherapy or radiation therapy.
decubitus position	Lying down position, on the back.
decubitus ulcer [707.xx]	Usually occurring over bony prominences, a pressure injury from constantly lying in one position that prevents blood flow to the tissues. The epidermis and then dermis break down and slough off, resulting in a shallow or deep wound.
deep tendon reflexes	Tapping briskly on a tendon causes an involuntary, automatic contraction of the muscle connected to that tendon. This tests whether the muscular-nervous pathway is functioning normally. A
deep vein thrombosis [453.xx]	A blood clot in one of the deep veins of the lower leg when blood pools in the veins and forms a clot. Sometimes a thrombus becomes an embolus that travels through the circulatory system until it becomes trapped and blocks the blood flow in a small artery of the brain, heart, or lungs. [*see also*: cerebrovascular accident, pulmonary embolism] A

A = Abbreviations Section   F = Figures Section   L = Laboratory Section   S = Synonyms Section
Sx (Symptoms)   Dx (Diagnosis)   Tx (Treatment)

Dx H&P. Imaging studies to visualize the lungs. [*see also*: ventilation-perfusion scan]

Tx Anticoagulants to thin the blood and prevent more clots from forming. Sometimes localized thrombolytic drugs are given to dissolve the clot. A surgically inserted venous filter (Greenfield filter) may be placed in the vein to catch the clots before they get to the heart and lungs.

defecation	Process by which undigested food fiber and water are removed from the body in the form of a bowel movement. [*see also*: constipation, diarrhea, encopresis, feces, hematochezia, melena, meconium, steatorrhea]	S
defibrillator	A device used to generate an electrical shock (measured in joules) to the heart, through the use of paddles. [*see also*: automatic external defibrillator, automatic implantable cardiac defibrillator, cardioversion, conduction system, dysrhythmia]	
degenerative disease	Caused by the progressive destruction of cells due to disease or the aging process. Examples: Multiple sclerosis, loss of hearing.	
degenerative joint disease [715.xx]	Chronic inflammatory disease of the joints, particularly the large weight-bearing joints of the knees and hips, and joints that move repeatedly, such as the shoulders, neck, and hands. [*see also*: arthrodesis, arthrography, arthroscopy, bone scintigraphy, cartilage transplantation, corticosteroid injection]	A S
deglutition	Process of swallowing food. [*see also*: dysphagia, epiglottis, glossopharyngeal nerve, odynophagia]	S
delirium	Acute confusion, disorientation, and agitation due to toxic levels of body chemicals, drugs, or alcohol in the blood that affect the brain. These acute signs slowly subside as toxic levels of drugs or alcohol in the blood decrease. [*see also*: delirium tremens]	S
delirium tremens [291.xx]	Caused by withdrawal symptoms from alcoholic intoxication and includes restlessness, tremors of the hands, hallucinations, sweating, and increased heart rate. [*see also*: detoxification]	A S
delusional disorder [297.xx]	Continued false beliefs (delusions) concerning events of everyday life. These beliefs are fixed and unchanging despite the efforts of others to persuade or evidence showing otherwise. Common delusions: other people or even strangers are in love with you, your husband or wife is unfaithful, other people are trying to hurt or kill you (delusions of persecution, also known as paranoia), or you have the powers of a god or are a famous person (delusions of grandeur). [*see also*: schizophrenia]	
dementia [290.xx–294.xx]	Gradual but progressive deterioration of cognitive function due to old age or a neurologic disease process. There is a gradual decline in mental abilities. Disease of the brain in which many neurons in the cerebrum die, the cerebral cortex shrinks in size, and there is progressive deterioration in mental function. Alzheimer's is the most common type of dementia. [*see also*: Alzheimer's disease, electroencephalography, Huntington's chorea, incontinence, presenile dementia]	S
dendrite	Multiple branches at the beginning of a neuron that receive a neurotransmitter and convert it to an electrical impulse. [*see also*: neurotransmitter, synapse]	
densitometry	Bone density test that measures the bone mineral density to diagnose osteoporosis. The two types are a DEXA scan and QCT.	

[see also: bone density test, dual energy x-ray absorptiometry scan, osteoporosis, quantitative computerized tomography]

dentistry Medical specialty that deals with the teeth and gums.

deoxygenated Blood that contains low levels of oxygen and high levels of carbon dioxide. [see also: anoxia, arterial blood gases, cyanosis]

dependent personality [301.xx] Expects and wants to be told what to do and what to think. Patients are passive, have difficulty making decisions, and want others to take care of them and the details of their lives.

depersonalization [300.xx] Loss of connection between personal thoughts and a sense of self and the environment. Patients feel as if they are in a dream or watching a movie of themselves, and things feel unreal and strange. [see also: multiple personality]

depolarization Changing of the permeability of a muscle cell to allow potassium ions to flow out of the cell and sodium and calcium ions to flow into the cell. This is triggered by the electrical impulse from a nerve. [see also: conduction system]

depressed fracture [829.xx] Cranium is fractured inward toward the brain. [see also: fracture]

dermabrasion Uses a rapidly spinning wire brush or diamond surface to mechanically abrade (scrape away) the epidermis. [see also: chemical peel, exfoliation, laser skin resurfacing, microdermabrasion]

dermatitis [692.xx] Any disease condition involving inflammation of the skin. [see also: contact dermatitis]

dermatome Area of the skin that sends sensory information to one spinal nerve. [see also: shingles, spinal nerves]

dermatomyositis [710.xx] Inflammation of a muscle with a skin rash, along with localized swelling, tenderness, muscle weakness, and inflammation. Can be caused by injury or strain. [see also: muscle biopsy]

dermatoplasty Surgical procedure for any type of plastic surgery of the skin, such as skin grafting, removal of keloids, release of skin contractures, and so forth. [see also: body dysmorphic disorder, rhytidectomy, skin grafting]

dermis Layer of skin under the epidermis. It is composed of collagen and elastin fibers. It contains arteries, veins, nerves, sebaceous glands, sweat glands, and hair follicles. [see also: edema, elastin, follicle, laser skin resurfacing, sebaceous gland, sudoriferous gland]

detoxication Observation and medical assistance for an alcohol-addicted or drug-addicted patient undergoing withdrawal. Drugs are given, as needed, to minimize withdrawal symptoms and prevent seizures. [see also: delirium tremens, seizures]

dextroscoliosis [737.xx] Abnormal, excessive, C-shaped or S-shaped lateral curvature of the spine to the patient's right. The back is said to have a scoliotic curvature. Scoliosis can be congenital but most often the cause is unknown. [see also: kyphosis, kyphoscoliosis, levoscoliosis, scoliosis]

diabetes insipidus [253.xx] Hyposecretion of antidiuretic hormone (ADH). Causes excessive amounts of water to be excreted in the urine. Symptoms include weakness, thirst (due to water loss and dehydration), and increased intake of fluids. [see also: antidiuretic hormone, posterior pituitary gland, syndrome of inappropriate ADH]   **A** **L**

　　Dx　H&P. I&O to keep track of volume and loss, laboratory studies to determine metabolic function and levels of electrolytes. MRI, CT scan to visualize organs that may contain tumors causing the problem. [*see also*: ADH stimulation test]

Tx Hormones to replace low levels of ADH. IV fluids and electrolytes to restore fluid balance. Vasopressors may be necessary if blood volume depletes enough to cause cardiovascular problems. Depending on the cause, surgical intervention may be necessary, either to relieve the pressure on the pituitary gland or to remove the tumor.

diabetes mellitus
[250.xx]

Hyposecretion of insulin. There is an elevated level of glucose in the blood (hyperglycemia). Excess glucose in the blood is excreted in the urine (glycosuria). If blood glucose levels remain high, there is increased urine production and the patient drinks often (polydipsia). The patient also feels hungry and eats often (polyphaiga) because the glucose in the blood cannot enter the cells without insulin. [*see also*: amputation, brittle diabetic, diabetic ketoacidosis, diabetic nephropathy, diabetic neuropathy, diabetic retinopathy, gestational diabetes, glucose tolerance test, ketonuria]

A
L
S

<u>Type 1</u>: An autoimmune response that may be triggered by a viral infection or an inherited genetic predisposition. There is destruction of the beta cells of the islets of Langerhans in the pancreas. The pancreas secretes little or no insulin. Can begin in childhood or adolescence. [*see also*: autoimmune diseases]

<u>Type 2</u>: Caused by decreased function of the beta cells and decreased amounts of insulin coupled with a decreased number of insulin receptors on the cell membranes. Begins in middle age with a gradual onset. Risk factors include obesity and a family history of diabetes. [*see also*: hyperinsulinism]

<u>Gestational diabetes</u>: Temporary disorder of glucose metabolism that occurs only during pregnancy. Increased levels of estradiol and progesterone block the action of insulin. Low levels of insulin lead to high levels of unmetabolized glucose in the mother's blood. These high levels of glucose cross the placenta and cause the fetus to grow too rapidly. [*see also*: diabetes mellitus, estradiol, growth abnormalities, polyhydramnios, progesterone]

Dx H&P. Laboratory tests of fasting blood sugar and glucose tolerance test to check for elevated levels of glucose in the blood. Urinalysis to check for elevated levels of glucose and ketones in the urine.

A
L

Tx Diet modification. Injected insulin (type 1 diabetes) or oral antidiabetic drug (type 2 diabetes). Long-term monitoring of glucose blood levels by patient (glucose self-testing) and by periodic hemoglobin A_{1c} laboratory blood test.

**diabetic
ketoacidosis**
[250.xx]

Excessive amounts of ketones in the blood. When there is no insulin to metabolize glucose, the body turns to other sources of energy like fat or protein. Body fat contains the most calories per gram, but body fat does not metabolize cleanly and leaves ketones, an acidic byproduct. Large amounts of ketones lower the pH of the blood to the point that chemical reactions in the body cannot occur and the patient becomes unconscious (diabetic coma).

A
L

Dx Lab tests to determine metabolic processes, ABGs to monitor the pH and cause of acidosis.

Tx The patient's blood sugar is frequently monitored. May be placed on continuous insulin until the condition is brought

A = Abbreviations Section   **F** = Figures Section   **L** = Laboratory Section   **S** = Synonyms Section
Sx (Symptoms)   **Dx** (Diagnosis)   **Tx** (Treatment)

under control. Supportive measures are taken and the patient is monitored for complications.

diabetic nephropathy [583.xx]
Progressive damage to the glomeruli because of diabetes mellitus. It causes degenerative changes, fibrosis, and scarring in the nephrons of the kidneys because of the local effects of biochemical imbalances of diabetes. The tiny arteries of the glomerulus harden because of accelerated arteriosclerosis throughout the body. [*see also*: arteriosclerosis, diabetes mellitus, renal failure]

diabetic neuropathy [250.xx]
A chronic, slowly progressive condition that affects the peripheral nerves, causing a decreased or abnormal sensation in the extremities in diabetic patients because of nerve damage due to demyelinization of the nerves. [*see also*: diabetes mellitus, impotence, paresthesia]   L

diabetic retinopathy [362.xx]
Chronic, progressive condition, with degenerative changes of the retina of the eye in diabetic patients because of the local effects of biochemical imbalances of diabetes. There is formation of new, abnormally fragile blood vessels that contain microaneurysms that leak, forming exudates on the retina. The vessels also rupture and hemorrhage easily, causing intraocular hemorrhage. [*see also*: fluorescein angiography, scotoma]

dialysis
Medical procedure to remove waste products from the blood of patients in renal failure. [*see also*: continuous ambulatory peritoneal dialysis, continuous cycling peritoneal dialysis, hemodialysis, peritoneal dialysis, renal failure]

diaphoresis [780.xx]
Profuse sweating caused by an underlying condition such as myocardial infarction, hypertension, hyperthyroidism, hypoglycemia, or narcotic drug withdrawal. [*see also*: angina pectoris, hypoglycemia, perspiration, pheochromocytoma, sudoriferous gland]   L S

diaphragm
Muscular sheet that divides the thoracic cavity from the abdominal cavity. Nerve impulses from the phrenic nerve cause the diaphragm to contract and move inferiorly to expand the thoracic cavity during inspiration. [*see also*: Heimlich maneuver, hiatal hernia, muscular dystrophy, phrenic nerve]

diaphysis
The straight shaft of a long bone.   F

diarrhea [787.xx]
Abnormally frequent and loose, watery stools. [*see also*: defecation, feces, hyperparathyroidism]   L S

diastole
Resting period between contractions. It is when the heart fills with blood. [*see also*: systole]

dietetics
Medical specialty that deals with nutrition, nutrients, and diet.

differentiation
Process by which embryonic cells assume different shapes and function in different parts of the body. [*see also*: anaplasia, grading, undifferentiated]

digestion
Process of mechanically and chemically breaking down food into nutrients that can be used by the body. [*see also*: amylase, lipase, peptidase, protease]

digital rectal examination
Medical procedure to palpate the prostate gland. A gloved finger inserted into the rectum is used to feel the prostate gland for signs of tenderness, nodules, hardness, or enlargement. This examination should be done yearly in men over age 40. [*see also*: benign prostatic hypertrophy, fecal occult blood test, prostatitis]   A

digital subtraction angiography
Radiologic procedure in which radiopaque contrast dye is injected into a blood vessel. Two x-ray images are obtained, first without contrast and then after contrast has been injected. A computer compares the two images and digitally "subtracts" or removes   A

A = Abbreviations Section   F = Figures Section   L = Laboratory Section   S = Synonyms Section
Sx (Symptoms)   Dx (Diagnosis)   Tx (Treatment)

the images of the soft tissues, bones, and muscles, leaving just the image of the arteries. [*see also*: angiography, arteriography]

dilated cardiomyopathy
The left ventricle is dilated and the myocardium is so stretched that it can no longer contract to pump blood. [*see also*: echocardiography, radionuclide ventriculography]

dilated funduscopy
Medical procedure to examine the posterior cavity of the eye. Mydriatic eye drops are used to dilate the pupil. An ophthalmoscope is used to examine the retina from all angles. The physician dials in the correct lens that produces a sharp image while compensating for both his visual defects and those of the patient. [*see also*: posterior cavity]

dilation
The act of opening or widening.
Reproductive: Widening of the cervical os from 0 to 10 cm during labor to allow passage of the fetal head. [*see also*: cervix, crowning, incompetent cervix]
Vascular: Widening of vessels due to physiological responses or medications. Causes decreased blood pressure. [*see also*: vasoconstriction, vasodilation]

dilation and curettage   A
Surgical procedure to remove abnormal tissue from inside the uterus. The cervix is dilated with progressively larger dilators inserted into the cervical os. A tenaculum is used to grasp and hold the cervix. Then a curet is inserted to scrape the endometrium. Alternatively, a vacuum aspirator is inserted to suction out pieces of endometrium. This procedure is performed for abnormal uterine bleeding or suspected uterine cancer. Also used to perform a therapeutic abortion or remove the products of conception following a spontaneous, but incomplete, abortion. [*see also*: elective abortion, miscarriage]

diplopia [368.xx]   S
Two visual fields are seen rather than one fused image. Can be caused by ambylopia, by tumor or trauma that increases the intracranial pressure, or by multiple sclerosis that affects nerve conduction to the visual cortex in the brain. [*see also*: papilledema]

diskectomy
Surgical excision of part or all of the herniated nucleus pulposus from an intervertebral disk. This relieves pressure on the adjacent dorsal nerve roots and relieves the pain. [*see also*: intervertebral disk, laminectomy, sciatica]

dislocation [830.xx–839.xx]
Displacement of the end of a bone from its normal position within a joint. Usually caused by injury or trauma. [*see also*: avascular necrosis]

displaced fracture [829.xx]
Broken bone ends are pulled out of their normal anatomical alignment. [*see also*: fracture]

dissecting aneurysm [441.xx]
Area of dilation and weakness in the wall of an artery that enlarges by tunneling between the layers of the artery wall. With each heartbeat, the weakened artery wall balloons outward. Aneurysms can rupture without warning. [*see also*: aneurysm]

Dx Angiogram to visualize the vessel, CBC to detect blood loss, monitor vital signs to show body status and potential complications. [*see also*: angiography]

Tx Surgical graft to repair the aneurysm, medications to control possible underlying causes such as hypertension.

disseminated intravascular coagulation [286.xx]   A
Severe disorder of clotting in which multiple small thrombi are   L
formed throughout the body. These blood clots use up platelets and fibrinogen from the plasma to the extent that there is spontaneous bleeding from the nose, mouth, IV sites, and incisions.

A = Abbreviations Section   **F** = Figures Section   **L** = Laboratory Section   **S** = Synonyms Section
Sx (Symptoms)   **Dx** (Diagnosis)   **Tx** (Treatment)

DIC can be triggered by severe injuries, burns, cancer, or systemic infections. [*see also*: burns, coagulation, hepatitis, postpartum hemorrhage, septicemia, transfusion reaction]

Dx   Lab studies, specifically clotting factors. Other tests will be performed to help determine the underlying cause. [*see also*: clotting factors]

Tx   Treat the underlying cause of DIC. Even though the patient is bleeding, the administration of anticoagulation therapy is necessary to stop the blood clot formation from robbing the body of the platelets and fibrinogen. Depending on the severity, blood products may be administered.

distal
Pertaining to away from the point of origin, particularly of an arm or leg.

distal convoluted tubule
Tubule of the nephron that begins at the loop of Henle. It empties into the collecting duct. Reabsorption takes place there. [*see also*: proximal convoluted tubule]

diverticulitis
[562.xx]
Area where the mucosa has been forced out through small defects in the wall of the colon. The feces become trapped inside a diverticular sac, which causes inflammation, infection, abdominal pain, and fever. [*see also*: colon]

Dx   H&P. Barium enema, endoscopy to visualize the intestine. [*see also*: barium enema, double contrast enema]

Tx   A high-fiber diet to prevent constipation and the trapping of feces. Medications are given to treat the underlying symptoms and infections that occur as a result of the disease. If severe enough, surgery may be required to drain the sac or even remove of part of the intestine. [*see also*: bowel resection and anastomosis]

dopamine
Neurotransmitter between neurons in the limbic system or hypothalamus. [*see also*: Parkinson's disease, substantia nigra]   S

Doppler ultrasonography
Uses ultra high-frequency sound waves emitted by an ultrasound transducer placed over an artery and Doppler technology to create an audible sound of blood flow through an artery. [*see also*: color flow duplex ultrasonography]

dorsal
Pertaining to the posterior of the body, particularly the back.

dorsal nerve roots
Group of spinal nerve roots that enter the posterior (dorsal) part of the spinal cord and carry sensory nerve impulses from the body to the spinal cord. [*see also*: diskectomy, laminectomy, myelography, pain management, sciatica, spinal nerves, ventral nerve roots]

dosimetry
Process of measuring the amount of radiation exposure as detected by a film badge and measured by a dosimeter. [*see also*: film badge]

double contrast enema
Barium contrast dye is instilled into the rectum. It outlines the colon and rectum and shows diverticula and abnormalities in the bowel wall. The barium is removed and then air is instilled as a second contrast. Fluoroscopy and individual radiographs are done to document the results of the procedure. [*see also*: barium enema]   S

Down syndrome
[758.xx]
Congenital genetic defect in which there are three of chromosome 21, instead of the normal two. This defect affects every cell in the body, but the most obvious functional limitation is mild-to-severe mental retardation. Persons with Down syndrome also have characteristic facial features with a thick, protruding   L

	tongue and short fingers with a single transverse palmar crease. [*see also*: chromosome studies]	
drug screening	Urine or blood test performed to detect any individual who is using illegal, addictive, or performance-enhancing drugs.	
dual energy x-ray absorptiometry scan	Radiologic procedure that uses two x-ray beams with different energy levels to create a two-dimensional image. It measures the bone mineral density (BMD) to determine if demineralization from osteoporosis has occurred and can detect as little as 1% loss of bone. The heel or wrist bone can be tested, but the hip and spine bones give more accurate results. [*see also*: densitometry, osteoporosis]	S
ductus arteriosus [747.xx]	Temporary, small blood vessel in the fetal heart that connects the pulmonary artery to the aorta. It should close when the baby is born. [*see also*: patent ductus arteriosus]	
duodenum	First part of the small intestine. It secretes cholecystokinin, a hormone that stimulates the gallbladder and pancreas to release bile and digestive enzymes. [*see also*: barium swallow, cholecystokinin, common bile duct, gastric bypass, lipase, pylorus]	F
Dupuytren's contracture [728.xx]	Progressive disease in which the fascia of the palm of the hand becomes thickened and shortened, causing a contracture and flexion deformity of the fingers. [*see also*: contracture, fasciectomy]	
dura mater	Tough, outermost layer of the meninges. The dura mater lies just beneath the bones of the cranium and within the foramen of each vertebra. [*see also*: epidural space, meninges, subdural hematoma]	F
dwarfism [259.xx]	Hyposecretion of growth hormone during childhood and puberty. Causes a lack of growth and short stature but with normal body proportions. [*see also*: anterior pituitary gland, hypopituitarism, gigantism, growth hormone]	S
dysentery [006.xx]	Bacterial infection caused by an unusual strain of *Escherichia coli*. Symptoms include watery diarrhea mixed with blood and mucus.	
dysfunctional uterine bleeding [626.xx]	Sporadic menstrual bleeding without a true menstrual period. Occurs in conjunction with anovulation. Estradiol causes the endometrium to thicken and slough off from time to time, but it never reaches its full thickness because there is no ovulation and no corpus luteum to make progesterone. [*see also*: anovulation, endometrial ablation, metorrhagia, oligomenorrhea]	A
dyskinesia [322.xx]	Abnormal motions due to difficulty controlling the voluntary muscles. Attempts at movement turn into tics, muscle spasms, muscle jerking, or slow, wandering, purposeless writhing of the hand, in which some muscles of the fingers are flexed and others are extended. [*see also*: ataxia, Huntington's chorea, Tourette's syndrome]	
dyslexia [784.xx]	Caused by an abnormality in the areas of the cerebrum that process visual images, particularly moving images (as the eye moves quickly across the page). This causes difficulty reading and writing words even though visual acuity and intelligence are normal. Tends to run in families and is more prevalent in left-handed persons and in males.	
dysmenorrhea [625.xx]	Painful menstruation. During menstruation, the uterus releases prostaglandin to constrict blood vessels in the uterine wall and prevent excessive bleeding. Abnormally high levels of prostaglandin cause cramping and temporary ischemia of the myometrium, both of which cause pain. Other causes can include pelvic inflammatory disease (PID), endometriosis, or uterine fibroids.	

A = Abbreviations Section   F = Figures Section   L = Laboratory Section   S = Synonyms Section
Sx (Symptoms)   Dx (Diagnosis)   Tx (Treatment)

dyspareunia
[302.xx; 625.xx]

Painful or difficult sexual intercourse or postcoital pain.
♀: Can be caused by the hymen being across the vaginal introitus, infections of the vagina, cervix, or uterus, pelvic inflammatory disease, endometriosis, or retroflexion of the uterus. [*see also*: endometriosis, pelvic inflammatory disease]

♂: Can be caused by a penile or prostatic infection, chordee of the penis, or phimosis. [*see also*: chordee, phimosis]

dyspepsia [536.xx]

Indigestion or epigastric pain that may be accompanied by gas or nausea.   S

dysphagia [787.xx]

Difficult or painful eating or swallowing. [*see also*: deglutition]   S

dysphasia
[438.xx; 784.xx]

Difficulty speaking or understanding words. Can be the result of head trauma, a stroke, brain disease, or dementia. [*see also*: aphasia]

dysplasia
[622.xx]

Resulting from chronic irritation and inflammation, a condition of atypical cells that are abnormal in size, shape, or organization, but have not yet become cancerous. [*see also*: cervical dysplasia, genital warts, Papanicolaou smear]

dysplastic nevus
[216.xx]

A mole (nevus) with irregular edges and variations in color. It can develop into malignant melanoma. [*see also*: nevus]

dyspnea [786.xx]

Difficult, labored, or painful respiration due to lung disease.   S
Dyspnea on exertion (DOE) can occur after minimal activity in patients with severe chronic obstructive pulmonary disease. [*see also*: paroxysmal nocturnal dyspnea, orthopnea, tachypnea]

dysrhythmia
[427.xx]

Any type of irregularity in the rate or rhythm of the heart. Dysrhythmias includes bradycardia, tachycardia, heart block, flutter, and fibrillation. [*see also*: automatic implantable cardiac defibrillator, cardioversion, conduction system, electrocardiography, electrophysiology study, Holter monitor, radiofrequency catheter ablation, stress test] [*see also the following abnormal rhythms*: bradycardia, fibrillation, flutter, heart block, left bundle branch block, premature contraction, right bundle branch block, sick sinus syndrome, tachycardia]

dysthymia [300.xx]

Chronic, mild-to-moderate depression. [*see also*: Beck Depression Inventory]

dystocia
[660.xx]

Any type of difficult or abnormal labor and delivery. [*see also*: abruptio placentae, assisted delivery, breech birth, eclampsia, ectopic pregnancy, failure to progress, incompetent cervix, induction of labor, malpresentation of the fetus, miscarriage, placenta previa, preeclampsia, premature rupture of membranes, uterine inertia]

dysuria [788.xx]

Difficult or painful urination, which can be due to many factors, such as kidney stones and cystitis. [*see also*: cystitis, sexually transmitted diseases, urination]

E

ecchymosis [782.xx]

A hemorrhage under the skin that is 3 cm in diameter or larger. [*see also*: bruise, hemorrhage]

echocardiography

Uses ultra high-frequency sound waves emitted by an ultrasound   S
transducer placed on the chest. The sound waves bounce off the contracting and relaxing heart, creating echoes that are changed into an image by a computer. [*see also*: color flow duplex ultrasonography, Doppler ultrasonography, transesophageal echocardiography]

A = Abbreviations Section   F = Figures Section   L = Laboratory Section   S = Synonyms Section
Sx (Symptoms)   Dx (Diagnosis)   Tx (Treatment)

eclampsia [642.xx] — A seizure or coma during pregnancy, usually after the 20th week of pregnancy, not associated with cerebral conditions. The cause is unknown. [*see also:* dystocia, preeclampsia]   **L**

ectopic pregnancy [633.xx] — Implantation of a fertilized ovum anywhere in the abdomen other than in the uterus, but most commonly in the fallopian tube. Occurs more readily if the fallopian tube has scar tissue or a blockage in it. The patient has a positive pregnancy test, but there is abdominal tenderness as the fallopian tube swells from the developing embryo. The tube can bleed and suddenly rupture, causing severe blood loss and shock. [*see also:* dystocia, menorrhagia, salpingectomy]   **S**

ectopic sites — Areas of tissue within the heart that can generate weak electrical impulses but are not part of the normal conduction system of the heart. [*see also:* atrial tachycardia, conduction system, radiofrequency catheter ablation, sick sinus syndrome, supraventricular tachycardia]

ectropion [374.xx] — Weakening of connective tissue in the lower eyelid in older patients. The lower eyelid turns outward, exposing the conjunctiva and causing dryness and chronic conjunctivitis. [*see also:* conjunctiva, presbyopia, xerophthalmia]

eczema [690.xx] — Oily areas are interspersed with patches of dry, scaly skin and dandruff. There can also be erythema and crusty, yellow exudates. It often appears after illness or stress, but can also be caused by environmental or food allergies.   **S**

edema — Excessive amounts of fluid move from the blood into the dermis or subcutaneous tissue and cause swelling. Localized areas of edema occur with inflammation, allergic reactions, and infections. Large areas of edema occur with cardiovascular or urinary system diseases. [*see also:* congestive heart failure, nephrotic syndrome, pulmonary edema]

effacement — Thinning of the cervical wall, measured in percentages from 0% to 100%. [*see also:* cervix]

efferent nerves — Nerves that carry motor nerve impulses from the brain or spinal cord to the body. [*see also:* afferent nerves]

ejaculatory duct — Duct that collects semen from both the vas deferens and the seminal vesicles and empties into the urethra during ejaculation. [*see also:* semen]   **F**

elastin — Elastic, yellow protein fibers in the dermis.

elective abortion — Medical procedure for planned termination of a pregnancy at any time during gestation. All products of conception are removed from the uterus with suction. [*see also:* dilation and curettage, hydatidiform mole]

electrocardio-graphy — Diagnostic procedure that records the electrical activity of the heart during contractions and rest. A 12-lead EKG records 12 different leads that show the electrical activity between different combinations of electrodes to give an electrical picture of the heart from 12 different angles. Samples of each of these 12 tracings are mounted on a backing. [*see also:* asystole, conduction system, dysrhythmia]   **A**

electrodesiccation — Medical procedure that involves the use of electrical current to remove a nevus, wart, skin tag, or small malignant lesion. The electrical current passes through an electrode that is touched to or inserted into the skin or lesion and causes the intracellular contents to evaporate. [*see also:* curettage, electrosection, electrosurgery, fulguration]

electroen-cephalography	Diagnostic procedure to record the electrical activity of the brain. **A** Multiple electrodes are placed on the scalp overlying the specific lobes of the brain. There are four types of normal brain waves (named for letters of the Greek alphabet: alpha, beta, delta, and theta). The patterns of brain waves in each of the two hemispheres of the cerebrum are compared for symmetry. Differences between the two hemispheres suggest a tumor or injury. The presence of abnormal waves suggests encephalopathy or dementia. Brain waves during an epileptic seizure show specific patterns that are used to diagnose the particular type of epilepsy. In order to induce an epileptic seizure during the EEG, the patient may look at flashing lights or have a sleep-deprived EEG recording. An EEG is also done as part of a polysomnography to diagnose sleep disorders and also as part of evoked potential testing. [*see also:* epilepsy, evoked potential testing, polysomnography, seizures]
electrolytes	Substances that have a positive or negative charge and conduct electricity when dissolved in a solution. Excess amounts in the blood are removed by the kidneys. Examples: sodium (Na^+), potassium (K^+), chloride (Cl^-), calcium (Ca^{++}), and bicarbonate (HCO_3^-).
electromyography	Diagnostic procedure to diagnose muscle disease or nerve **A** damage. A needle electrode, inserted into a muscle, records electrical activity as the muscle contracts and relaxes. The electrical activity is displayed as waveforms on a screen and recorded on paper. [*see also:* carpal tunnel syndrome, Guillain-Barré syndrome, Lou Gehrig's disease, myasthenia gravis, nerve conduction study]
electrophoresis	Immunoglobulin electrophoresis determines the amounts of immunoglobulins in the blood. A sample of serum is placed in a gel. An electric current causes the immunoglobulins to become charged and move toward a positive or negative electrode. Each immunoglobulin travels a different distance and direction through the gel, depending on its size and charge, and appears as a spike in a different area on the graph paper. The size of the spike corresponds to how much immunoglobulin is present. [*see also:* leukemia, multiple myeloma]
electrophysiology study	Diagnostic procedure to map the heart's conduction system in **A** patients with arrhythmias. While an EKG is performed, catheters are inserted into the femoral vein and the subclavian vein. X-rays are used to guide the catheters to the heart. The catheters send out electrical impulses to stimulate the heart and try to induce an arrhythmia to pinpoint where the arrhythmias are originating from in the heart. [*see also:* conduction system, dysrhythmia]
electrosection	Medical procedure that involves the use of electrical current to remove a nevus, wart, skin tag, or small malignant lesion. The electrical current passes through a wire loop electrode that is used to cut tissue. [*see also:* electrodesiccation, electrosurgery, fulguration]
electroshock therapy	Uses an electrical current and electrodes on the head to produce **A** seizures (convulsions). Patients are given sedative and muscle **S** relaxant drugs to make them unconscious and relaxed. The seizure lasts about one minute and the patient awakens within one hour. Used to treat severe depression and schizophrenia. ECT relieves symptoms more quickly than antidepressant drugs (that can take up to a month to become effective). [*see also:* major depression, schizophrenia]

A = Abbreviations Section   **F** = Figures Section   **L** = Laboratory Section   **S** = Synonyms Section
Sx (Symptoms)   **Dx** (Diagnosis)   **Tx** (Treatment)

electrosurgery	Medical procedure that involves the use of electrical current to remove a nevus, wart, skin tag, or small malignant lesion. The electrical current passes through an electrode and causes the intracellular contents to evaporate. [*see also*: electrodesiccation, electrosection, fulguration]
embryo	The fertilized ovum is an embryo from 4 days after fertilization through 8 weeks of gestation. Then it becomes a fetus. [*see also*: amniotic fluid, fetus, growth abnormalities, hydatidiform mole, zygote]
emesis [787.xx]	The expelling of food from the stomach through the mouth. [*see also*: hematemesis, hyperemesis gravidarum, migraine headache, morning sickness, regurgitation] L S
emotion	Intense state of feelings. [*see also*: affect, amygdaloid body, hypothalamus, limbic system, mood, Thematic Apperception Test]
emphysema [492.xx]	Chronic, irreversibly damaged alveoli that become large air spaces that trap air in the lungs. [*see also*: chronic obstructive pulmonary disease] L
emulsification	Process performed as bile breaks down large fat droplets into smaller droplets with more surface area. [*see also*: bile, lipase]
en bloc resection	Surgical procedure to excise a tumor and surrounding structures, which are removed as one block of tissue.
encapsulated	Having a capsule or enveloping structure around it. Benign tumors have a capsule; cancerous tumors do not.
encephalitis [323.xx]	Inflammation of the brain caused by a virus. [*see also*: cerebrospinal fluid examination, electroencephalography]
encopresis [307.xx; 787.xx]	Repeated passage of stool into the clothing in a child older than age 5 who does not have a gastrointestinal illness, mental retardation, or a disability. [*see also*: defecation]
endocarditis [421.xx]	Inflammation and bacterial infection of the endocardium and the valves. This occurs in patients who already have a structural defect of the valves or heart. Bacteria from an infection elsewhere in the body travel through the blood, are trapped by the structural defect, and cause infection. Acute endocarditis causes a high fever and shock, while subacute bacterial endocarditis (SBE) causes fever, fatigue, and aching muscles. [*see also*: chordae tendineae, echocardiography, endocardium, valves] L
endocardium	Innermost layer of the heart. It covers the inside of the heart chambers and valves. [*see also*: chordae tendineae, endocarditis, epicardium, myocardium, pericardium]
endocrine system	Body system that includes organs and glands that secrete hormones into the blood. They produce and release hormones that direct other body organs.
endometrial ablation	Surgical procedure that uses heat or cold to destroy the endometrium. A laser, hot fluid in a balloon, or an electrode with electrical current is inserted into the uterus. Alternatively, a cryoprobe is inserted to freeze the endometrium. Used to treat dysfunctional uterine bleeding. [*see also*: dysfunctional uterine bleeding]
endometriosis [617.xx]	Endometrial tissue in abnormal places. The endometrium sloughs off during menstruation but is forced upward through the fallopian tubes and out into the pelvic cavity because the uterus is in retroflexion. The endometrial tissue can implant itself on the walls of the ovaries, uterus, and pelvic cavity. These tissue implants remain alive and sensitive to hormones. During each menstrual

cycle, they thicken and slough off, forming more implants with old blood and tissue debris in the pelvic cavity. They also form adhesions between the internal organs. [see also: adhesions, endometrium, salpingitis]

Dx   H&P. Imaging tests to visualize the tissue and its location. [see also: culdoscopy, dysmenorrhea, dyspareunia]

Tx   Medications for pain. Surgical intervention is the most common treatment, used to remove the tissue and sometimes the entire organ, if necessary.

endometrium   Innermost layer of the uterine wall. Composed of a specialized mucous membrane that contains many glands. It lines the uterine cavity. [see also: dilation and curettage, endometrial ablation, estradiol, intrauterine cavity, menstruation, uterine fibroid]   F

endoplasmic reticulum   Organelle that consists of a network of channels that transport materials within the cell. Also the site of protein, fat, and glycogen synthesis.

endorphins   Neurotransmitter between neurons in the hypothalamus, thalamus, or brainstem. Endorphins are the body's own natural pain relievers.

endoscopic retrograde cholangiopancre-atography   Radiologic procedure that uses a contrast dye to outline the bile ducts. An endoscope is passed through the mouth and into the duodenum. A catheter is passed through the endoscope, and the contrast dye is injected into the lower end of the common bile duct. An x-ray is taken to identify stones in the gallbladder and biliary ducts or thickening of the gallbladder wall. The pancreatic duct is also visualized. [see also: bile ducts, cholangiography]   A

endoscopic sinus surgery   Surgical procedure that uses an endoscope to examine the nose, sinuses, or throat. It can remove tissue and fluid for analysis or perform a biopsy. [see also: endoscopy]

endoscopy   Surgical procedure that uses a fiberoptic endoscope to examine a body cavity for signs of abnormal tissues or tumors. Grasping and cutting instruments can be inserted through the endoscope to perform biopsies. [see also: arthroscopy, bronchoscopy, endoscopic sinus surgery, laparoscopy]

endothelium   Smooth innermost layer of the wall of a blood vessel. [see also: arteriosclerosis]   S

endotoxin   Toxic substance produced by some bacteria. It acts as a poison in the body and can cause decreased blood pressure. [see also: tumor necrosis factor]

endotracheal intubation   Medical procedure that inserts an endotracheal tube (ETT) between the vocal cords in the larynx and into the trachea in order to establish an airway for the patient to breathe through or to manually or mechanically ventilate the patient.

end-stage renal disease [586.xx]   The final, irreversible stage of chronic renal failure in which there is little or no remaining kidney function. [see also: renal failure]   A

engagement   The top of the uterine fundus lowers as the fetal head drops into position within the mother's pelvis in anticipation of birth. [see also: fundal height]   S

enhanced   Roentgenography, CT scan, or MRI scan that uses a contrast dye to enhance anatomic details. If no contrast dye is used, the image is said to be unenhanced. [see also: barium, gadolinium, magnetic resonance imaging]

enucleation   Surgical procedure to remove the eye from the orbit because of trauma or tumor.

A = Abbreviations Section   F = Figures Section   L = Laboratory Section   S = Synonyms Section
Sx (Symptoms)   Dx (Diagnosis)   Tx (Treatment)

enuresis [788.xx]
Involuntary urination. It is only considered a disease in older children or adults who should have voluntary bladder control. [*see also*: encopresis, nocturnal enuresis, voiding]

environmental disease
Caused by exposure to external substances. Examples: Allergies to pollen or skin cancer from the sun.

enzyme
Substance that breaks the chemical bonds that hold food molecules together. The name of an enzyme usually ends in -*ase*. The action of an enzyme in breaking down food is known as chemical digestion. [*see also*: amylase, enzyme-linked immunosorbent assay, lactase, leukocyte esterase, lipase, Lou Gehrig's disease, pepsin, protease, renin]

enzyme-linked immunosorbent assay
Involves the use of two antibodies to determine if a patient's immune system has encountered a particular antigen. The first antibody will bind to the antigen, forming a complex. The second antibody will react to an enzyme in the formed complex. Used to assist in diagnosing HIV, lupus erythematosis, Lyme disease, or syphilis. [*see also*: antigen, OraSure, p24 antigen test, viral load test, Western blot]   **A**

eosinophil
A type of leukocyte. It is classified as a granulocyte because granules in its cytoplasm stain bright pink to red with eosin dye. The nucleus has two lobes. It is a phagocyte that eats foreign cells, such as pollen, animal dander, and parasites. [*see also*: complete blood count]   **A F L S**

ependymal cells
Specialized cells that line the walls of the ventricles and spinal canal and produce cerebrospinal fluid. [*see also*: cerebrospinal fluid, hydrocephalus]

epicardium
Inner membrane of the double-layered pericardium. It covers the myocardium of the heart. [*see also*: endocardium, myocardium, pericardium]

epidermis
Thin, outermost layer of skin. The most superficial part of the epidermis consists of dead cells filled with keratin. The deepest part (basal layer) contains constantly dividing cells and melanocytes. [*see also*: dermabrasion, exfoliation, laser skin resurfacing]

epididymis
Long, coiled tube on the outer wall of each testis. It receives spermatozoa from the seminiferous tubules, stores them, and destroys defective spermatozoa. [*see also*: epididymis]   **F**

epididymitis [604.xx]
Inflammation and infection of the epididymis. Caused by a bacterial urinary tract infection or sexually transmitted diseases such as gonorrhea or *Chlamydia*. [*see also*: bacteriuria, sexually transmitted disease, urinary tract infection]

epidural
Local anesthesia produced by injecting an anesthetic drug into the epidural space between vertebrae in the lower back. This numbs the abdomen, perineum, and legs. Commonly used in labor to decrease labor pain. Epidural anesthesia is not given until the cervix is more than 4 cm dilated to prevent prolonging labor. [*see also*: anesthesia]

epidural space
Area between the dura mater and the vertebral body.

epigastric region
One of nine regions on the surface of the anterior abdominal area. It is centered and superior to the umbilical region. [*see also*: hypochondriac region, hypogastric region, inguinal region, lumbar region, quadrant, umbilical region]

epiglottis
Lidlike structure that seals the larynx when food is swallowed and directs food into the esophagus. [*see also*: deglutition]   **F**

A = Abbreviations Section   **F** = Figures Section   **L** = Laboratory Section   **S** = Synonyms Section
Sx (Symptoms)   **Dx** (Diagnosis)   **Tx** (Treatment)

epilepsy [345.xx]   Recurring condition in which a group of neurons in the brain   S
spontaneously sends out electrical impulses in an abnormal,
uncontrolled way. Impulses spread from neuron to neuron,
causing altered consciousness and abnormal muscle movements.
The type and extent of the symptoms depend on the number and
location of the affected neurons. [*see also*: aura, eclampsia,
postictal state, status epilepticus]

> **Dx**   Evidence of the seizure. PET scan and EEG to locate the
> focal point in the brain. [*see also*: electroencephalography;
> *see also the following types of seizures*: absence (petit mal),
> complex partial (psychomotor), simple partial (focal motor),
> and tonic-clonic (grand mal)]

> **Tx**   Medications to control the seizures.

epinephrine   Neurotransmitter for the sympathetic nervous system. It increases   A
the heart rate to prepare for exercise or the "flight or fight"   S
response. Secreted by the adrenal medulla in response to
stimulation by nerves of the sympathetic nervous system. [*see
also*: adrenal medulla, pheochromocytoma, sympathetic nervous
system, vanillylmandelic acid]

epiphysis   The widened end of a long bone. Each end contains the
epiphysial plate where bone growth takes place. [*see also*:
avascular necrosis]

episiotomy   Surgical incision in the posterior edge of the vagina to prevent a
spontaneous tear during delivery of the baby's head. Spontaneous
vaginal tears usually have ragged tissue edges that are difficult to
suture and can extend into the rectum, causing incontinence.
[*see also*: perineum, rectum]

epispadias [752.xx]   Congenital condition in which the female urethral meatus is
incorrectly located near the clitoris, or the male urethral meatus
is incorrectly located on the upper surface of the shaft of the
penis rather than at the tip of the glans penis. [*see also*:
hypospadias, urethroplasty]

epistaxis [784.xx]   Sudden, sometimes severe, bleeding from the nose. Due to   S
irritation or dryness of the nasal mucosa and the rupture of a
small artery just beneath the mucous membrane. It can also be
caused by trauma to the nose.

epithelium   Category that includes the skin and all of its structures that cover
the external surface of the body, but also includes the mucous
membranes that line the walls of internal cavities that connect to
the outside of the body. [*see also*: cervical dysplasia, dermis, epidermis]

erythema   Reddish discoloration of the skin. It can be confined to one area
[695.xx]   of local inflammation or infection, or it can affect large areas of
the skin surface, as in sunburn. [*see also*: systemic lupus
erythematosus]

erythrocyte   A red blood cell. Erythrocytes contain hemoglobin and carry   F
oxygen and carbon dioxide to and from the lungs and cells of the   S
body. [*see also*: anemia, anisocytosis, antigen, blood, blood smear,
fibrin, heme, hemoglobin, hemolytic reaction, poikilocytosis,
polycythemia vera, sickle cell anemia, spleen]

erythropoietin   Hormone secreted by the kidneys when the number of red blood   A
cells decreases. It stimulates the bone marrow to produce more   L
red blood cells. [*see also*: blood transfusion, urinary system]

eschar   A thick, crusty scar of necrotic tissue that forms on a third-degree
burn. It traps fluid released by the burn tissue, delays healing,

A = Abbreviations Section   F = Figures Section   L = Laboratory Section   S = Synonyms Section
Sx (Symptoms)   **Dx** (Diagnosis)   **Tx** (Treatment)

and can become the site of an infection. It is commonly removed to promote healing. [*see also*: third-degree burn]

esophagus   Flexible, muscular tube that moves food from the pharynx to the stomach. [*see also*: gastroesophageal reflux, heartburn, hiatal hernia, peristalsis, varices]   F

esotropia [378.xx]   Medial deviation of one or both eyes. Also known as cross-eye. [*see also*: amblyopia, convergence, exotropia, strabismus]   S

essential hypertension [401.xx]   The most common type of hypertension, one in which the exact cause of the elevated blood pressure is not known. [*see also*: hypertension]

estradiol   Most abundant and biologically active of the female sex hormones. It is secreted by the follicles of the ovary. During puberty, it causes the development of the female sex characteristics. It causes the endometrium to thicken during the menstrual cycle. After ovulation, it is secreted by the corpus luteum. During pregnancy, it is secreted by the placenta. [*see also*: corpus luteum, gestational diabetes mellitus, hyperemesis gravidarum, infertility, menopause, morning sickness, precocious puberty]

estrogen receptor assay   Cytology test performed on breast tissue that has already been diagnosed as malignant. This test looks for a large number of estrogen receptors on the tumor cell membranes. If present, this means that the tumor requires estrogen (estradiol) in order to grow and that chemotherapy drugs that block estrogen would cause the tumor cells to die. [*see also*: receptor assays]

ethmoid sinuses   Groups of small air cells in the ethmoid bone, which is located between the nose and the eye. [*see also*: pansinusitis]

eupnea   A normal rate and rhythm of breathing.

eustachian tube   Tube that connects the middle ear to the nasopharynx and equalizes the air pressure in the middle ear. [*see also*: otitis media, tonsillitis]   F

euthyroidism   State of normal functioning of the hormones of the thyroid gland.

eversion   Turning a body part outward and toward the side. Opposite of inversion.

evertor   Muscle that produces eversion when it contracts.

evoked potential testing   Diagnostic procedure in which an EEG is used to record changes in brain waves that occur following various stimuli presented to evoke (stimulate) a response. Used to evaluate the potential ability of a particular nervous pathway to conduct nerve impulses. [*see also*: electroencephalography]

excisional biopsy   An incision is made to expose the suspected cancer, and the entire tumor is removed along with a surrounding margin of normal tissue. [*see also*: biopsy]

excoriation   Superficial injury from a sharp object such as a fingernail or thorn that creates a linear scratch in the skin. [*see also*: abrasion]

exenteration   Surgical procedure to excise the tumor as well as all the nearby organs. Used to treat widely metastatic cancer in the abdominopelvic cavity. [*see also*: metastasis]

exfoliation   Normal process of constant shedding of dead skin cells from the most superficial part of the epidermis. [*see also*: chemical peel, epidermis, exfoliative cytology]

exfoliative cytology   Cytology test that uses the cells in body secretions or cells that are scraped or washed from the body. The sample is examined

under the microscope to look for abnormal or cancerous cells.
[*see also*: Papanicolaou smear]

exhibitionism [302.xx]	Obtaining power, control, and sexual arousal by exposing the genital area in public areas to strangers and seeing their reactions.
exocrine gland	Type of gland that secretes substances through a duct. [*see also*: cystic fibrosis, sebaceous glands, sudoriferous glands]
exophthalmos [376.xx]	Pronounced outward bulging of the anterior surface of the eye with a startled, staring expression. If just one eye is affected, it often has a tumor behind it. If both eyes are affected, the patient usually has hyperthyroidism. [*see also*: Graves' disease, hyperthyroidism]
exotropia [378.xx]	Lateral deviation of one or both eyes. Also known as wall-eye. S [*see also*: amblyopia, convergence, esotropia, strabismus]
expectoration	The process of coughing up sputum from the lungs. [*see also*: cough, hemoptysis, intercostal muscles]
exploratory laparotomy	Surgical procedure that uses an abdominal incision to widely open the abdominopelvic cavity so that it can be visually and/or physically explored.
expressive aphasia [315.xx]	Loss of the ability to express thoughts verbally because of injury S to the area of the brain that deals with language and the interpretation of sounds and symbols. [*see also*: aphasia]
extension	Straightening and extending a joint to increase the angle between two bones or two body parts. Opposite of flexion.
extensor	Muscle that produces extension when it contracts.
external	Pertaining to near or on the outside surface of the body or an organ.
external auditory canal	Passageway from the external ear to the middle ear. It contains A glands that secrete cerumen. [*see also*: cerumen] F S
external auditory meatus	Opening at the entrance to the external auditory canal. [*see also*: external auditory canal]
external beam radiotherapy	Beams of radiation are generated by a machine outside the body and directed at the site of a cancerous tumor. Linear accelerators are used to increase the energy of the radiation so that it can penetrate more deeply into the body. [*see also*: conformal radiotherapy]
external cephalic version	Medical procedure to manually correct a breech or other A malpresentation prior to delivery. The physician puts hands on the mother's abdominal wall and manipulates the position of the fetus. [*see also*: malpresentation of the fetus]
external fixation	Surgical procedure used to treat a complicated fracture. An external fixator orthopedic device has metal pins that are inserted in the bone on either side of the fracture and connected to a metal frame immobilizing the fracture. To lengthen a congenitally short leg, the device has screws that are turned each day to pull the bone and lengthen it. [*see also*: open reduction and internal fixation]
external genitalia	♀: Labia majora, labia minora, clitoris, vaginal introitus, Bartholin's glands, urethral glands, and Skene's glands. ♂: Scrotum, testes, and penis.
extracapsular cataract extraction	An incision is made in the sclera to remove the lens, but the posterior lens capsule is left in place. The central part of the lens is removed and replaced with an artificial intraocular lens implant. The implant folds to pass through the incision and then unfolds

within the capsule. [*see also*: aphakia, cataract extraction, phacoemulsification]

extracorporeal shock wave lithotripsy	Medical or surgical procedure that uses sound waves to break up a kidney stone or bone. A S Renal: After an x-ray pinpoints the location of the stone, a lithotriptor generates sound waves that break up the stone. [*see also*: percutaneous ultrasonic lithotripsy] Skeletal: Used to break up bony spurs and treat other minor but painful skeletal problems of the foot.
extremity	An arm or a leg. S
eye patching	Medical procedure in which the eye is covered with a soft bandage and a hard outer shield after eye trauma or eye surgery. Also, a normal eye can be patched to treat amblyopia. [*see also*: amblyopia]

F

facial nerve	Cranial nerve VII. Sense of taste. Control of salivary and lacrimal glands. Movement of face and scalp muscles. [*see also*: Bell's palsy]
failure of lactation [676.xx]	Hyposecretion of prolactin from the anterior pituitary gland causes a lack of development of lactiferous glands in the breasts during puberty, with a resulting inability of the breasts to produce milk or to produce sufficient milk for breastfeeding after the baby is born. [*see also*: lactation, prolactin, oxytocin]
failure to progress [661.xx]	Cessation of or prolonging of labor. The cervix does not dilate and efface, and the head of the fetus does not progress through the birth canal. [*see also*: cephalopelvic disproportion, cesarean section, dystocia, induction of labor, malpresentation of the fetus] S
fallopian tube	Narrow tube that is connected at one end to the uterus. The other end, which is not directly connected to the ovary, has a funnel-shaped infundibulum and fingerlike fimbriae that draw an ovum into its lumen. [*see also*: broad ligament, culdoscopy, ectopic pregnancy] F S
family therapy	Involves the entire family, not just the patient. The focus is on relationships and conflicts between family members. What family members say to each other, how they say it, and how they act toward each other can be dysfunctional. The family often labels one family member as the troublemaker, while others can do no wrong. Unless corrected, these fixed roles inhibit changing and adopting more appropriate behaviors.
fascia	Thin connective tissue sheet around each muscle or groups of muscles. It merges into and becomes part of the tendon. [*see also*: compartment syndrome, Dupuytren's syndrome, muscle]
fascicle	A bundle composed of many muscle fibers surrounded by fascia.
fasciectomy	Surgical procedure to partially or totally remove the fascia causing contractures. [*see also*: Dupuytren's contracture, fascia]
fasciotomy	Surgical procedure to cut into the fascia around a muscle and release pressure from built-up blood and tissue fluid. [*see also*: compartment syndrome, fascia]
fasting blood sugar	Blood test that measures the level of glucose after the patient has fasted (not eaten) for at least 12 hours. Used to evaluate the function of the pancreas. [*see also*: diabetes mellitus] A
fecal occult blood test	Diagnostic test to detect occult blood in the feces. A sample of feces is placed on paper and mixed with the chemical reagent guaiac. If blood is present, the guaiac will turn the paper blue. [*see also*: digital rectal examination] A

A = Abbreviations Section   **F** = Figures Section   **L** = Laboratory Section   **S** = Synonyms Section
Sx (Symptoms)   **Dx** (Diagnosis)   **Tx** (Treatment)

fecalith [560.xx]	Hardened feces that become a stone-like mass. [*see also*: constipation, diverticulitis]	
feces	Formed, solid waste composed of undigested food, fiber, and water that is eliminated from the body. [*see also*: defecation, diverticulitis]	S
femoral artery	Major artery that carries blood to the upper leg. [*see also*: cardiopulmonary bypass, coronary angiography, percutaneous coronary angioplasty, transarterial chemoembolization, uterine artery embolization]	F
ferritin	Blood chemistry test that indirectly measures the amount of iron stored in the body by measuring the small amount that is always present in the blood. [*see also*: iron deficiency anemia]	A S
fertilization	The act of a spermatozoon uniting with an ovum.	S
fetal distress [768.xx]	Lack of oxygen to the fetus because of decreased blood flow through the placenta or umbilical cord. The fetus develops bradycardia and passes meconium because of the stress from decreased levels of oxygen. [*see also*: meconium aspiration, prolapsed cord]	
fetishism [302.xx]	Obtaining sexual arousal from objects rather than a person.	
fetus	The embryo becomes a fetus beginning at 9 weeks of gestation and until the moment of birth.	
fibrillation [427.xx]	Arrhythmia in which there is a very fast, uncoordinated quivering of the myocardium. It can affect the atria or ventricles. Ventricular fibrillation is a life-threatening emergency in which the heart is unable to pump blood; this can progress to cardiac arrest. [*see also*: asystole, cardioversion, defibrillator]	
fibrin	Fiber strands formed by the activation of clotting factors. Fibrin traps erythrocytes to form a blood clot. [*see also*: clotting factors]	
fibrinogen	Blood clotting factor I. [*see also*: clotting factors, disseminated intravascular coagulation]	S
fibrocystic disease [610.xx]	Benign condition in which numerous, fluid-filled cysts of various sizes form in one or both breasts. The sizes of the cysts can change, usually in response to hormone levels, and are painful and tender. [*see also*: mammary glands]	
fibromyalgia [729.xx]	Caused by injury or trauma, pain is located at specific, small trigger points along the neck, back, or hips. The trigger points are very tender to the touch and feel firm.	S
	Dx Only on the H&P. There is no diagnostic test to perform.	
	Tx Because of the diversity of pain and its locations, treatment plans are designed for a specific patient. [*see also*: trigger point injections]	
film badge	Small, flat container that holds an unexposed piece of x-ray film that detects the total amount of a healthcare worker's exposure to radiation or radioactive substances. [*see also*: dosimetry]	
filtration	Process in which water and substances in the blood are pushed through the pores of the glomerulus in the nephron of the kidney. The resulting fluid is known as filtrate. [*see also*: glomerulus, reabsorption]	
fimbriae	Fingerlike projections on the ends of the fallopian tubes that create currents to draw an ovum into the fallopian tube. [*see also*: fallopian tube, ectopic pregnancy]	
fine-needle biopsy	Surgical procedure that uses a very fine needle inserted into a tumor. The fluid or tissue inside the tumor is aspirated into the	

A = Abbreviations Section   F = Figures Section   L = Laboratory Section   S = Synonyms Section
Sx (Symptoms)   **Dx** (Diagnosis)   **Tx** (Treatment)

attached syringe and then tested in the lab to determine if the tumor is benign or malignant.

first-degree burn
[948.xx–949.xx]
Involves only the epidermis. Heat (fire, hot objects, steam, boiling water), electrical current (lightning, electrical outlets or cords), chemicals, or radiation or x-rays (sunshine or prescribed radiation therapy) can injure superficial or deep tissues. [see also: burns]

first-degree heart block
[426.xx]
Arrhythmia in which electrical impulses are delayed in traveling from the SA node to the Purkinje fibers. [see also: conduction system, heart block]

fissure
Deep division that runs anterior to posterior through the cerebrum and divides it into right and left hemispheres. [see also: cerebrum]

flaccid paralysis
[359.xx]
After an injury to the spinal cord, the absence of nerve impulses causes muscles to lose their tone and firmness and eventually atrophy. [see also: paraplegia, quadriplegia, spastic paralysis]

flagellum
The long tail on a spermatozoon that propels it, making it motile. [see also: infertility, spermatozoon]

flank
Area of the back between the ribs and the pelvis that overlies the kidneys.

flashers and floaters
Flashers are brief bursts of bright light that occur when the vitreous humor pulls on the retina. Floaters are clumps, dots, or strings of collagen molecules that form in the vitreous humor because of aging. [see also: retinal detachment, vitreous humor]

flatulence
[787.xx]
Presence of excessive amounts of flatus (gas) in the stomach or intestines. [see also: flatus]   S

flatus
Gas produced by bacteria that inhabit the large intestine or by some foods. [see also: dyspepsia, flatulence]   S

flexion
Bending of a joint to decrease the angle between two bones or two body parts. Opposite of extension.

flexor
Muscle that produces flexion when it contracts.

fluorescein angiography
Diagnostic procedure in which fluorescein, an orange fluorescent dye, is injected intravenously. The dye travels to the retinal artery in the eye. It glows fluorescent green on flash photography of the retina. It reveals retinal microaneurysms, leaking, and hemorrhages. [see also: diabetic retinopathy]

fluorescein staining
Diagnostic procedure in which fluorescein, a fluorescent dye, is applied topically to the cornea. A blue light is used to examine the eye, and corneal abrasions and ulcers will fluoresce (glow). [see also: corneal abrasion]

fluoroscopy
Uses a continuous x-ray beam to capture the motion of internal organs after the administration of a radiopaque contrast dye. A fluorescent screen acts like a TV monitor to display a series of changing images. [see also: double contrast enema, barium swallow]

flutter [427.xx]
Arrhythmia in which there is a very fast but regular rhythm (250 beats per minute) of the atria or ventricles. The chambers of the heart do not have time to completely fill with blood before the next contraction. Flutter can progress to fibrillation. [see also: cardioversion, conduction system, fibrillation]

Foley catheter
Sometimes referred to as a Foley, this catheter is an indwelling tube that drains urine continuously. It has an expandable balloon tip that keeps it positioned in the bladder. [see also: condom catheter, straight catheter, suprapubic catheter]

A = Abbreviations Section   F = Figures Section   L = Laboratory Section   S = Synonyms Section
Sx (Symptoms)   Dx (Diagnosis)   Tx (Treatment)

folic acid anemia [281.xx]

Caused by a deficiency of folic acid in the diet. Commonly seen in patients who are malnourished, those who have malabsorption diseases, and pregnant women. The erythrocytes are abnormally large and very immature. [*see also*: anemia, anisocytosis]

L

follicle

Skin: Site where a hair is formed. The follicle is located in the dermis. [*see also*: acne vulgaris, blepharitis, boil, folliculitis, pilonidal sinus]

Reproductive: Mass of cells with a hollow center. It holds an oocyte before puberty and a maturing ovum after puberty. The follicle ruptures at the time of ovulation and becomes the corpus luteum. [*see also*: corpus luteum, estradiol, follicle-stimulating hormone, luteinizing hormone, polycystic ovary syndrome]

follicle-stimulating hormone

Follicle-stimulating hormone is released from the anterior pituitary gland. [*see also*: anterior pituitary gland]

♀: It causes a follicle in the ovary to enlarge and produce a mature ovum. FSH also stimulates the follicles to secrete estradiol, which causes the development of the female sex characteristics.

♂: It causes the seminiferous tubules of the testes to enlarge during puberty. [*see also*: follicle]

A
S

folliculitis [704.xx]

Inflammation or infection of the hair follicle. It occurs after shaving, plucking, or removing hair with hot wax. [*see also*: boil]

fontanels

Soft, flexible areas on a newborn's head between the bones of the cranium. In these areas, the brain is only covered with dura mater and skin. Fontanels allow the cranium to expand as the baby's brain grows.

S

foramen

A hole in a bone: foramen magnum in the cranium, vertebral foramen in a vertebra, and obturator foramen in each ischium.

foramen ovale

Temporary, oval-shaped opening in the interatrial septum of the fetal heart. It should close when the baby is born.

fornix

Neurologic: Tract of nerves that joins all the parts of the limbic system. [*see also*: limbic system]

S

Reproductive: Area of the superior part of the vagina that lies behind and around the cervix.

fovea

Small depression in the center of the macula. This area has the greatest visual acuity and lies directly opposite the pupil. [*see also*: macula]

F

fractionation

The total dose of external beam radiation to be given to a patient is divided into smaller doses (fractions of the total dose) that are given each day to decrease the occurrence of side effects of radiation therapy.

fracture [829.xx]

Broken bone due to an accident, injury, or disease process. Fractures are classified according to the way in which the bone breaks and whether or not the skin is pierced with a bony fragment.

A

Types of fractures: Closed, Colles', comminuted, compound, compression, depressed, displaced, greenstick, hairline, oblique, open, nondisplaced, pathologic, spiral, and transverse. [*see also*: avascular necrosis, bone graft, bone scintigraphy, cast]

fraternal twins

The ovary releases two ova that are fertilized by different spermatozoa. [*see also*: identical twins, polyhydramnios]

S

freckle

Benign, pigmented, flat macule that develops after sun exposure. Freckles contain groups of melanocytes.

A = Abbreviations Section   F = Figures Section   L = Laboratory Section   S = Synonyms Section
Sx (Symptoms)   Dx (Diagnosis)   Tx (Treatment)

frequency [788.xx]	Urinating often, usually in small amounts. Can be caused by a kidney stone, enlargement of the prostate gland, overactive bladder, or a urinary tract infection. [*see also*: urination]
frontal lobe	Lobe of the cerebrum that predicts future events and consequences. Exerts conscious control over the skeletal muscles. Contains the gustatory cortex for the sense of taste. **F**
frontal sinuses	Pair of sinuses above each eyebrow in the frontal bone of the skull. [*see also*: pansinusitis] **F**
frozen section	Cytology test that involves freezing a tissue specimen obtained from a biopsy. Freezing the tissue distorts some of the architecture, and so a permanent section is also done using a paraffin-like substance to make the tissue firm.
FSH assay and LH assay	Blood test that measures the levels of follicle-stimulating hormone (FSH) and luteinizing hormone (LH). Used to evaluate the function of the anterior pituitary gland, ovaries, and testes.
fugue [300.xx]	Impulsive flight from one's life and familiar surroundings after a traumatic event. The patient begins a new life in a new location and functions normally but later is unable to remember anything that occurred during this time.
fulguration	Medical procedure that involves the use of electrical current to remove a nevus, wart, skin tag, or small malignant lesion. The electrical current passes through an electrode that is held away from the skin and transmits a spark to the skin surface that causes the intracellular contents to evaporate. [*see also*: electrodesiccation, electrosection, electrosurgery]
fundal height	The distance in centimeters from the top of the symphysis pubis to the top of the uterine fundus. It is a general indication of fetal growth. **F**
fundus	Round, dome-like part of an organ that is opposite its opening. **F**

G

gadolinium	Contrast medium used in MRI scans. It is a metallic element that responds to a magnetic field. [*see also*: magnetic resonance imaging]
galactorrhea [676.xx]	Hypersecretion of prolactin, sometimes from an adenoma of the anterior pituitary gland. The patient has secretion of milk from the breasts, even though the patient is not pregnant. The high levels of prolactin also cause cessation of the menstrual cycle by inhibiting secretion of FSH and LH. [*see also*: prolactin] **S**
gallbladder	Small, dark green sac posterior to the liver that stores and concentrates bile. When stimulated by cholecystokinin from the duodenum, it contracts and releases bile into the common bile duct that empties into the duodenum. [*see also*: bile, bile ducts, celiac trunk, cholangiography, cholecystectomy, hydroxyimino-diacetic acid scan] **F** **S**
gallium-67	Given intravenously for nuclear medicine imaging of many different areas of the body to detect inflammation, infection, and benign or cancerous tumors. Gallium is a soft, silvery metal that is liquid at room temperature.
gamete	A cell (ovum or spermatozoon) that has 23 chromosomes instead of the usual 46 chromosomes like other cells of the body. [*see also*: ovum, spermatozoon, zygote]
gamma ray	Form of subatomic radiation emitted from a radioactive substance. [*see also*: radioactive substance] **S**

ganglion [727.xx]   Semisolid or fluid-containing cyst that develops on a tendon, often on the wrist, hand, or foot. A ganglion is clearly visible as a rounded lump under the skin that may or may not be painful.   **S**

    Dx   H&P.

    Tx   Sometimes it goes away without intervention. Aspiration to remove the fluid, or surgery to resect the entire ganglion. Medications to treat the pain, swelling, and underlying symptoms, if necessary. [see also: ganglionectomy]

ganglionectomy   Surgical procedure to remove a ganglion from a tendon.

gangrene [785.xx]   Necrosis of the tissue with subsequent bacterial invasion and decay. [see also: amputation, necrosis]   **L**
S

gastrectomy   Surgical procedure to remove part of the stomach, usually because of a cancerous tumor.

gastric analysis   Diagnostic test to determine the amount of hydrochloric acid in the stomach. An NG tube is inserted, and a sample of gastric juices is collected. Then a drug is given to stimulate acid production, and another sample is collected.

gastric bypass   Surgical procedure to treat severely obese patients. Staples are placed in the stomach to make a small stomach pouch. The pouch is then anastomosed to the jejunum. This bypasses the duodenum, where most fats are absorbed. [see also: gastroplasty]   **S**

gastrins   Hormones produced by the stomach that stimulate the release of hydrochloric acid and pepsinogen in the stomach. [see also: hydrochloric acid, pepsinogen]

gastritis [535.xx]   Acute or chronic inflammation of the stomach due to eating spicy foods, excess acid production, or a bacterial infection.

gastroenteritis [009.xx; 558.xx]   Acute inflammation or infection of the stomach and intestines.   **S**

gastroesophageal reflux disease [530.xx]   Chronic inflammation and irritation of the esophagus due to the backward flow of stomach acid into the esophagus. [see also: barium swallow, cardiac sphincter]   **A**
S

gastrointestinal system   Body system that includes the oral cavity, pharynx, esophagus, stomach, small and large intestines, and the accessory organs of the liver, gallbladder, and pancreas. Its function is to digest food and remove undigested wastes from the body.   **A**
S

gastroplasty   Surgical procedure to treat severely obese patients. Staples are placed in the stomach to make a small stomach pouch. A gastroplasty can be combined with a gastric bypass. [see also: gastric bypass]   **S**

gastrostomy   Surgical procedure to create a permanent opening from the abdominal wall into the stomach to insert a gastrostomy tube, a permanent feeding tube. [see also: jejunostomy, percutaneous endoscopic gastrostomy]

gaze testing   Medical procedure to test the extraocular muscles. The patient follows the physician's finger from side to side and up and down. Conjugate gaze is when both eyes move together as a unit. Dysconjugate gaze is when the eyes do not move together. [see also: convergence]

gene   An area on a chromosome that contains all the DNA information needed to produce one type of protein molecule.   **S**

genetic mutation   Damage to the DNA molecule that deletes genes, reverses the normal order of genes, or breaks off gene segments from one   **S**

chromosome and inserts them in another chromosome. [*see also*: translocation]

genital herpes
[054.xx]

A sexually transmitted skin infection caused by the herpes virus. **S**
Vesicles form in the genital area and rupture, releasing clear fluid
that forms crusts. These lesions tend to recur during illness and
stress. [*see also*: herpes]

Sx Vesicular lesions on the anus, penis, perineum, scrotum,
vagina, or vulva. When the blisters break, they become skin
ulcers. There may be flu-like symptoms or no symptoms
at all.

Dx Culture grown from swab of lesion, polymerase chain
reaction test. [*see also*: Tzanck test]

Tx No known cure. Topical and oral antiviral drugs shorten
the duration of each outbreak and the number of outbreaks.

genital organs Male and female internal and external genitalia.

genital warts
[178.xx]

A sexually transmitted disease caused by the human papilloma- **S**
virus (HPV). Certain strains cause genital warts; other strains
cause dysplasia of the cervix, which can lead to cervical cancer.
[*see also*: cervical dysplasia, sexually transmitted disease]

Sx Itching, flesh-colored, irregular lesions that are raised and
cauliflower-like. Women may also have a vaginal discharge.

Dx Visual examination. In women, a Pap smear can assist in
diagnosis. [*see also*: Papanicolaou smear]

Tx Topical chemicals. Sometimes cryosurgery, cautery, or lasers
are used to remove the warts. [*see also*: cryosurgery, laser
surgery, electrodesiccation]

genitalia External and internal organs and structures of the male and female
genital and reproductive systems.

genu valgum
[736.xx]

Congenital deformity in which, beginning at the knees, the lower **S**
legs are bent outward. Also known as knock-knee. [*see also*:
genu varum]

genu varum
[736.xx]

Congenital deformity in which, beginning at the knees, the lower **S**
legs are bent toward the midline. Also known as bowleg.
[*see also*: genu valgum]

gestation Period of time from the moment of fertilization of the ovum
until birth.

**gestational
diabetes mellitus**
[648.xx]

Temporary disorder of glucose metabolism that occurs only during **A**
pregnancy. Increased levels of estradiol and progesterone block
the action of insulin, which metabolizes glucose. Low levels of
insulin lead to high levels of unmetabolized glucose in the mother's
blood. These high levels of glucose cross the placenta and cause
the fetus to grow too rapidly. [*see also*: diabetes mellitus, estradiol,
growth abnormalities, polyhydramnios, progesterone]

gigantism [253.xx] Hypersecretion of growth hormone during childhood and puberty. **S**
Causes all the bones and tissues to grow continuously. [*see also*:
acromegaly, dwarfism, hyperpituitarism]

**Glasgow
Coma Scale**

Numerical scale that measures the depth of a coma. The scores **A**
range from 3 to 15 and are the sum of individual scores for eye
opening, motor response, and verbal response following a painful
stimulus.

glaucoma [365.xx] Increased intraocular pressure because aqueous humor cannot
circulate freely. Can progress to blindness. [*see also*: anisocoria,

aqueous humor, closed-angle glaucoma, gonioscopy, hyphema, open-angle glaucoma, scotoma, tonometry]

glenoid fossa
Shallow depression in the scapula where the head of the humerus articulates to form the shoulder joint.   S

global amnesia
[300.xx; 437.xx; 780.xx]
Total loss of long-term memory due to trauma or disease of the hippocampus. All memories are lost. [*see also:* anterograde amnesia, retrograde amnesia]

global aphasia
[438.xx; 784.xx]
Patients with both expressive and receptive aphasia. Loss of the ability to express thoughts verbally or understand the spoken or written word. Caused by injury to the area of the brain that deals with language and the interpretation of sounds and symbols. [*see also:* aphasia]   S

globins
Chains of protein molecules in hemoglobin. [*see also:* antibodies, hemoglobin]

glomerulonephritis
[580.xx; 582.xx]
Complication that develops following an acute infection. The immune system produces antibodies that combine with the infectious agent forming antigen–antibody complexes that clog the pores of the glomeruli. [*see also:* albuminuria, chronic renal failure]   L

glomerulus
Network of intertwining capillaries within Bowman's capsule in the nephron. [*see also:* Bowman's capsule, filtration, nephron, nephrotic syndrome]

glossitis [529.xx]
Inflammation of the tongue. Caused by irritation from food, an infection, or vitamin B deficiency. [*see also:* gustatory cortex]

glossopharyngeal nerve
Cranial nerve IX. Sensation in the mouth. Movement of the throat muscles for swallowing. Controls the salivary glands.   S

glottis
V-shaped structure of mucous membranes and vocal cords within the larynx.

glucagon
Hormone secreted by alpha cells in the islets of Langerhans in the pancreas. It breaks down glycogen to form glucose. [*see also:* glucose, glycogen, pancreas, somatostatin]

glucocorticoids
Group of hormones secreted by the adrenal cortex. [*see also:* cortisol]   S

glucose
A simple sugar found in foods and in the blood. It is produced when the hormone glucagon breaks down glycogen.   S

glucose tolerance test
Blood and urine tests that measure the level of glucose. Used to evaluate the function of the pancreas. After the patient has fasted for 12 hours, blood and urine specimens are obtained. Then the patient either drinks glucose or it is given intravenously. Blood and urine specimens are obtained every hour for four hours after the glucose administration. Normally, the blood glucose returns to normal within one to two hours. High blood and urine levels of glucose indicate diabetes mellitus. [*see also:* diabetes mellitus]   A S

gluten enteropathy
[579.xx]
A food allergy to the gluten in wheat, in which the tissues of the small intestine are damaged by the allergic response. [*see also:* allergic reaction]   S

glycogen
The form that glucose (sugar) takes when it is stored in the liver and skeletal muscles. [*see also:* Cushing's disease/syndrome, endoplasmic reticulum, glucose]

glycosuria [271.xx; 790.xx–791.xx]
Glucose in the urine, an indication of elevated blood sugar levels seen in diabetes mellitus. [*see also:* diabetes mellitus]   L S

glycosylated hemoglobin
Blood test that measures the A_{1C} fraction of hemoglobin in red blood cells. Hemoglobin A_{1C} binds with glucose. Because   S

A = Abbreviations Section   F = Figures Section   L = Laboratory Section   S = Synonyms Section
Sx (Symptoms)   Dx (Diagnosis)   Tx (Treatment)

red blood cells only live about 12 weeks, the hemoglobin A_{1C} result indicates the average level of blood glucose during the previous 12 weeks. Used to monitor how well diabetic patients are controlling their blood sugar levels with diet and drugs. [*see also*: brittle diabetic, diabetes mellitus]

Golgi apparatus   Organelle that consists of curved, stacked membranes that process and store intracellular hormones and enzymes. Also makes lysosomes and the digestive enzymes they contain.   S

goiter [240.xx–242.xx; 246.xx]   Chronic and progressive enlargement of the thyroid gland. Mild-to-moderate thyroid gland enlargement is known as thyromegaly. The physician can feel enlargement on physical examination even before it becomes visible. Causes of goiter and thyromegaly include a lack of iodine in the soil and the diet, an adenoma or nodule growing in the thyroid gland, or an autoimmune disease such as Hashimoto's thyroiditis or Graves' disease. [*see also*: autoimmune diseases, Graves' disease, Hashimoto's thyroiditis, thyroiditis]   S

gonadotropins   Category of hormones that stimulate the male and female gonads. Includes FSH and LH. [*see also*: follicle-stimulating hormone, luteinizing hormone]

gonads   The sex glands. In females, the ovaries; in males, the testes.

goniometry   Medical procedure in which a protractor-like device (goniometer) is used to measure the angle and degrees of a joint's range of movement (ROM).   S

gonioscopy   Diagnostic procedure for glaucoma. It uses a slit lamp with a special lens that illuminates the trabecular meshwork. [*see also*: glaucoma, slit lamp examination]

gonorrhea [098.xx; 647.xx]   A sexually transmitted disease caused by *Neisseria gonorrhoeae*, a gram-negative diplococcus bacterium. *Neisseria gonorrhoeae* is also known as gonococcus (GC).   S

    Sx   ♂: Painful urination. Thick yellow urethral discharge (gonococcal urethritis). Some men have no symptoms.

        ♀: Half of infected women have no symptoms. Painful urination. Thick yellow vaginal discharge.

    Dx   Gram-stained smear of discharge shows characteristic intracellular diplococci under the microscope. Culture grown from a swab of discharge.

    Tx   Oral antibiotic drugs.

gout [274.xx]   Metabolic disorder where excessive levels of uric acid in the blood can cause sudden, severe pain as uric acid moves from the blood into the soft tissues and forms masses of crystals. [*see also*: uric acid]   L S

    Dx   H&P. Serum uric acid levels are drawn, and sometimes joint fluid will be aspirated and tested for the presence of uric acid. [*see also*: arthocentesis, metabolic panel, metabolism]

    Tx   Preventive education to decrease the number of attacks. If medication is needed, it is based on three different approaches: anti-inflammatory drugs, pain relief, and addressing underlying metabolic problems causing the gout.

grading   Medical procedure that classifies cancer by how well differentiated the cells appear under the microscope. Normal cells appear well differentiated and characteristic of that tissue type. Poorly differentiated or undifferentiated cells lack evidence of specialization and appear immature and embryonic. The greater the number of undifferentiated cells, the poorer the prognosis.

graft-versus-host disease
Immune reaction originating from the donor tissue or organ (graft) against the patient (host). This may cause a rash and fever, or it can be severe enough to cause death. [*see also*: allograft, xenograft]   **A**

granulocyte
Category of leukocytes with large granules in the cytoplasm. Includes neutrophils, eosinophils, and basophils.

Graves' disease [242.xx]
The most common form of hyperthyroidism. This is an auto-immune disease in which the body produces antibodies that stimulate TSH receptors on the thyroid gland, increasing the production of thyroid hormones. [*see also*: autoimmune disease, exophthalmos, hyperthyroidism]   **L S**

Dx H&P. Lab test to evaluate thyroid hormone levels and thyroid function. A thyroid scan is performed to visualize the thyroid. [*see also*: radioactive iodine uptake and thyroid scan, thyroid function tests]

Tx Medications to treat the underlying symptoms. Antithyroid drugs may also be prescribed to block the thyroid hormones. Radioactive iodine may be administered to destroy the hyperactive cells. Surgery for removal of thyroid tissue may be considered.

gray matter
Areas of gray tissue in the brain and spinal cord that are composed of cell bodies and dendrites.   **F**

great vessels
Collective phrase for the aorta (the largest artery), the superior and inferior venae cavae (the largest veins), and the pulmonary arteries and veins.

greenstick fracture [829.xx]
Bone is broken only on one side. Occurs most often in children. [*see also*: fracture]

group therapy
Provides simultaneous therapy to several patients who have a similar mental illness such as anxiety, depression, or being a victim of sexual abuse. Group members share experiences and insights and provide feedback and emotional support to each other.

growth abnormalities
Many factors affect the growth rate of the embryo and fetus. Maternal illness, malnutrition, and smoking can make the fetus small. Diabetes mellitus in the mother can make the fetus large. [*see also*: intrauterine growth retardation, gestational diabetes]   **A S**

growth hormone
Blood test that measures the level of growth hormone (GH). Used to evaluate the function of the anterior pituitary gland. Growth hormone stimulates all of the body tissues to grow. [*see also*: acromegaly, anterior pituitary gland, dwarfism, gigantism, somatostatin]

Guillain-Barré syndrome [357.xx]
Caused by a triggering event of an infection, stress, or trauma, the body makes antibodies against myelin. There is acute inflammation of the peripheral nerves, with interruption of nerve conduction. Once the swelling subsides, the syndrome does not recur, and the patient recovers some or all neurological function. [*see also*: antibodies, myelin]   **L S**

Dx H&P. The symptoms and their progression help to direct the diagnosis. A lumbar puncture will show high levels of protein, but few or no inflammatory cells. An EMG will be slowed and, when combined with other factors, will help with the diagnosis. [*see also*: cerebrospinal fluid examination, electromyelography, nerve conduction study]

A = Abbreviations Section   **F** = Figures Section   **L** = Laboratory Section   **S** = Synonyms Section
Sx (Symptoms)   **Dx** (Diagnosis)   **Tx** (Treatment)

Tx	Depends on the type and progression of symptoms. In some, this may be a medical emergency and require resuscitative measures and mechanical ventilation. Plasmapheresis is often performed to remove the toxic substances from the blood. Medications will also be given to treat the underlying symptoms. [*see also*: endotracheal intubation, plasmapheresis]
gustatory cortex	Area in the frontal lobe of the cerebrum that receives and analyzes sensory nerve impulses from the tongue and taste receptors.
gynecologic examination	Medical procedure to physically examine the female external and internal genitalia. Performed with the patient supine in the dorsal lithotomy position.
gynecomastia [611.xx]	Enlargement of the male breasts. In the male, some androgens secreted by the adrenal cortex are converted to estradiol (a female hormone). Most of the androgen male hormone testosterone is secreted by the testes . Any increase in the secretion of androgens from the adrenal cortex or decrease in the secretion of testosterone from the testes upsets the balance of androgens/testosterone. When the relative amount of estradiol is increased, it causes the male breasts to enlarge. Caused by puberty, aging, surgical removal of the testes, or estrogen drug treatment for prostate cancer. **S**
gyrus	One of many large, elevated folds of brain tissue on the surface of the cerebrum with smaller folds on the cerebellum. In between each gyrus is a sulcus (groove). Plural: gyri. [*see also*: sulcus]

H

hairline fracture	Very thin break line with the bone pieces still together. [*see also*: fracture]
half-life	Length of time it takes for half of the atoms in an amount of a radioactive substance to emit gamma rays or positrons (to decay) and become stable.
Hashimoto's thyroiditis [245.xx]	An autoimmune disorder in which the body forms antibodies against its own thyroid gland. The thyroid becomes inflamed and enlarged. Over time, the patient develops hypothyroidism as thyroid tissue is destroyed and replaced by fibrous tissue. [*see also*: antithyroglobulin antibodies, autoimmune disease, hypothyroidism]
haustra	Pouches in the wall of the large intestine that expand or contract to accommodate varying amounts of food.
hay fever [477.xx]	Occurring in the spring or fall and coinciding with the blooming of certain trees and plants. In response to an inhaled antigen, the immune response releases histamine, producing nasal stuffiness, sneezing, rhinorrhea, hypertrophy of the turbinates with red, edematous, and boggy mucous membranes, and postnasal drip. **L** **S**
health	Optimum state of physical, mental, spiritual, and social well-being.
heart	Organ that pumps blood through the body. [*see also*: autonomic nervous system, cardiac tamponade, cardiomegaly, cardiomyopathy, cardiopulmonary bypass, cardiopulmonary resuscitation, cardiovascular system, conduction system, congestive heart failure, coronary artery disease, diastole, ductus arteriosus, echocardiography, endocardium, epicardium, foramen ovale, myocardial infarction, myocardium, pericardium, systole, valve] **F**

A = Abbreviations Section   **F** = Figures Section   **L** = Laboratory Section   **S** = Synonyms Section
Sx (Symptoms)   **Dx** (Diagnosis)   **Tx** (Treatment)

heart block [426.xx]	Arrhythmia in which electrical impulses cannot travel normally from the SA node to the Purkinje fibers. [see also: conduction system, first-degree heart block, second-degree heart block, third-degree heart block, and right and left bundle branch block]
heartburn [787.xx]	Temporary inflammation of the esophagus due to reflux of stomach acid. [see also: Campylobacter-like organism test, cardiac sphincter] S
Heimlich maneuver	Medical procedure to assist a choking victim with an airway obstruction. The rescuer stands behind the victim and places a fist on the victim's abdominal wall just below the diaphragm, grasps the fist with the other hand and, with both hands, gives a sudden push inward and upward. This generates a burst of air that pushes the obstruction into the mouth, where it can be expelled.
helix	Rim of tissue and cartilage that forms the C shape of the external ear.
hemangioma [228.xx]	Congenital growth composed of a mass of superficial and dilated blood vessels on the skin. S
hemarthrosis [719.xx]	Blood in the joint cavity from blunt trauma or a penetrating wound. It also occurs spontaneously in hemophiliac patients. [see also: arthrocentesis, arthroscopy]
hematemesis [578.xx]	Vomiting of new or old blood from bleeding in the stomach or esophagus. [see also: emesis, melena]
hematochezia [569.xx]	Blood in the stool. [see also: defecation] S
hematoma	An elevated, localized collection of blood under the skin. [see also: hemorrhage]
hematopoiesis	Process by which blood cells are formed in the red bone marrow. S
hematuria [599.xx; 791.xx]	Blood in the urine. Can be caused by a kidney stone, cystitis, or bladder cancer. In addition, menstrual blood can contaminate a urine specimen. [see also: interstitial cystitis, urination]
heme	Molecule in hemoglobin that contains iron and gives erythrocytes their red color. S
hemianopia [368.xx]	Loss of one half of the visual field (right or left, top or bottom). [see also: peripheral vision, scotoma] S
hemiparesis [438.xx]	Muscle weakness on one side of the body. [see also: cerebrovascular accident]
hemiplegia [438.xx]	Paralysis on one side of the body. [see also: cerebrovascular accident]
hemisphere	One half of the cerebrum. The right hemisphere recognizes patterns and three-dimensional structures (including faces) and the emotions of words. The left hemisphere deals with mathematical and logical reasoning, analysis, and interpreting sights, sounds, and sensations. The left hemisphere is active in reading, writing, and speaking. [see also: cerebrum]
hemodialysis	Medical procedure to remove waste products from the blood of patients in renal failure through the use of a fistula or a shunt in the patient's arm. A fistula is created by surgically joining an artery and vein. Over a few weeks, the vein enlarges enough to accommodate two needles, one that removes blood and sends it to the dialysis machine and another that receives purified blood from the dialysis machine and returns it to the body. [see also: continuous ambulatory peritoneal dialysis, continuous cycling peritoneal dialysis, dialysis, peritoneal dialysis]

A = Abbreviations Section   F = Figures Section   L = Laboratory Section   S = Synonyms Section
Sx (Symptoms)   Dx (Diagnosis)   Tx (Treatment)

hemoglobin	Substance in an erythrocyte that binds to oxygen and carbon dioxide. Made of a heme molecule and globin chains.	A L
hemophilia [286.xx]	Inherited genetic abnormality of a gene, causing a lack or a deficiency of a specific clotting factor. When injured, hemophiliac patients continue to bleed for long periods of time. [*see also*: blood dyscrasia, clotting factors]	L S

> **Dx** H&P. Lab tests to determine clotting factor abnormalities.
>
> **Tx** Lifestyle changes to reduce the risk of bleeding. Transfusions to replace the missing clotting factors.

hemoptysis [786.xx]	The coughing up of blood-tinged sputum. [*see also*: expectoration]	
hemorrhage	Loss of a large amount of blood, externally or internally. Usually caused by trauma to the large arteries in the skin or internal organs or disease that erodes into a large artery. [*see also*: contusion, ecchymosis, hematoma, petechia]	L
hemorrhoid-ectomy	Surgical procedure to remove hemorrhoids from the rectum or around the anus.	
hemorrhoids [455.xx]	Swollen, protruding veins in the rectum (internal hemorrhoids) or on the perianal skin (external hemorrhoids). [*see also*: hemorrhoidectomy]	S
hemostasis	The cessation of bleeding after the formation of a blood clot.	
hemothorax [860.xx]	Presence of blood in the thoracic cavity, usually from trauma. [*see also*: chest tube insertion]	
hemotympanum [385.xx]	Blood in the middle ear space behind the tympanic membrane. It can be caused by infection or trauma (head trauma, a slap to the ear, or a nearby explosion). [*see also*: myringotomy, tympanic membrane]	
hepatitis [070.xx]	Inflammation and infection of the liver caused by the hepatitis virus. [*see also*: alpha fetoprotein, disseminated intravascular coagulation, hepatomegaly]	L S
hepatomegaly [789.xx]	Enlargement of the liver due to liver damage from cirrhosis, hepatitis, or cancer. [*see also*: alpha fetoprotein, hepatitis]	S
Her2/neu	Cytology test that detects a gene that affects the prognosis and treatment options for cancer of the bladder, breast, and ovary. A tumor that is Her2/neu positive is an aggressive tumor that is resistant to hormone therapy and some chemotherapy drugs.	
hereditary disease	Caused by an inherited or spontaneous mutation in the genetic material of a cell. Examples: Down syndrome, sickle cell disease.	
heredity	Genetic inheritance passed on from the DNA of the father and mother to the child. Genetic mutations that cause cancer can be inherited.	
hernia [550.xx–553.xx]	Protrusion of an organ from its cavity or space. Hernias are named according to their location. [*see also*: hiatal hernia, incisional hernia, inguinal hernia, omphalocele, rectocele, umbilical hernia, ventral hernia, vesicocele]	
herniorrhaphy	Surgical procedure that uses sutures to close a defect in a muscle wall where there is a hernia. [*see also*: hernia]	
herpes [054.xx]	Skin infection caused by the herpes virus causing vesicles that rupture, releasing clear fluid that forms crusts. [*see also*: cold sores, genital herpes, herpes whitlow, shingles, Tzanck test]	S
herpes whitlow [054.xx]	A herpes simplex infection at the base of the fingernail caused by contact with herpes simplex type 1 of the mouth or type 2 of the	

genitals. The virus enters through a small tear in the cuticle. [*see also*: herpes, onychomycosis, paronychia]

hesitancy [788.xx]	Inability to initiate a normal stream of urine. There is dribbling, and the urinary stream has a decreased caliber. The volume of urine passed is less, and urine may remain in the bladder. Can be caused by blockage of the urethra by a kidney stone, a urinary tract infection, or an enlarged prostate gland. [*see also*: nephrolithiasis, prostatitis, urination]
heterophil antibody test	Rapid test for mononucleosis that uses the patient's serum mixed with horse erythrocytes. If the patient has infectious mononucleosis, heterophil antibodies in the patient's serum will cause the horse's erythrocytes to clump. **S**
hiatal hernia [553.xx]	Weakness in the diaphragm, the muscular wall between the thoracic and abdominopelvic cavities. This allows the esophagus or stomach to slide through and balloon into the thoracic cavity. [*see also*: barium swallow] **S**
hilum	Area of an organ where blood vessels and nerves enter. **S**
hippocampus	Irregular, curved area within each temporal lobe that controls long-term memory and compares past and present emotions and experiences. [*see also*: amnesia]
hirsutism [704.xx]	The presence of excessive, dark hair on the forearms and over the upper lip of a woman. [*see also*: adrenogenital syndrome] **S**
histamine	Released by basophils. It dilates blood vessels and increases blood flow to damaged tissue. It also allows protein molecules to leak out of blood vessels into the tissue, which produces redness and swelling. [*see also*: allergic reaction, basophil, immunoglobulin E, pruritus]
Hodgkin's lymphoma [201.xx]	Occurs most often in young adults and is discovered on physical examination as a painless, enlarged cervical lymph node in the neck. [*see also*: non-Hodgkin's lymphoma, splenomegaly] **S**
	Dx H&P. The definitive diagnosis comes with a biopsy of lymph tissue showing the presence of Reed-Sternberg cells. The number of these cells increases as the disease progresses.
	Tx An individual plan is established by the patient's oncologist. Radiation and chemotherapy are used, sometimes alone or in combination with each other.
Holmes Social Readjustment Rating Scale	Assigns point values to various stressors (negative and positive life events) to measure the total amount of stress in a patient's life.
Holter monitor	Diagnostic procedure during which the patient's heart rate and rhythm are continuously monitored for 24 hours or longer. The patient wears electrodes attached to a small, portable ECG monitor (carried in a vest or placed in a pocket). The patient also keeps a diary of activities, meals, and symptoms. This procedure is used to document infrequently occurring arrhythmias and to link them to activities or symptoms such as chest pain. [*see also*: conduction system, dysrhythmia]
homeostasis	State of equilibrium of the internal environment of the body, including fluid balance, acid–base balance, temperature, metabolism, and so forth, to keep all the body systems functioning optimally.
hormone	Chemical messenger of the endocrine system that is secreted by a gland or organ and travels through the blood. [*see also*: adrenocorticotropic hormone, aldosterone, antidiuretic hormone,

calcitonin, cholecystokinin, cortisol, erythropoietin, estradiol, follicle-stimulating hormone, gastrin, glucagon, growth hormone, human chorionic gonadotropin, insulin, luteinizing hormone, melanocyte-stimulating hormone, melatonin, norepinephrine, oxytocin, progesterone, prolactin, somatostatin, testosterone, thyroid-stimulating hormone, thyroxine, triiodothyronine]

hormone testing

Blood test to determine the levels of FSH and LH from the anterior pituitary gland, estradiol and progesterone from the ovaries (in females), and testosterone from the testes (in males). Used to diagnose infertility problems. [see also: antisperm antibody test]

human chorionic gonadotropin

A hormone secreted by the chorion of the fertilized ovum. It stimulates the corpus luteum of the ovary to keep producing estradiol and progesterone, and this causes menstruation to cease for the duration of the pregnancy. [see also: corpus luteum]   A S

Blood Test: Detects this hormone, which is normally present during pregnancy but not at other times. Elevated levels of HCG can be seen in patients with cancer of the testes, choriocarcinoma, cirrhosis, duodenal ulcer, and inflammatory bowel disease. [see also: pregnancy test]

human immunodeficiency virus [042.xx]

The human immunodeficiency virus can be contracted through high-risk behavior, such as unprotected sexual intercourse, sharing needles, or contact with contaminated bodily fluids. With the advances in medications and early detection tests, HIV is becoming more manageable and is not the death sentence it once was. [see also: acquired immunodeficiency syndrome, enzyme-linked immunosorbent assay, OraSure, p24 antigen test, viral load test, Western blot]   A L

Huntington's chorea [333.xx]

Progressive inherited degenerative disease of the brain that begins in middle age. It is characterized by dementia with irregular spasms of the extremities and face (chorea), alternating with slow, writhing movements of the hands and feet (athetosis). [see also: bradykinesia, dementia, dyskinesia]   S

hyaline membrane disease [769.xx]

Difficulty inflating the lungs to breathe because of a lack of surfactant. This occurs in premature newborns. [see also: lecithin/sphingomyelin ratio, surfactant]   A S

hydatidiform mole disease [630.xx]

Abnormal union of an ovum and spermatozoon that produces hundreds of small, fluid-filled sacs but no embryo. The chorion produces HCG, so the patient has early signs of pregnancy. The hydatidiform mole grows more rapidly than a normal pregnancy, and the uterus is much larger than expected for the gestational age.   S

hydrocephalus [331.xx; 741.xx–742.xx]

Condition in which an excessive amount of cerebrospinal fluid is produced, or the flow of cerebrospinal fluid is blocked. The intracranial pressure builds up, distends the ventricles in the brain, and compresses the brain tissue. [see also: ependymal cells, ventriculoperitoneal shunt]   S

hydrochloric acid

Strong acid produced by the stomach. It breaks down food, kills microorganisms on food, and converts pepsinogen to pepsin. [see also: gastric analysis, gastrin, pepsinogen]

hydronephrosis [591.xx]

Enlargement of the kidney due to constant pressure from backed-up urine in the ureter, because of an obstructing stone or stricture. [see also: benign prostatic hypertrophy, nephrolithiasis]   S

hydrosalpinx [614.xx]

Inflammation of the fallopian tube, where the inflammation fills the tube with tissue fluid. [see also: fallopian tube]

A = Abbreviations Section   F = Figures Section   L = Laboratory Section   S = Synonyms Section
Sx (Symptoms)   Dx (Diagnosis)   Tx (Treatment)

hydroxyimino-diacetic acid scan	Nuclear medicine procedure that uses scintigraphy and the radiopharmaceutical technetium-99m as a tracer to create an image of the gallbladder. The technetium is attached to a carrier molecule (HIDA or hydroxyiminodiacetic acid). [see also: gallbladder]	A S
hymen	Elastic membrane that partially or completely covers the inferior end of the vaginal canal. [see also: dyspareunia]	S
hyperaldos-teronism [255.xx]	Hypersecretion of aldosterone. Caused by an adenoma in the adrenal cortex. It can also be caused by hypersecretion of adrenocorticotropic hormone from an adenoma in the anterior pituitary gland. [see also: aldosterone]	L S
hypercapnia [786.xx]	Abnormally high level of carbon dioxide (CO_2) in the arterial blood. [see also: arterial blood gases, cyanosis, deoxygenated]	
hypercholes-terolemia [272.xx]	An elevated level of cholesterol in the blood. [see also: arteriosclerosis, hyperlipidemia, lipid profile, metabolic panel, myocardial infarction]	S
hyperemesis gravidarum [643.xx]	Nausea and excessive vomiting during the first trimester of pregnancy that causes weakness, dehydration, and fluid and electrolyte imbalance. Thought to be due to elevated estradiol and progesterone levels. [see also: emesis, estradiol, morning sickness, progesterone]	S
hyperesthesia [782.xx]	Condition in which there is an abnormally heightened awareness and sensitivity to touch and increased response to painful stimuli. [see also: complex regional pain syndrome]	S
hyperinsulinism [251.xx]	Hypersecretion of insulin. Caused by a tumor in the pancreas or by insulin resistance syndrome (IRS), in which receptors on body cells show resistance and do not allow insulin to bring glucose into the cell to be metabolized. The pancreas secretes large amounts of insulin to overcome the resistance. When the pancreas can no longer secrete large amounts of insulin, the patient develops type 2 diabetes mellitus. [see also: diabetes mellitus type 2]	
hyperkinesis	An abnormally increased amount of muscle movements. Can be a side effect of some drugs. [see also: ataxia, bradykinesia]	S
hyperlipidemia [272.xx]	Elevated levels of lipids (fats) in the blood. Lipids include cholesterol and triglycerides. [see also: hypertriglyceridemia, lipid profile, xanthelasma, xanthoma]	L S
hyperopia [367.xx]	Light rays from a far object focus correctly on the retina, creating a sharp image. However, light rays from a near object come into focus posterior to the retina, creating a blurred image. Also known as farsightedness. [see also: myopia]	S
hyperpara-thyroidism [252.xx]	Hypersecretion of parathyroid hormone caused by an adenoma in the parathyroid glands. The calcium level in the blood becomes very high as the bones lose calcium and become demineralized and prone to fracture. Excess calcium in the blood is excreted in the urine and can form kidney stones. [see also: calcium, nephrolithiasis, parathyroidectomy]	L
hyperpituitarism [253.xx]	Hypersecretion of one or all of the hormones from the anterior pituitary gland. Caused by a benign tumor in the pituitary gland. [see also: anterior pituitary gland, gigantism]	
hypersensitivity	Individually unique response to an allergen that provokes an allergic response in some people. [see also: allergic reaction]	
hypertension [401.xx–406.xx]	Elevated blood pressure. Normal blood pressure readings in an adult are less than 120/80 mm Hg. [see also: arteriosclerosis,	A

A = Abbreviations Section   F = Figures Section   L = Laboratory Section   S = Synonyms Section
Sx (Symptoms)   Dx (Diagnosis)   Tx (Treatment)

chronic renal failure, congestive heart failure, dissecting aneurysm, essential hypertension, pheochromocytoma, portal hypertension, preeclampsia, secondary hypertension]

hyperthyroidism
[242.xx]

Hypersecretion of T_3 and T_4 thyroid hormones. Caused by an adenoma or a nodule in the thyroid gland or by hypersecretion of TSH from an adenoma in the anterior pituitary gland. There is thyroid enlargement that can be felt on palpation of the neck. [see also: Graves' disease, thyroid storm]

L
S

hypertri-glyceridemia
[272.xx]

An elevated level of triglycerides in the blood. [see also: hyperlipidemia, lipid profile]

hyphema
[364.xx]

Blood in the anterior chamber of the eye. Caused by trauma or increased intraocular pressure. [see also: anterior chamber, glaucoma]

hypnosis

Places the patient in a sleep-like trance. The therapist makes suggestions that are incorporated in the patient's subconscious mind and later acted upon consciously to some degree. Used to treat anxiety and phobias and to help patients stop smoking or lose weight. [see also: phobia, psychoanalysis]

hypoaldosteronism
[255.xx]

Hyposecretion of aldosterone. Rare condition caused by an inherited genetic abnormality of the adrenal cortex. [see also: chronic renal failure, heart block]

hypochondriac region

Two of nine regions on the surface of the anterior abdominal area. The right and left hypochondriac regions are inferior to the lower edges of the anterior right and left ribs. [see also: epigastric region, hypogastric region, inguinal region, lumbar region, quadrant, umbilical region]

hypochondriasis
[300.xx]

Preoccupation with and misinterpretation of minor bodily sensations with the fear that these indicate disease. Patients are convinced they have a serious illness and make frequent trips to the doctor despite medical evidence and reassurance to the contrary.

hypogastric region

One of nine regions on the surface of the anterior abdominal area. It is centered and inferior to the umbilical region. [see also: epigastric region, hypochondriac region, inguinal region, lumbar region, quadrant, umbilical region]

hypoglossal nerve

Cranial nerve XII. Movement of the tongue.

S

hypoglycemia
[251.xx]

Low levels of glucose in the blood. Caused by diabetics who take an antidiabetic pill or inject insulin but then miss a meal, or it can occur in nondiabetic patients who are dieting or fasting. The patient experiences a headache, dizziness, sweating, shakiness, and tunnel vision. If left untreated, hypoglycemia can progress to insulin shock and then coma as the blood glucose level becomes too low to support brain activity. [see also: diabetes mellitus]

hypokalemia
[276.xx]

Decreased amounts of potassium in the blood. Can be caused by diuretic drugs that cause the kidney to excrete excessive amounts of urine (and potassium). [see also: dysrhythmia, myalgia]

S

hypopara-thyroidism
[252.xx]

Hyposecretion of parathyroid hormone. Sometimes caused by the accidental removal of the parathyroid glands during a thyroid-ectomy. The calcium level in the blood becomes very low, causing irritability of the nerves and skeletal muscle cramps or sustained muscle spasm (tetany). [see also: calcium, parathyroid glands]

L

hypopharynx	Most posterior portion of the throat, from the base of the tongue to the entrances of the esophagus and trachea.	F
hypopituitarism [253.xx]	Hyposecretion of one or all of the hormones of the anterior pituitary gland. Caused by an injury or a defect in the pituitary gland itself. [*see also:* anterior pituitary gland, panhypopituitarism]	L
hypospadias [752.xx]	The male urethral meatus is incorrectly located on the underside of the shaft of the penis rather than at the tip of the glans penis. [*see also:* chordee, epispadias, urethroplasty]	S
hypotension [458.xx]	Blood pressure lower than 90/60 mm Hg, usually because of a loss of blood volume. [*see also:* anaphylactic shock, orthostatic hypotension]	L
hypothalamus	Area in the center of the brain just below the thalamus that coordinates the activities of the pons and medulla oblongata. It controls heart rate, blood pressure, respiratory rate, body temperature, sensations of hunger and thirst, emotions, bodily responses to emotions, and the circadian rhythm. It also produces hormones, regulates the sex drive, and contains the feeding and satiety centers. Functions as part of the "fight or flight" response of the sympathetic nervous system.	
hypothyroidism [244.xx]	Hyposecretion of T_3 and T_4. Caused by thyroiditis, drugs prescribed to treat hyperthyroidism, or by hyposecretion of TSH from the anterior pituitary gland. Characterized by fatigue, decreased body temperature, dry hair and skin, constipation, and weight gain; or, if severe, by myxedema, with swelling of various parts of the body, tingling in the hands and feet, an enlarged heart, bradycardia, an enlarged tongue, slow speech, and mental impairment. [*see also:* congenital hypothyroidism]	L
hypoxemia [799.xx]	Abnormally low level of oxygen in the arterial blood. In comparison, hypoxia is a low level of oxygen at the cellular level. [*see also:* anoxia, arterial blood gases]	S
hysterectomy	Surgical procedure to remove the uterus. Can be performed with a laparoscope through an abdominal incision or through the vagina. A total hysterectomy involves removing both the uterus and cervix. [*see also:* oophorectomy, salpingectomy]	
hysterosalpin-gography	Radiologic procedure in which radiopaque contrast dye is injected through the cervix into the uterus. It coats and outlines the uterus and fallopian tubes and shows narrowing, scarring, and blockage. This test is done as part of an infertility workup. [*see also:* infertility]	A

I

iatrogenic disease	Caused by medicine or treatment given to the patient. Examples: Wrong drug given to patient, surgery performed on the wrong leg.	
identical twins	The initial division of a zygote, a fertilized ovum, creates two separate, but identical, developing embryos. [*see also:* fraternal twins, polyhydramnios, zygote]	S
idiopathic disease	Having no identifiable cause.	
idiopathic cardiomyopathy [425.xx]	A condition of the heart muscle that includes heart enlargement and heart failure. The cause of the enlargement and failure of the heart muscle is unknown. [*see also:* cardiomyopathy, echocardiography, radionuclide ventriculography]	
ileum	Third and last part of the small intestine. It connects to the cecum of the large intestine. [*see also:* Crohn's disease, mesentery]	F

ileus [560.xx]	Abnormal absence of peristalsis in the small and large intestines.	S
immune response	Coordinated effort between the blood and lymphatic system to identify and destroy invading microorganisms or cancerous cells produced within the body. [*see also*: active immunity, complement proteins, passive immunity]	
immunoglobulin A	Antibody present in body secretions (tears, saliva, mucus, and breast milk). It gives passive immunity to a breastfeeding infant. [*see also*: passive immunity]	A
immunoglobulin D	Antibody present on the surface of B cells. It stimulates the B cell to become a plasma cell. [*see also*: B cell]	A
immunoglobulin E	Antibody present on the surface of basophils. It causes them to release histamine and heparin during inflammatory and allergic reactions. [*see also*: basophils, radioallergosorbent test]	A
immunoglobulin G	Antibody that is produced by plasma cells the second time a specific pathogen enters the body; IgG forms the basis for active immunity. Smallest in size, but most abundant of all the immunoglobulins. During pregnancy, it crosses the placenta to the fetus and provides passive immunity. [*see also*: active immunity, immunoglobulin M, pathogen]	A
immunoglobulin M	Antibody that is produced by plasma cells during the initial exposure to a pathogen. IgM also reacts to incompatible blood types during a blood transfusion. Largest of the immunoglobulins. [*see also*: immunoglobulin G, pathogen]	A
impotence [302.xx; 607.xx]	Inability to achieve or sustain an erection of the penis. Can be caused by cardiovascular disease that impedes blood flow to the penis, a neurological disease that impairs sensory stimuli and innervation, a low level of testosterone, the side effects of drugs, or psychological factors. [*see also*: penile implant, priapism]	S
in situ	Area where the cancerous cell first formed and is still contained in that area. [*see also*: primary site, secondary site]	
incentive spirometry	Medical procedure to encourage patients to breathe deeply. A spirometer is a portable plastic device with a mouthpiece and balls that move as the patient inhales forcefully.	
incision and drainage	Medical procedure to treat a cyst or abscess. A scalpel is used to make an incision, and the fluid or pus inside is removed or allowed to drain out. [*see also*: abscess, boil]	A
incisional biopsy	An incision is made to expose the suspected cancer, and part (but not all) of the tumor is removed for analysis. [*see also*: biopsy]	S
incisional hernia [553.xx]	A weakness in the muscles of the abdominal wall that allows loops of intestine to balloon outward, occurring along the suture line of a prior surgical incision. [*see also*: hernia]	
incompetent cervix [761.xx]	Spontaneous dilation of the cervix during the second trimester of pregnancy, but without uterine contractions; this can result in spontaneous abortion of the fetus. [*see also*: cerclage, dystocia, miscarriage]	
incontinence [788.xx]	Inability to voluntarily keep urine in the bladder. Can be caused by a spinal cord injury, surgery on the prostate gland, unconsciousness, stress, or mental conditions such as dementia. [*see also*: bladder neck suspension, cystometry, overactive bladder, urination]	
indium-111	Indium is a soft, silvery metal. Given intravenously for nuclear medicine imaging of many different areas of the body to detect cancerous tumors. Indium-111 is combined with a hormone that is	

attracted to cancerous cells of the endocrine system, or it can be combined with a monoclonal antibody that is attracted to cancerous cells of the ovary or colon. [see also: carcinoma]

induction of labor
Medical procedure to begin labor by administering an oxytocin drug. This is done when the mother is past her estimated due date or when the health of the mother or fetus necessitates delivery. [see also: amniotomy, dystocia, Nägele's rule]

infectious disease
Caused by a pathogen (disease-causing microorganism such as a bacterium, virus, or fungus). A communicable disease is an infectious disease that is transmitted by direct contact with another person, animal, or insect. Examples: Gonorrhea (a sexually transmitted disease), rabies from an animal bite.

inferior
Pertaining to the lower half of the body or a position below an organ or structure. Opposite of superior. [see also: transverse plane]

infertility
[608.xx; 628.xx]
Failure to conceive after at least one year of regular intercourse.
♀: Imbalance or lack of estradiol or progesterone. (It can also be caused by a lack of FSH and LH from the anterior pituitary gland.) There is a lack of ovulation, abnormal menstruation, or history of miscarriage. [see also: anovulation, hormone testing, hysterosalpingography, pelvic inflammatory disease]
♂: Hyposecretion of testosterone, damage to the testes from mumps or infection, abnormalities of the spermatozoa, failure of one or both of the testes to descend into the scrotum before birth, or surgical removal of a testis because of cancer. [see also: antisperm antibody test, cryptorchism, oligospermia, semen analysis, varicocele]

inflammatory bowel disease
Chronic inflammation of various parts of the small and large intestine. There are two types of inflammatory bowel disease: Crohn's disease and ulcerative colitis. [see also: Crohn's disease, ulcerative colitis] A

influenza [487.xx]
Acute viral infection of the upper respiratory tract that some-times also involves the lungs. L S

infundibulum
Funnel-shaped end of the fallopian tube. It collects an ovum from the ovary and channels it into the fallopian tube.

inguinal canal
Passageway in the groin area through which the testes travel as they descend from the abdomen to the scrotum. The open canal closes snugly around the spermatic cord at birth or shortly thereafter. [see also: cryptorchism] F

inguinal hernia
[550.xx]
A weakness in the muscles of the abdominal wall that allows loops of intestine to balloon outward, occurring in the groin region. In a male patient with an inguinal hernia, the intestines travel through the inguinal canal and into the scrotum. [see also: hernia]

inguinal region
Two of nine regions on the surface of the anterior abdominal area. The right and left inguinal regions are inferior to the right and left lumbar regions. [see also: epigastric region, hypochondriac region, hypogastric region, lumbar region, quadrant, umbilical region] S

inhibition
Action of a hormone to prevent an organ or gland from secreting its hormones. [see also: galactorrhea, somatostatin]

insulin
Hormone secreted by the beta cells of the islets of Langerhans in the pancreas. It transports glucose to the cells. [see also:

A = Abbreviations Section   F = Figures Section   L = Laboratory Section   S = Synonyms Section
Sx (Symptoms)   Dx (Diagnosis)   Tx (Treatment)

diabetes mellitus, diabetic ketoacidosis, gestational diabetes, hyperinsulinism, pancreas, somatostatin]

intake and output Nursing procedure that documents the patient's total amount of fluid intake and the total amount of fluid output. Used to monitor a patient's fluid balance. **A**

integumentary system Body system that includes the skin, hair, nails, sweat glands, and oil glands. It perceives pain, touch, and temperature; protects the internal organs from infection and trauma; and regulates body temperature by sweating.

intercostal muscles Muscles of the chest that work in pairs to spread the ribs apart during inspiration and move the ribs together during expiration, coughing, and sneezing. [see also: cough, expectoration] **F**

interferon Substance released by macrophages that have engulfed a virus. It stimulates normal body cells to produce an antiviral substance that prevents the virus from entering them to reproduce.

interleukin Substance released by macrophages that stimulates B cell and T cell lymphocytes and activates natural killer cells. It also produces fever. [see also: B cell]

intermittent explosive disorder [312.xx] Sudden, explosively violent, unprovoked attacks of rage that are out of proportion to the stress experienced. Patients always place the blame on other people or circumstances for making them angry. Involves assault, battery, and is often associated with domestic violence. During a psychiatric interview, this patient is asked if he has any homicidal ideations about actually killing someone.

internal genitalia ♀: Ovaries, fallopian tubes, uterus, cervix, and vagina.

♂: Vas deferens, seminal vesicles, ejaculatory ducts, and prostate gland.

internal radiotherapy An implant placed near the tumor that contains a radioactive substance that emits radiation. [see also: brachytherapy, interstitial radiotherapy, intracavitary radiotherapy, transarterial chemoembolization]

interstitial cells Special cells between the seminiferous tubules of the testes that secrete testosterone. [see also: luteinizing hormone, testosterone]

interstitial cystitis [595.xx] A chronic and progressive infection of the bladder in which the mucosal lining becomes extremely irritated and red, often with bleeding. [see also: cystitis, hematuria, pyelonephritis, urinary tract infection]

interstitial radiotherapy Radioactive implants (needles, wires, capsules, or pellets [seeds]) are inserted into the tumor or into the tissue around the tumor. [see also: internal radiotherapy, intracavitary radiotherapy, transarterial chemoembolization]

interventional radiology Uses CT, MRI, or ultrasonography to guide the insertion of a needle (such as in amniocentesis) for a biopsy, or for other procedures (such as percutaneous coronary angioplasty). [see also: magnetic resonance imaging]

intervertebral disk Circular disk between two vertebrae. It consists of an outer wall of fibrocartilage and an inner gelatinous substance, the nucleus pulposus, that acts as a cushion. [see also: diskectomy, laminectomy, myelography, sciatica, spondylolisthesis] **F**

intracavitary radiotherapy Radioactive implants are inserted into a body cavity near the tumor. [see also: internal radiotherapy, interstitial radiotherapy, transarterial chemoembolization]

intrauterine cavity	Hollow cavity inside the uterus, which is lined with endometrium. [*see also*: endometrium]	F
intrauterine growth retardation [764.xx]	Many factors affect the growth rate of the embryo and fetus. Maternal illness, malnutrition, and smoking can make the fetus small for gestational age (SGA). [*see also*: lecithin/sphingomyelin ratio]	A
intravenous cholangiography	Contrast dye is injected intravenously. It travels through the blood to the liver and is then excreted with bile into the gallbladder. It outlines the gallbladder and stones and shows thickening of the gallbladder wall. [*see also*: cholangiography]	A
intraventricular hematoma [431.xx; 772.xx]	Localized collection of blood that forms within one of the ventricles in the brain because of the rupture of an artery or vein. [*see also*: aneurysm, cerebrovascular accident, subdural hematoma]	
introitus	The entrance to the vagina from the outside of the body. [*see also*: crowning, uterine prolapse, vagina]	
intussusception [560.xx]	Telescoping of one segment of intestine into the lumen of an adjacent segment.	
invasive	Characteristic of cancerous tumors. They penetrate and destroy the normal cells around them, compromising tissue functions.	
inversion	Turning a body part inward. Opposite of eversion.	
invertor	Muscle that produces inversion when it contracts.	
involution	Process by which the uterus gradually shrinks in size after childbirth. [*see also*: postpartum depression]	
iodinated contrast dye	Radiopaque contrast dye that contains iodine, a chemical element with a high atomic weight that makes it opaque on an x-ray.	
iodine-123	Given intravenously for nuclear medicine imaging of the thyroid gland. Iodine is a purple-black, shiny crystalline solid that is a trace element in the soil. The body uses iodine to produce thyroid hormones.	
ion	A positively or negatively charged atom.	
iris	Colored ring of tissue whose muscles contract or relax to change the size of the pupil in its center. [*see also*: anisocoria, closed-angle glaucoma, iritis, miosis, mydriasis, open-angle glaucoma, slit-lamp examination]	F
iritis [364.xx]	Inflammation or infection of the iris. Can be caused by infection in the eye or another part of the body, allergy, trauma, or an autoimmune disease. [*see also*: autoimmune disease]	
iron deficiency anemia [280.xx]	Caused by a deficiency of iron in the diet. Also caused by increased loss of iron due to menstruation, hemorrhage, or chronic blood loss. The erythrocytes are small in size and pale in color. [*see also*: anemia, anisocytosis, ferritin, total iron binding capacity]	L
irritable bowel syndrome [564.xx]	Disorder of the function of the colon, although the mucosa of the colon never shows any visible signs of inflammation. [*see also*: colon]	A S
	Dx The symptoms vary, making a definitive diagnosis difficult. Some base a diagnosis on the Rome II criteria. An endoscopy will also be performed to visualize the GI tract. [*see also*: endoscopy]	

Tx	Medications for the disease and to treat the underlying symptoms.
ischemic phase	Days 27–28 of the menstrual cycle when the corpus luteum degenerates into a white scar and progesterone production ceases. The endometrium sloughs off to begin menstruation. The menstrual cycle consists of the menstrual phase, proliferative phase, secretory phase, ovulation, and ischemic phase.

J

jaundice [774.xx]	Yellowish discoloration of the skin and whites of the eyes. Associated with liver disease. The liver cannot process bilirubin, and high levels of unconjugated bilirubin in the blood move into the tissues and color the skin yellow. [*see also*: neonatal jaundice, scleral icterus]	L S
jejunostomy	Surgical procedure to create a permanent opening from the abdominal wall into the jejunum through which to insert a permanent feeding tube. [*see also*: percutaneous endoscopic gastrostomy]	
jejunum	Second part of the small intestine. [*see also*: mesentery]	F
jock itch [110.xx]	Skin infection occurring in the groin and perineum caused by a microscopic fungus that feeds on epidermal cells. [*see also*: tinea]	S
joint	Area where two bones come together. There are three types of joints: suture, symphysis, and synovial.	
joint replacement surgery	Surgical procedure to replace a joint that has been destroyed by inflammation. A prosthesis takes the place of part of the bones in the joint. Done on hips, knees, ankles, shoulders, elbows and the small joints of the fingers. [*see also*: arthrodesis, bursitis, cartilage transplantation, prosthesis]	S

K

Kaposi's sarcoma [176.xx]	Cancer that arises from connective tissue or lymph nodes. Tumors on the skin are elevated, irregular, and dark reddish-blue. This was once a relatively rare malignancy, but is now commonly seen in AIDS patients. [*see also*: acquired immunodeficiency syndrome]	A
karyotype	Cytology test used to examine chromosomes under the microscope. A photograph of the karyotype is studied to look for chromosomal deletions or translocations. [*see also*: chromosome]	
keloid [701.xx]	A very firm, abnormally large scar that is bigger than the original injury. It is due to an overproduction of collagen fibers. Unlike a scar, a keloid does not fade or decrease in size over time.	
keratin	Hard protein found in the cells of the outermost part of the epidermis and in the nails.	
ketonuria [791.xx]	Ketone bodies in the urine. Ketones are waste products produced when fat is metabolized. Patients with diabetes mellitus metabolize fat for energy because they cannot metabolize glucose. Also seen in malnourished patients. [*see also*: diabetes mellitus, folic acid anemia]	S
kidney	Organ of the urinary system that produces urine. [*see also*: acute tubular necrosis, blood urea nitrogen, creatinine, erythropoietin, hydronephrosis, KUB x-ray, nephrectomy, nephrolithiasis, nephroblastoma, nephroptosis, polycystic kidney disease, pyelonephritis, renal colic, renal failure]	F
kleptomania [312.xx]	Overwhelming impulse to steal things, usually that have little or no value. These things are not stolen out of anger or revenge,	

and the patient sometimes even secretively returns them. Unlike shoplifting, the patient does not steal in order to obtain something without paying for it.

krypton-81m   A gas that is inhaled for nuclear medicine imaging of the lung. Krypton is a colorless, odorless gas that is present in trace amounts in the atmosphere.

KUB x-ray   Radiologic procedure that x-rays the kidneys (K), ureters (U), and bladder (B). It is used to find kidney stones or as a preliminary x-ray before performing a pyelogram.   A

kyphoscoliosis [737.xx]   Complex, abnormal curvature of the spine with components of both kyphosis and scoliosis. [see also: dextroscoliosis, kyphosis, levoscoliosis, scoliosis]

kyphosis [737.xx]   Abnormal, excessive, posterior curvature of the thoracic spine. The spine is said to have a kyphotic curvature. [see also: dextroscoliosis, kyphoscoliosis, levoscoliosis, lordosis, scoliosis]   S

L

labia   A pair of fleshy lips covered with pubic hair (the labia majora) and a small, thin, inner pair of lips (the labia minora) that partially cover the clitoris, urethral meatus, and vaginal introitus in the female. [see also: external genitalia].

labyrinthitis [386.xx]   Bacterial or viral infection of the semicircular canals of the inner ear, causing severe vertigo.   S

laceration   Deep, penetrating wound with cleanly cut or torn, ragged skin edges.

lacrimal gland   Gland located near the superior-lateral aspect of the eye. It produces and releases tears through the lacrimal ducts. [see also: lacrimal sac, xerophthalmia]   S

lacrimal sac   Small structure that collects tears as they drain from the medial aspect of the eye. It empties into the nasolacrimal duct. [see also: dacryocystitis, lacrimal gland]

lactase   Digestive enzyme from villi in the small intestine. It breaks down lactose, the sugar in milk. [see also: villi]   S

lactate dehydrogenase   Found in many different cells, including the heart. LDH levels begin to rise 12 hours after a myocardial infarction. An elevated LDH can corroborate elevated CK-MB results but cannot be the sole basis for diagnosing a myocardial infarction. [see also: cardiac enzymes]   L

lactation   Production of colostrum and then breast milk by the mammary glands after childbirth. The let-down reflex is the release of milk from the breasts in response to crying or sucking by the newborn. [see also: colostrum, failure of lactation, mastitis, prolactin, oxytocin]   S

lactiferous lobules   Clusters of milk-producing glands throughout the breast that produce and secrete milk after the birth of a baby. The milk flows from them through the lactiferous ducts to the nipple. [see also: failure of lactation, oxytocin]

laminectomy   Surgical excision of the lamina (the flat area of the arch of the vertebra). Removal of this bony segment relieves pressure on the dorsal nerve roots and relieves pain from a herniated nucleus pulposus. [see also: diskectomy, sciatica]

laparoscopy   Surgical procedure to visualize the inside of the abdominal cavity and organs. A small incision is made near the umbilicus, and

A = Abbreviations Section   **F** = Figures Section   **L** = Laboratory Section   **S** = Synonyms Section
Sx (Symptoms)   **Dx** (Diagnosis)   **Tx** (Treatment)

	carbon dioxide gas is used to inflate the abdominal cavity. A fiberoptic scope is then inserted through the incision. Grasping and cutting instruments can be inserted through the scope, if needed. [*see also*: appendicitis, cholecystectomy, exploratory laparotomy, hysterectomy, myomectomy]	
large intestine	Organ of absorption between the small intestine and the anal opening. Includes the cecum, appendix, colon, rectum, and anus. [*see also*: flatus, haustra, ileus, inflammatory bowel disease]	S F
laryngitis [464.xx; 467.xx]	Hoarseness or complete loss of the voice, difficulty swallowing, and cough due to swelling and inflammation of the larynx. Caused by a bacterial or viral infection.	
larynx	Triangular structure in the anterior neck (visible as the laryngeal prominence or Adam's apple) that contains the vocal cords and is a passageway for inhaled and exhaled air. [*see also*: epiglottis, glottis, laryngitis, radical neck dissection, stridor, vocal cords]	F
laser photocoagulation	Surgical procedure to seal leaking or hemorrhaging retinal blood vessels or to reattach a detached retina. Light from the laser creates heat that coagulates the tissues. If there is blood in the vitreous humor, the light from the laser cannot reach the retina, and a vitrectomy must be done first to remove the vitreous humor and replace it with a synthetic substitute. [*see also*: retinopexy, retinal detachment]	
laser skin resurfacing	Uses a computer-controlled laser to vaporize the epidermis and some of the dermis. This promotes the regrowth of smooth skin. [*see also*: chemical peel, dermabrasion, exfoliation, skin resurfacing]	S
laser surgery	Medical procedure that uses pulses of laser light to remove birthmarks, tattoos, superficial blood vessels of acne rosacea, and unwanted hair. A tunable laser has a specific wavelength of light that only reacts with certain colors (the dark red of a birthmark, the black pigment of a tattoo, and so forth) to break up that color and the structure that contains it. Surrounding tissue is unharmed. [*see also*: genital warts, nevus]	
lateral	Pertaining to the side of the body, the side of an organ or structure, going in from the side or going to the side. Opposite of medial. [*see also*: midsagittal plane]	A
lateral epicondylitis [726.xx]	Inflammation and pain of the extensor and supinator muscles where their tendons originate on the lateral epicondyle of the humerus by the elbow joint. [*see also*: cumulative trauma disorder, medial epicondylitis]	S
lead apron	Shielding apron worn by radiologic personnel to protect themselves from radiation exposure, or by patients to shield parts of the body that are not being x-rayed.	
lecithin/ sphingomyelin ratio	Lecithin is a component of surfactant that keeps the alveoli from collapsing with each breath. Sphingomyelin levels are higher until the fetal lungs are mature, and then lecithin levels become higher than sphingomyelin by 2:1. This test is done during late pregnancy to determine the maturity of the fetal lungs. [*see also*: amniocentesis, hyaline membrane disease, intrauterine growth retardation, surfactant]	A
left bundle branch block [426.xx]	Arrhythmia in which the electrical impulses from the AV node do not travel down the left bundle of His. [*see also*: dysrhythmia, right bundle branch block]	A
left-sided congestive heart	In left-sided congestive heart failure, the left ventricle is unable to adequately pump blood, and blood backs up into the lungs,	

failure [428.xx]	causing pulmonary edema, which can be seen on a chest x-ray. [*see also*: cor pulmonale, congestive heart failure, pulmonary edema]
legally blind [369.xx]	Patients whose best visual acuity is 20/200 even with corrective lenses. [*see also*: blindness]
Legionnaire's disease [482.xx]	Severe, sometimes fatal, bacterial infection that begins with flu-like symptoms, body aches and fever, followed by severe pneumonia with possible liver and kidney degeneration. [*see also*: adult respiratory distress syndrome]
leiomyoma [218.xx]	Benign, smooth muscle neoplasm. [*see also*: myomectomy, uterine fibroid] **S**
lens	Clear, hard disk in the internal eye. The muscles of the ciliary body **F** change the lens shape to focus light rays on the retina. [*see also*: accommodation, aphakia, aqueous humor, cataract, cilliary body, extracapsular cataract extraction, hyperopia, myopia, phacoemulsification, presbyopia, slit-lamp examination]
lens capsule	Clear membrane that envelops the lens in the eye.
lesion	Any area of visible damage on the skin, whether it is from **S** disease or injury.
leukemia [204.xx–207.xx]	Cancer of the leukocytes (white blood cells). The excessive numbers **S** of leukocytes crowd out other cells in the bone marrow. Patients have anemia (from too few erythrocytes), easy bruising and hemorrhages (from too few thrombocytes), fever, and susceptibility to infection (from too many immature leukocytes). Leukemia is named according to the type of leukocyte that is most prevalent and whether the onset of symptoms is acute or chronic. [*see also*: leukocyte, pancytopenia, splenomegaly, thrombocytopenia]
	Dx H&P. Lab tests to determine the level of WBCs. A bone marrow aspiration and biopsy will confirm the diagnosis. [*see also*: blood smear, bone marrow testing, electrophoresis]
	Tx An individualized plan may include chemotherapy or radiation therapy. A bone marrow transplant may be considered. [*see also*: bone marrow transplant, chemotherapy, radiation therapy]
leukocyte	A white blood cell. There are five different types of mature **F** leukocytes: neutrophils, eosinophils, basophils, lymphocytes, **S** and monocytes. [*see also*: leukemia]
leukocyte esterase	Urine test to detect esterase, an enzyme associated with leukocytes and a urinary tract infection. This dipstick test gives a quick result so that antibiotic drugs can be started immediately. At the same time, a urine specimen is sent for culture and sensitivity.
leukoplakia	Benign, thickened, white patch on the mucous membrane; it can become cancerous. Most commonly found in the mouth (caused by tobacco use), it can also be found in the cervix, esophagus, penis, or vagina. It can also be caused by an Epstein-Barr virus infection in AIDS patients. [*see also*: mononucleosis]
levoscoliosis [739.xx; 754.xx]	Abnormal, excessive, C-shaped or S-shaped lateral curvature of the spine to the patient's left. The back is said to have a scoliotic curvature. Scoliosis can be congenital, but most often the cause is unknown. [*see also*: dextroscoliosis, kyphosis, kyphoscoliosis, scoliosis]
ligament	Fibrous bands that hold two bone ends together in a synovial joint. [*see also*: sprain, tendon]

A = Abbreviations Section   **F** = Figures Section   **L** = Laboratory Section   **S** = Synonyms Section
Sx (Symptoms)   **Dx** (Diagnosis)   **Tx** (Treatment)

limbic lobe — Curved, encircling area of the brain that includes the medial edges of the two cerebral hemispheres and extends into the temporal lobes. **S**

limbic system — Related structures in the brain that control emotion, mood, memory, motivation, and behavior and link the conscious to the unconscious mind. The limbic system consists of the thalamus, hypothalamus, hippocampus, amygdaloid bodies, and fornix. [see also: amygdaloid body, dopamine, fornix, serotonin]

limbus — Border between the transparent edge of the cornea and the white, fibrous sclera of the eye.

linea nigra — Melanocyte-stimulating hormone can become active during pregnancy and cause a dark, hyperpigmented line on the skin of the abdomen from the umbilicus to the pubis. [see also: chloasma]

lingual tonsils — Lymphoid tissue located on both sides of the base of the tongue in the hypopharynx. [see also: tonsillitis] **F**

lipase — Digestive enzyme from the pancreas. It breaks down fat globules in the duodenum into fatty acids. [see also: bile, chyme, digestion, emulsification, pancreas]

lipid profile — Blood test that provides a comprehensive picture of the levels of cholesterol and triglycerides and their lipoprotein carriers in the blood: HDL, LDL, and VLDL. [see also: hypercholesterolemia, hyperlipidemia, hypertriglyceridemia] **L**

lipocyte — Cell in the subcutaneous layer of the skin that stores fat. **S**

lipoma [214.xx] — Benign growth composed of adipose tissue from the subcutaneous layer. It causes a soft, rounded, nontender elevation of the skin. [see also: adipose tissue] **S**

liposuction — Surgical procedure to remove excessive adipose tissue deposits, usually from the abdomen, hips, legs, or buttocks. A suction cannula removes the fat through small incisions. Ultrasonic-assisted liposuction uses ultrasonic waves to break up the fat before it is removed. [see also: adipose tissue] **S**

lithogenesis — Process of forming stones which are composed of magnesium, calcium, or uric acid crystals. [see also: cholelithiasis, extracorporeal shock wave lithotripsy, nephrolithiasis, renal colic, sialolithiasis] **S**

liver — Largest solid organ in the body. It produces bile. [see also: alpha fetoprotein, bile, bile ducts, carcinoembryonic antigen, cirrhosis, glycogen, hepatitis, hepatomegaly, jaundice, Reye's syndrome] **F**

lobe — The divisions of an organ visible on its outer surface, such as the lobes of the liver, lungs, and brain. **F**

local reaction — Allergic reaction that takes place on a certain area of the skin that was exposed to an allergen. [see also: allergen, allergic reaction]

lochia — Small amounts of blood, tissue, and fluid that are discharged from the uterus after childbirth. [see also: products of conception]

loop of Henle — Tubule of the nephron that is U-shaped. It begins at the proximal convoluted tubule and ends at the distal convoluted tubule. Reabsorption takes place there.

lordosis [737.xx] — Abnormal, excessive, anterior curvature of the lumbar spine. The spine is said to have a lordotic curvature. [see also: kyphosis, scoliosis] **S**

Lou Gehrig's disease [335.xx] — Chronic, progressive disease of the motor nerves of the spinal cord. There is no damage to the sensory nerves, so sensation remains intact. Some cases are caused by the lack of an enzyme, which is an inherited defect, but in most cases the cause is not known. **S**

A = Abbreviations Section   F = Figures Section   L = Laboratory Section   S = Synonyms Section
Sx (Symptoms)   Dx (Diagnosis)   Tx (Treatment)

Dx	H&P. Progressive muscle weakness. Tests on the muscles and nerves are performed. [*see also:* cerebrospinal fluid examination, electromyography, nerve conduction study]
Tx	No known cure. Treatment is supportive, treating the symptoms and providing comfort.

lumbar region

Two of nine regions on the surface of the anterior abdominal area. The right and left lumbar regions are positioned at the same level as the lumbar area of the back and to either side of the umbilical region. [*see also:* epigastric region, hypochondriac region, hypogastric region, inguinal region, quadrant, umbilical region]

lumen

Central open area throughout the length of a tube or duct.

Digestive: Open channel inside the tubular structures of the gastrointestinal tract, such as the esophagus, small intestine, and large intestine.

Pulmonary: Central opening inside the trachea, bronchus, or bronchiole through which air flows.

Vascular: Central opening inside a blood vessel through which blood flows.

lumpectomy

Surgical procedure to excise a small cancerous tumor without taking any surrounding tissue. [*see also:* mastectomy]

lung

Organ of respiration that contains alveoli. [*see also:* adult respiratory distress syndrome, alveolus, aspiration pneumonia, asthma, atelectasis, bronchus, chronic obstructive pulmonary disease, congestive heart failure, cor pulmonale, cystic fibrosis, dyspnea, emphysema, expectoration, hyaline membrane disease, lecithin/sphingomyelin ratio, lung resection, pleura, pneumoconiosis, pneumothorax, pulmonary embolism, pulmonary function tests, pyothorax, respiration, thoracentesis, thoracotomy, tuberculosis, ventilation-perfusion scan] **F**

lung resection

Surgical procedure to remove a part or all of a lung. A wedge resection removes a small wedge-shaped piece of tissue from one lobe. A segmental resection removes a large piece or segment of one lobe. A lobectomy removes an entire lobe. A pneumonectomy removes an entire lung. [*see also:* thoracotomy]

lunula

Whitish half-moon visible under the proximal portion of the nail plate. It is the visible tip of the nail root. **S**

luteinizing hormone

Hormone secreted by the anterior pituitary gland. [*see also:* FSH assay and LH assay, hormone testing, infertility, precocious puberty, progesterone, puberty] **A S**

♀: Triggers ovulation. It stimulates the corpus luteum to secrete estradiol and progesterone. [*see also:* corpus luteum, menopause, ovaries]

♂: Stimulates the interstitial cells of the testes to secrete testosterone. [*see also:* oligospermia, testes]

Lyme disease
[088.xx]

Arthritis caused by a bacterium in the bite of an infected deer tick. If untreated, Lyme disease can cause severe fatigue and affect the nervous system and the heart. [*see also:* enzyme-linked immunosorbent assay] **S**

lymph

Fluid that flows through the lymphatic system. [*see also:* lymphatic system]

---

lymph node biopsy

Surgical process that uses a fine needle to aspirate material from a lymph node. The lymph node may also be completely removed by doing an excisional biopsy. [see also: lymph nodes]

lymph node dissection

Surgical procedure to remove several or all of the lymph nodes in a lymph node chain during extensive cancer surgery. Involved lymph nodes represent metastasis of the cancer from its original site. [see also: lymph nodes, modified radical mastectomy]

lymph nodes   F

Small, encapsulated pieces of lymphoid tissue located along the lymphatic vessels. Lymph nodes filter and destroy invading microorganisms and cancerous cells present in the lymph. [see also: breast self-examination, cystectomy, Kaposi's sarcoma, lymph node biopsy, lymph node dissection, lymphadenopathy, prostatectomy, radical mastectomy, radical resection, sentinel node biopsy, testicular self-examination, TNM system]

lymphadenopathy
[785.xx]

Enlarged lymph nodes due to bacteria or cancer. The lymph nodes trap cancerous cells that break away from the site of the original tumor. The lymph node itself then becomes a site of cancer. Chains of lymph nodes in the neck, axillae, and groin regions are common sites of enlargement. [see also: lymph nodes]

lymphangio-graphy

Radiologic procedure in which a radiopaque contrast dye is injected into a lymphatic vessel. X-rays are taken as the dye travels through the lymphatic vessels and lymph nodes. Used to demonstrate enlarged lymph nodes, lymphomas, and areas of blocked lymphatic drainage. [see also: lymphatic vessels]

lymphatic system   F

Body system that includes a network of lymphatic vessels, circulating lymph fluid, lymph nodes, the lymphoid organs (thymus, spleen), and lymphoid tissues (tonsils and adenoids, appendix, and Peyer's patches). Also includes the blood cells lymphocytes and macrophages. [see also: appendix, carcinoma, immune response, lingual tonsils, lymph nodes, lymphatic vessels, lymphocyte, palatine tonsils, pharyngeal tonsils, spleen]

lymphatic vessels

Vessels that begin as capillaries carrying lymph, continue through lymph nodes, and empty into the right lymphatic duct or the thoracic duct. [see also: lymphangiography, lymphedema, metastasis]

lymphedema
[457.xx]

Generalized swelling of an arm or a leg that occurs after surgery when a chain of lymph nodes has been removed. Tissue fluid in that area cannot drain into the lymphatic vessels at the normal rate, and this causes edema. [see also: lymphatic vessels]

lymphocyte   A
F
L

Second most abundant leukocyte, but the smallest in size. It is classified as an agranulocyte, and the cytoplasm is only a thin ring that edges the round nucleus. Lymphocytes in the red bone marrow become NK cells or B lymphocytes that produce antibodies. Lymphocytes in the thymus become T lymphocytes. [see also: agranulocyte, B cell, complete blood count, interleukin, leukocyte, lymphoma, natural killer cells, T cell, thymus]

lymphoma
[200.xx–208.xx]

Cancerous tumor of lymphocytes in the lymph nodes or lymphoid tissue. A lymphoma that originates in a lymph node should not be confused with metastasis to a lymph node from a primary site of cancer located elsewhere in the body. [see also: bone marrow testing, non-Hodgkin's lymphoma, Hodgkin's lymphoma, radiation therapy]

lysosome

Organelle that consists of a small sac with digestive enzymes in it. It destroys pathogens that invade the cell. [see also: Golgi apparatus]

A = Abbreviations Section   **F** = Figures Section   **L** = Laboratory Section   **S** = Synonyms Section
Sx (Symptoms)   **Dx** (Diagnosis)   **Tx** (Treatment)

M

macrophage	Another name for a monocyte because it is able to engulf large numbers of cells and cellular debris. [*see also*: B cell, interferon, interleukin, monocyte, tumor necrosis factor]	**S**
macula	Dark yellow-orange area with indistinct edges in the retina. [*see also*: fovea, macular degeneration]	**F**
macular degeneration [362.xx]	Chronic, progressive loss of central vision as the macula degenerates. In dry macular degeneration, the macula deteriorates with age. In wet macular degeneration, abnormal blood vessels grow under the macula. They are fragile and leak, causing the macula to lift away from the retina. [*see also*: macula, scotoma]	
macule	A discolored small spot on the skin that is not elevated. Characteristic of some conditions, like smallpox and purpura.	
magnetic resonance imaging	The use of a magnetic field and radiowaves to align the protons in atoms and then cause them to vibrate and emit energy as a signal. Produces individual images as "slices" through the body, as well as a composite three-dimensional view. The noniodinated contrast dye gadolinium can also be used to enhance the image. [*see also*: arthrography, enhanced, gadolinium, interventional radiology, myelography]	**A**
major depression [296.xx]	Chronic, severe symptoms of depression with apathy, hopelessness, helplessness, worthlessness, crying, insomnia, lack of pleasure in any activity, increased or decreased appetite, inability to make decisions or concentrate, fatigue, and slowed movements. During the psychiatric interview, a depressed patient is asked if he has suicidal ideation or suicide attempts. [*see also*: Beck Depression Inventory, electroshock therapy, postpartum depression]	
malignant melanoma [172.xx]	Arises from melanocytes in the epidermis. It grows quickly and metastasizes to other parts of the body. [*see also*: dysplastic nevus]	
malingering	Exhibiting factitious medical or psychiatric symptoms in order to get a tangible reward, like narcotic drugs or disability payments. Patients are aware that they are lying and know exactly what they want to achieve from their deceptions.	**S**
malpresentation of the fetus [652.xx]	Birth position in which the presenting part of the fetus is not the head. If the fetus is in a transverse lie, the shoulder or arm is the presenting part. [*see also*: breech birth, dystocia]	**S**
	Dx Physical examination, ultrasound to determine presentation. [*see also*: colposcopy]	
	Tx External cephalic version (after 37 weeks' gestation), delivery either vaginally or by cesarean section. [*see also*: external cephalic version]	
mammaplasty	Surgical procedure to change the size, shape, or position of the breast. [*see also*: augmentation mammaplasty, reconstructive mammaplasty, reduction mammaplasty]	**S**
mammary glands	The breasts. A female sexual characteristic that develops during puberty. The breasts contain fatty tissue and lactiferous glands and ducts. The breasts provide milk to nourish the baby after birth. The skin fold beneath each breast is known as the inframammary crease. [*see also*: fibrocystic disease, lactation]	**S**
mammography	Radiologic procedure that uses x-rays to produce an image of the breast to detect tumors. The breast is compressed between two flat surfaces to decrease its thickness and increase the quality of the image. [*see also*: xeromammography]	

A = Abbreviations Section   **F** = Figures Section   **L** = Laboratory Section   **S** = Synonyms Section
Sx (Symptoms)   **Dx** (Diagnosis)   **Tx** (Treatment)

manic-depressive disorder [296.xx]	Chronic mood swings between mania and depression. Patients with mania are hyperactive, with limitless energy and extreme happiness. Gradually, their thoughts get out of control, and they are unable to concentrate and show increasingly poor judgment and recklessness. After an episode of mania, the patient swings abruptly into severe depression. [*see also:* cyclothymia]	S
	Dx Depends on the type (bipolar I or bipolar II). The manic episodes, depressive episodes, and mixed episodes are mapped to determine their frequency, supplemented with the DSM-IV criteria. [*see also:* Beck Depression Inventory]	
	Tx Psychological or psychiatric intervention. [*see also:* psychotherapy]	
Mantoux test	Screening test used to determine if a patient has been exposed to tuberculosis recently or in the past. An intradermal injection of PPD (purified protein derivative), part of the bacterium *Mycobacterium tuberculosis*, is given. A raised skin reaction after 48 to 72 hours indicates antibodies to the bacterium because of prior exposure. A positive Mantoux test is followed up with a chest x-ray to confirm whether or not active tuberculosis is present.	
masochism [302.xx]	Obtaining sexual arousal through abuse, pain, humiliation, or bondage that is deliberately done by another person. [*see also:* sadism]	
mastectomy	Surgical resection of all or part of the breast to excise a malignant tumor. [*see also:* lumpectomy, mammography, modified radical mastectomy, prophylactic mastectomy, radical mastectomy, total mastectomy]	
mastication	Process of chewing, during which the teeth and tongue work together to tear, crush, and grind food. This is the first part of the process of mechanical digestion.	S
mastitis [611.xx]	Inflammation or infection of the breast. Caused by milk engorgement in the breast or an infection, usually due to the bacterium *Staphylococcus aureus*. The affected breast is red and swollen and the patient has a fever.	
maxillary sinuses	Largest of the sinuses. Pair of sinuses on either side of the nose in the maxillary bone. [*see also:* pansinusitis]	
meconium	Thick, sticky, greenish-black stool that is the first stool passed by a newborn baby. [*see also:* meconium aspiration]	
meconium aspiration [770.xx]	Fetal distress causes the fetus to pass meconium into the amniotic fluid. The meconium gets in the mouth and nose of the fetus and is inhaled at birth, causing severe respiratory distress. [*see also:* fetal distress]	
medial	Pertaining to the middle of the body or the middle of an organ or structure. Opposite of lateral. [*see also:* midsagittal plane]	
medial epicondylitis [726.xx]	Inflammation and pain of the flexor and pronator muscles of the forearm where their tendons originate on the medial epicondyle of the humerus by the elbow joint. [*see also:* cumulative trauma disorder, lateral epicondylitis]	S
mediastinum	Central area within the thoracic cavity that lies between the lungs. It contains the esophagus, heart, great vessels, thymus, trachea, and other structures not related to the respiratory system.	
medulla oblongata	Most inferior part of the brainstem that joins to the spinal cord. It relays nerve impulses from the cerebrum to the cerebellum. It	F

	contains the respiratory center. Cranial nerves IX through XII originate there. [*see also*: anencephaly, brainstem]
medullary cavity	Long cavity in the center of a long bone. It contains yellow bone marrow (fatty tissue).
megakaryocyte	Very large cell whose cytoplasm breaks away at the edges to form individual thrombocytes. [*see also*: thrombocyte] **F**
meiosis	Process by which a spermatocyte reduces the number of chromosomes in its nucleus to 23, or half the normal number, to create gametes. [*see also*: mitosis, oogenesis, spermatozoon]
melanocyte-stimulating hormone	Hormone secreted by the anterior pituitary gland. It stimulates melanocytes in the skin to produce the pigment melanin during pregnancy. [*see also*: chloasma, linea nigra] **A**
melatonin	Hormone secreted by the pineal body. It maintains the 24-hour wake–sleep cycle known as the circadian rhythm. [*see also*: pineal gland, seasonal affective disorder] **S**
melena [578.xx]	Dark, tarry stools that contain digested blood due to bleeding in the esophagus or stomach. [*see also*: defecation]
menarche [256.xx]	The first monthly menstruation at the onset of puberty. [*see also*: menstruation]
Ménière's disease [386.xx]	Edema of the semicircular canals with destruction of the cochlea, causing hearing loss, tinnitus, and vertigo. It can be triggered by head trauma or middle ear infections. [*see also*: audiometry, conductive hearing loss, mixed hearing loss, nystagmus, sensorineural hearing loss]
meninges	Three separate membranes that envelop and protect the entire brain and spinal cord. The meninges include the dura mater, arachnoid, and pia mater. [*see also*: meningitis, meningocele, spina bifida] **F**
meningitis [047.xx; 320.xx–322.xx]	Inflammation of the meninges of the brain or spinal cord by a bacterial or viral infection.
	Dx H&P. The patient will have pain with inability to touch the chin to the chest. A lumbar puncture will be performed to determine the cause and analyze the cerebrospinal fluid. [*see also*: cerebrospinal fluid examination]
	Tx Medications to treat the cause, antivirals or antibiotics, and other medications to treat the symptoms.
meningocele [349.xx; 741.xx–742.xx]	Congenital abnormality of the neural tube in which the vertebrae form incompletely and there is protrusion of the meninges through the defect. [*see also*: alpha fetoprotein, neural tube defect, spina bifida]
meniscus	Crescent-shaped cartilage pad found in some synovial joints such as the knee. [*see also*: torn meniscus]
menometro-rrhagia [626.xx]	Excessive menstrual flow during menstruation or at other times of the month. Can cause anemia. [*see also*: menorrhagia]
menopause [627.xx]	Hyposecretion of estradiol. Caused by the aging process in which the ovaries secrete progressively less estradiol. As the hypothalamus senses low estradiol levels, it stimulates the anterior pituitary gland to secrete FSH and LH to stimulate the ovary, which causes hot flashes. [*see also*: estradiol, menstruation, perimenopausal period]
menorrhagia [627.xx]	An excessive amount of menstrual flow, or menstrual flow that lasts longer than 7 days. Can cause anemia. Caused by a hormone **S**

imbalance, uterine fibroids, or endometriosis. [*see also*: menometrorrhagia, menstruation, metrorrhagia, oligomenorrhea]

menses	A monthly menstrual period. [*see also*: menstruation]	S
menstrual cycle	A 28-day cycle that consists of the menstrual phase, proliferative phase, secretory phase, ovulation, and ischemic phase. [*see also*: menstruation]	
menstrual phase	Days 1–6 of the menstrual cycle when the endometrial lining of the uterus is shed. The menstrual cycle consists of the menstrual phase, proliferative phase, secretory phase, ovulation, and ischemic phase.	
menstruation [625.xx–626.xx]	Process in which the endometrium of the uterus is shed each month, causing a flow of blood and tissue through the vagina. Under the influence of estradiol, the endometrium thickens in preparation to receive a fertilized ovum. If the ovum is not fertilized, the endometrium is again shed to begin another menstrual cycle. [*see also*: amenorrhea, cold sores, dysfunctional uterine bleeding, dysmenorrhea, human chorionic gonadotropin, iron deficiency anemia, menarche, menometrorrhagia, menopause, menorrhagia, menses, menstrual cycle, metrorrhagia, oligomenorrhea, precocious puberty, premenstrual dysphoric disorder, premenstrual syndrome]	
mesentery	Thick sheet of peritoneum that supports the jejunum and ileum within the abdominal cavity. [*see also*: peritoneum]	
messenger RNA	RNA that duplicates DNA information in the nucleus and carries that information to the ribosome.	
metabolic panel	A metabolic panel includes many individual chemistry tests performed at the same time on the serum of the blood. These include albumin, alkaline phosphatase, ALP, ALT, AST, BUN, Ca^{++}, Cl^-, CO_2, creatinine, direct bilirubin, gamma GT, glucose, LDH, phosphorus, K^+, Na^+, total bilirubin, total cholesterol, total protein, and uric acid.	L S
metabolism	Process of using oxygen and glucose to produce energy for cells. Metabolism also produces byproducts such as carbon dioxide and other waste products. [*see also*: blood, bone scintigraphy, carbon dioxide, gout, homeostasis, metabolic panel, positron emission tomography scan, triiodothyronine, urea, uric acid]	
metastases	Process by which cancerous cells break off from a tumor and move through the blood vessels or lymphatic vessels to other sites in the body. [*see also*: carcinoma, carcinomatosis, exenteration, lymph node dissection, malignant melanoma, pathologic fracture, scintigraphy, secondary site, TNM system]	A L S
metrorrhagia [626.xx]	Excessive bleeding at a time other than menstruation. This can be caused by a tubal pregnancy or uterine cancer. [*see also*: dysfunctional uterine bleeding, ectopic pregnancy, menstruation]	
microderm-abrasion	Uses aluminum oxide crystals to abrade and remove the epidermis to produce smoother skin. [*see also*: dermabrasion]	
microglia	Cells that move, engulf, and destroy pathogens anywhere in the central nervous system.	S
microscope	Instrument used to examine very small structures.	
microscopic	Very small in size. A microscope is used to view tissues, cells, and structures that cannot be seen with the unaided eye.	

midsagittal plane	Plane that divides the body into right and left sections and creates a midline. [*see also*: coronal plane, oblique, projection, transverse plane]
migraine headache [346.xx]	Caused by a constriction of the arteries in the brain, followed by a sudden dilation. There is a sudden onset with severe, throbbing pain, often on just one side of the head. Usually accompanied by nausea and vomiting and sensitivity to light. [*see also*: cephalalgia, emesis, photophobia, scotoma] **S**
mineralocorticoids	Group of hormones secreted by the adrenal cortex. [*see also*: aldosterone]
mini mental status examination	Tests the patient's concrete and abstract thought processes and long- and short-term memory. The patient is asked to state his/her name, the date, and where he/she is. If the answers are all correct, the patient is said to be oriented to person, time, and place, or oriented x3. The patient is asked to perform simple mental arithmetic, recall objects or words, name the current and recent presidents, spell a word backwards, and give the meaning of a proverb. A full mental status examination is performed during psychiatric evaluations. **A**
miosis	Contraction of the iris muscle to decrease the size of the pupil and limit the amount of light entering the eye. [*see also*: anisocoria, mydriasis, pupillary response]
miscarriage [634.xx]	Loss of a pregnancy. An early spontaneous miscarriage usually occurs because of a genetic abnormality or poor implantation of the embryo within the endometrium. A later spontaneous miscarriage can occur because of preterm labor or an incompetent cervix. In a miscarriage, the embryo or fetus is expelled but the placenta and other tissue can remain in the uterus. [*see also*: dystocia, dilation and curettage, hydatidiform mole] **S**
mitochondria	Organelle that produces and stores ATP and then converts it to ADP to release energy for cellular activities.
mitosis	Process by which most body cells reproduce. The 46 chromosomes in the nucleus duplicate and then split, creating two identical cells, each with 46 chromosomes. The rate of cellular division is known as the mitotic rate. [*see also*: meiosis, oogenesis, spermatogenesis]
mitral valve	Heart valve located between the left atrium and the left ventricle. [*see also*: mitral valve prolapse, rheumatic heart disease, valve] **F** **S**
mitral valve prolapse [424.xx]	Structural abnormality in which the leaflets of the mitral valve do not close tightly. This can be a congenital condition or can occur if the valve is damaged by infection. There is regurgitation as blood flows backwards into the left atrium with each contraction. Slight prolapse is a common condition and does not require treatment. [*see also*: chordae tendineae, endocarditis] **A**
mixed hearing loss [389.xx]	A combination of both conductive and sensorineural hearing loss. [*see also*: audiometry, conductive hearing loss, sensorineural hearing loss, Rinne and Weber hearing tests]
modified radical mastectomy	Surgical resection of all or part of the breast to excise a malignant tumor. An axillary node dissection is also performed, and some of the axillary lymph nodes are removed. [*see also*: lymph node dissection, mastectomy]
Moh's surgery	Surgical procedure to remove skin cancer, particularly tumors with irregular shapes and depths. An operating microscope is used during the surgery to examine each layer of excised tissue.

A= Abbreviations Section   **F**= Figures Section   **L**= Laboratory Section   **S**= Synonyms Section
Sx(Symptoms)   **Dx**(Diagnosis)   **Tx**(Treatment)

	If the tissue shows cancerous cells, more tissue is removed until no trace of cancer remains.	
molding	Reshaping of the fetal cranium as it passes through the mother's pelvic bones during birth. [*see also*: cephalopelvic disproportion]	
moles	Darkly pigmented nevi that can be flat or elevated and often contain hairs. [*see also*: nevus]	
monocyte	Largest of the leukocytes. It is classified as an agranulocyte. The nucleus is shaped like a kidney bean. [*see also*: complete blood count]	A F L S
mononucleosis [075.xx]	Infectious disease caused by the Epstein-Barr virus (EBV). Often called "the kissing disease" because it commonly affects young adults and is transmitted through contact with saliva that contains the virus. [*see also*: leukoplakia, heterophil antibody test, splenomegaly]	A L S
mood	Prevailing, predominant emotion affecting a person's state of mind. [*see also*: cyclothymia, emotion, limbic system, postpartum depression, seasonal affective disorder]	
morning sickness [643.xx]	Nausea and vomiting during the first trimester of pregnancy. Thought to be due to elevated estradiol and progesterone levels. [*see also*: hyperemesis gravidarum]	S
Morton's neuroma [355.xx]	Benign tumor of the nerve around the metatarsophalangeal joint, between the ball of the foot and the toes, from repetitive damage to the nerve.	
motion sickness [994.xx]	Dysequilibrium with headache, dizziness, nausea, and vomiting caused by riding in a car, boat, or airplane. [*see also*: nausea, vertigo]	S
mucosa	The mucous membranes that are located in several different places within the body. [*see also*: aphthous stomatitis, *Campylobacter*-like organism test , candidiasis, Crohn's disease, diverticulitis, interstitial cystitis, irritable bowel syndrome, peptic ulcer disease, polyps, rugae, somatitis, varices, villi]	S
multidetector-row computerized axial tomography	Radiologic procedure that uses an x-ray beam controlled by a computer and moves around the body axis of a patient inside the CT scanner. Produces individual images as "slices," as well as a composite three-dimensional view. A multidetector-row CT scanner (MDCT) has an area (not just a row) of x-ray detectors and can quickly scan multiple "slices" simultaneously. [*see also*: computerized axial tomography, spiral computerized tomography]	A
multinucleated	Having many nuclei within one cell. A characteristic of skeletal muscle cells.	
multiple myeloma [203.xx]	Cancer of the plasma cells that produce antibodies. Multiple tumors in the bone destroy the red marrow and cause pain, fractures, and hypercalcemia. The abnormal plasma cells produce Bence Jones protein, an abnormal immunoglobulin that can be detected in the urine. [*see also*: B cell, Bence Jones protein, electrophoresis]	S
multiple personality [301.xx]	Loss of connection between the normally integrated functions of conscious thought, perception of the environment, identity, and memory. This is done in an effort to repress traumatic memories. Two or more distinct personalities are present, each with its own identity (made up of some facets of the original personality) and	

A = Abbreviations Section   F = Figures Section   L = Laboratory Section   S = Synonyms Section
Sx (Symptoms)   Dx (Diagnosis)   Tx (Treatment)

history. Each personality is capable of independent thoughts and actions and may be unaware of the other personalities.

multiple sclerosis
[340.xx]

Chronic, progressive, degenerative autoimmune disease in which the body makes antibodies against myelin. There is acute inflammation of the nerves and loss of myelin with interruption of nerve conduction in the brain and spinal cord, which eventually become scar tissue known as plaques. [see also: autoimmune disease, myelin]

A
L
S

Dx   H&P. Emphasis on neurological exam. A scanning MRI will detect the presence of plaques. A lumbar puncture will be performed to analyze the CSF. An EEG with evoked response is performed to test the time it takes for the patient to respond to stimuli. [see also: cerebrospinal fluid examination, neurogenic bladder, nystagmus]

Tx   There is no known cure. Some medications may decrease the frequency of attacks or slow the progression of the disease. Other medications are given for the underlying symptoms and to provide comfort.

Munchausen syndrome [301.xx]

Exhibiting factitious medical or psychiatric symptoms. Patients are aware that they are lying, but are unaware that their motivation is the desire for assistance, attention, compassion, pity, and being excused from the normal expectations of life. Patients are not concerned about the cost of multiple tests, treatments, or surgeries and, in fact, desire to have them.

Munchausen by proxy: Patient creates illness in another person, usually a child. The parent, usually the mother, makes up a medical history, induces physical symptoms with drugs, or contaminates laboratory tests. The parent vicariously lives the role of being sick while simultaneously enjoying attention as the sacrificing, loving caregiver.

murmur
[728.xx–785.xx]

Abnormal heart sound created by turbulence as blood leaks past a defective heart valve. Murmurs are described according to their volume (soft or loud), their sound, and when they occur during the cardiac cycle. [see also: chordae tendineae, valve]

muscle

Many muscle fascicles grouped together and surrounded by fascia. [see also: origin]

muscle biopsy

Surgical procedure that is performed to make a definitive diagnosis when muscle weakness could be caused by many different muscular diseases. An incision is made into the muscle and a piece of tissue is removed. Alternatively, a needle is inserted and some tissue is aspirated through the needle. [see also: atrophy, dermatomyositis, muscular dystrophy, necrosis, polymyositis]

muscle fiber

One muscle cell. So named because it stretches over a long distance.

muscle spasm

Painful but temporary condition with a sudden, severe, involuntary, and prolonged contraction of a muscle, usually in the legs. Often brought on by over-exercise. [see also: contraction, dyskinesia, pain management, spastic paralysis, temporomandibular joint syndrome]

S

muscle strain

Overstretching of a muscle, often due to physical overexertion, causing inflammation, pain, swelling, and bruising as capillaries in the muscle tear. There can be small tears in the muscle fibers. [see also: sprain]

S

muscle strength test

Medical procedure used to test the strength of certain muscle groups. Muscle strength (or motor strength) is measured on a

A = Abbreviations Section   F = Figures Section   L = Laboratory Section   S = Synonyms Section
Sx (Symptoms)   Dx (Diagnosis)   Tx (Treatment)

scale of 0–5, with 5 being normal strength and 0 being the inability to move the muscles being tested. [*see also*: physical therapy, rehabilitation exercises]

muscular dystrophy [359.xx]

Genetic inherited disease due to a mutation of the gene that makes the muscle protein dystrophin, which causes the muscles to weaken and then atrophy. Weakness of the diaphragm muscle and inability to breathe is the most frequent cause of death. [*see also*: creatine phosphokinase MM bands, muscle biopsy]

A L S

musculature

Group of skeletal muscles in one body part or the muscles in the body as a whole.

myalgia [729.xx]

Pain in one or more muscles due to injury or muscle disease. [*see also*: fibromyalgia, hypokalemia, pain management, polymyalgia]

S

myasthenia gravis [358.xx]

Abnormal and rapid fatigue of the muscles, particularly evident in the muscles of the face. The body produces antibodies against its own acetylcholine receptors located on muscle fibers. The antibodies destroy many of the receptors. [*see also*: acetylcholine, autoimmune disease, blepharoptosis]

L S

Dx H&P with an emphasis on the neurological exam. An EMG will be performed to evaluate the nerves. Lab tests will be performed to detect the presence of antibodies, but the definitive diagnosis is the injection of medications that increase acetylcholine in the body. [*see also*: acetylcholine receptor antibodies, electromyelography, Tensilon test]

Tx Medications to prolong the action of acetylcholine once it attaches to a receptor, and other medications to treat the symptoms. If the disease is advanced or severe enough, plasmapheresis may be performed to remove the antibodies. Thymectomy to remove the thymus. [*see also*: plasmapheresis, thymectomy]

mydriasis [379.xx]

Relaxation of the iris muscle to increase the size of the pupil and increase the amount of light entering the eye. [*see also*: anisocoria, miosis, pupillary response]

myelin

Fatty sheath around the axon of a neuron. It acts as an insulator to keep the electrical impulse intact. Myelin around the axons of neurons in the brain and spinal cord is produced by oligodendroglia cells. Myelin around the axons of the cranial and spinal nerves is produced by the Schwann cells. An axon with myelin is said to be myelinated. [*see also*: axon, diabetic neuropathy, Guillain-Barré syndrome, multiple sclerosis, oligodendroglia, Schwann cell, white matter]

myelocyte

Immature cell that comes from a myeloblast in the red bone marrow and develops into a neutrophil, eosinophil, or basophil.

F

myelography

Contrast dye is injected into the subarachnoid space at the level of the L3 and L4 vertebrae. It outlines the spinal cavity, spinal nerves, nerve roots, intervertebral disks, and shows tumors and herniated disks. Because myelograms can have the side effect of severe headache, a CT scan or MRI scan of the spine is often performed instead. [*see also*: magnetic resonance imaging]

myocardial infarction [410.xx; 412.xx]

Death of myocardial cells due to severe ischemia. The flow of oxygenated blood in a coronary artery is blocked by a blood clot or atherosclerosis. The patient may experience severe angina pectoris, may have mild symptoms like indigestion, or may have no symptoms at all (a silent MI). The infarcted area of myocardium

A L S

has necrosis. If the area of necrosis is small, it will eventually be replaced by scar tissue. If the area is large, the heart muscle may be unable to contract. [see also: arteriosclerosis, atherosclerosis]

Dx H&P. An EKG will be performed to demonstrate heart function. Depending on severity, an angiography may be performed to visualize the coronary arteries. Lab tests will be performed to determine heart damage. [see also: angina pectoris, cardiac catheterization, cardiac enzymes, lactate dehydrogenase]

Tx Medications to dissolve the clot and provide relief of symptoms. Angioplasty or stent placement may be performed. If severe enough, the patient may have bypass surgery. [see also: coronary artery bypass graft, percutaneous transluminal coronary angioplasty]

myocardial perfusion scan	Nuclear medicine procedure that combines a cardiac exercise stress test with intravenous injections of a radioactive tracer. The radioactive tracer collects in those parts of the myocardium that have the best perfusion. A gamma camera records gamma rays emitted by the radioactive tracer and creates a two-dimensional image of the heart. Areas of decreased uptake ("cold spots") on the image indicate poor perfusion from a blocked coronary artery. The artery must be about 70% blocked before any abnormality is evident on the image. Areas of no uptake indicate dead tissue from a previous myocardial infarction. [see also: stress test]
myocardium	Muscular wall of the heart. [see also: endocardium, epicardium, myocardium, pericardium] **F**
myofibril	Thin filament (actin) and thick filament (myosin) within the skeletal muscle fiber that give it its characteristic striated appearance. [see also: muscle fiber]
myomectomy	Surgical procedure to remove leiomyomata or fibroids from the uterus. This procedure can be done vaginally or through a laparoscope inserted into the abdomen. [see also: leiomyoma]
myometritis [615.xx]	Inflammation or infection of the myometrium. Associated with pelvic inflammatory disease. [see also: pyometritis]
myometrium	Smooth muscle layer of the uterine wall. It contracts during menstruation to expel the endometrial lining or during labor and delivery of the newborn. [see also: menstruation, myometritis] **F**
myopathy [359.xx]	Category that includes many different diseases of the muscles. [see also: cardiomyopathy, muscular dystrophy, myositis]
myopia [367.xx]	Light rays from a near object focus correctly on the retina, creating a sharp image. However, light rays from a far object come into focus anterior to the retina, creating a blurred image. People who suffer from myopia often half-close their eyelids and squint to improve their nearsightedness. [see also: hyperopia] **S**
myorrhaphy	Surgical procedure to suture together the torn ends of a muscle following an injury.
myositis [782.xx–729.xx]	Inflammation of a muscle with localized swelling and tenderness. Can be caused by injury or strain. [see also: dermatomyositis, polymyositis] **S**
myringotomy	Surgical procedure that uses a myringotome to make an incision in the tympanic membrane to drain fluid from the middle ear. For chronic middle ear infections, a ventilating tube can also be inserted through the incision to form a permanent opening into the middle ear known as a tympanostomy. [see also: hemotympanum]

N

Nägele's rule
Used to calculate the patient's due date or estimated date of birth (EDB). Often the patient does not remember when the date of the first day of her last menstrual period occurred, so the EDB is just an approximation. [see also: cesarean section, induction of labor]

nail plate   S
Hard, flat, protective covering over the distal end of each finger and toe. It is composed of dead cells that contain keratin. [see also: lunula, onychomycosis, paronychia]

nail root
Produces cells that form the lunula and nail plate. [see also: lunula, nail plate]

narcissistic personality [301.xx]   S
Exaggerated sense of self-worth and importance. Patients feel superior to others and believe they are entitled to be the center of attention and to receive compliments, admiration, and affection. They are angry, demanding, and manipulative if others receive more than they do. Their demand to be noticed can be emotional, dramatic, and done for its effect.

narcolepsy [347.xx]   S
Brief, involuntary episodes of falling asleep during the daytime while engaged in activity. The patient is not unconscious and can be aroused, but is unable to prevent falling asleep. [see also: polysomnography]

naris
One nostril, the opening into a nasal cavity.

nasal cavity   F
Hollow area inside the nose, formed by the facial bones and lined with mucosa. Inhaled air flows into it.

nasal polyp [471.xx]
Benign growth from the mucous membrane of the nose or sinuses. A single polyp or several polyps may grow large enough to limit the flow of air.

nasal septum
Wall of cartilage and bone that divides the right and left nostrils from each other.

nasolabial fold
Skin crease in the cheek from the nose to the corner of the mouth.

nasolacrimal duct
Tube that carries tears from the lacrimal sac to the inside of the nose. [see also: lacrimal sac]

nasopharynx   F
Uppermost portion of the throat where the posterior nares unite. The nasopharynx contains the openings for the eustachian tubes and the adenoids.

natural killer cell   A
Type of lymphocyte that matures in the red bone marrow and, without the help of antibodies or complement, recognizes and destroys pathogens.

nausea [787.xx]
An unpleasant, queasy feeling in the stomach that precedes the urge to vomit. [see also: dyspepsia, emesis, hyperemesis gravidarum, migraine headache, motion sickness, radiation therapy]

necrosis
Gray-to-black discoloration where tissue has died. [see also: acute tubular necrosis, avascular necrosis, cerebrovascular accident, gangrene, muscle biopsy, myocardial infarction, tuberculosis, tumor necrosis factor]

neonatal apnea [770.xx]
Temporary or permanent cessation of breathing in the neonate after birth. The immature central nervous system of a newborn fails to maintain a consistent respiratory rate, and there are occasional long pauses between periods of regular breathing.

neonatal jaundice [774.xx]
During gestation, the fetus has extra red blood cells that are no longer needed at birth. The immature newborn liver is not able to conjugate this much bilirubin (a breakdown product of red blood cells) and it builds up in the blood and causes jaundice. The more

premature the infant, the greater the chance of developing jaundice. [*see also*: jaundice]

neonate	Newborn from the time of birth until 1 year of age.
neoplasm	General word for any growing tissue that is not part of normal body structure or function. It is either malignant or benign. Malignant neoplasms are known as cancer. [*see also*: TNM system] **S**
neoplastic disease	Caused by the growth of benign or malignant tumors. Examples: Benign cyst, cancerous tumors of the skin.
nephrectomy	Surgical procedure to remove a diseased or cancerous kidney. Alternatively, a healthy kidney may be removed from a donor so that it can be transplanted into a patient with renal failure. [*see also*: allograft, renal failure]
nephroblastoma [189.xx]	Cancerous tumor of the kidney that occurs in children and arises from residual embryonic or fetal tissue. **S**
nephrolithiasis [592.xx]	Kidney stone formation in the urinary system that varies in size from microscopic to large enough to block the ureter or fill the renal pelvis. [*see also*: hydronephrosis, lithogenesis, renal colic] **L**

<table>
<tr><td></td><td>**Dx**</td><td>H&P. KUB or ultrasound to visualize the stones. Sometimes an intravenous urography or retrograde urography is performed to visualize the kidney. [*see also*: pyelography] **S**</td></tr>
<tr><td></td><td>**Tx**</td><td>Medications to treat the underlying symptoms. The patient's urine is strained to catch the stones so they can be analyzed. If the stones are large enough, the patient may undergo lithotripsy to crush them or surgery to excise them. [*see also*: extracorporeal shock wave lithotripsy, nephrolithotomy]</td></tr>
</table>

nephrolithotomy	Surgical procedure in which a small incision is made in the skin and an endoscope is inserted in a percutaneous approach into the kidney to remove a kidney stone embedded in the renal pelvis or calices.
nephron	Microscopic functional unit of the kidney. [*see also*: Bowman's capsule, glomerulus]
nephropexy	Surgical procedure to correct a kidney that is in an abnormally low position by suturing it back into anatomical position. [*see also*: nephroptosis]
nephroptosis [593.xx]	Abnormally low position of a kidney. It sometimes requires surgery, but more often is mentioned as an incidental finding seen on an x-ray. [*see also*: nephropexy]
nephrotic syndrome [581.xx]	Damage to the glomeruli allows albumin to leak into the urine, decreasing the amount of blood proteins. This changes the osmotic pressure of the blood and allows fluid to go into the tissues, producing edema in the extremities, and into the abdominal cavity, producing ascites. [*see also*: ascites, albuminuria] **L**
nerve	A bundle of individual neurons. [*see also*: neuron]
nerve conduction study	Medical procedure to measure the speed at which an electrical impulse travels along a nerve. An electrode is used to stimulate a peripheral nerve with an electrical impulse. Another electrode, a measured distance away, records how long it takes for the electrical impulse to reach it. This test is usually performed in conjunction with electromyography to help differentiate between weaknesses due to nerve disorders versus muscle disorders. [*see also*: carpal tunnel syndrome, Guillain-Barré syndrome, Lou Gehrig's disease, neuropathy] **S**

nervous system	Body system that consists of the brain, cranial nerves, spinal cord, spinal nerves, and other structures. Its purpose is to receive nerve impulses from the body and send nerve impulses to the body. Anatomically, it consists of the central nervous system and the peripheral nervous system. Physiologically, it consists of the somatic nervous system and the autonomic nervous system.
neural tube defect [741.xx; 751.xx–759.xx]	Congenital abnormality of the neural tube, an embryonic structure that develops into the fetal brain and spinal cord. [*see also*: meningocele, spina bifida]
neuralgia	Pain along the path of a nerve and its branches. It is caused by an injury and can be mild to severe in nature. [*see also*: causalgia, pain management, tic douloureux]
neuritis	Inflammation or infection of a nerve. [*see also*: neuropathy, polyneuritis]
neurofibro-matosis [237.xx]	Hereditary disease with multiple benign tumors that arise from the peripheral nerves. Most noticeable on the skin, but they can also be present anywhere on or in the body. They range in size from small nodules to large tumors. S
neurogenic bladder [596.xx]	Urinary retention due to a lack of innervation of the nerves of the bladder. Caused by a spinal cord injury, spina bifida, multiple sclerosis, or Parkinson's disease. The bladder must be catheterized intermittently because it does not contract to expel urine. [*see also*: cystometry, straight catheter]
neuroglia	Cells that hold neurons in place and perform specialized tasks. Includes astrocytes, ependymal cells, microglia cells, oligodendroglia cells, and Schwann cells.
neuroma	Benign tumor of a nerve or any of the specialized cells of the nervous system. [*see also*: acoustic neuroma, Morton's neuroma, neurofibromatosis]
neuromuscular junction	Area on a single muscle fiber where a nerve connects to it.
neuron	An individual nerve cell, the functional part of the nervous system. [*see also*: Alzheimer's disease, dementia, epilepsy, seizures]
neuropathy	General category for any type of disease or injury to a nerve. [*see also*: diabetic neuropathy, Guillain-Barré syndrome, nerve conduction study, shingles, syphilis]
neurotransmitter	Chemicals that relay messages from one neuron to another. [*see also*: acetylcholine, dopamine, endorphins, epinephrine, serotonin]
neutrophil	Most numerous type of leukocyte. It is classified as a granulocyte, but granules in its cytoplasm do not readily stain red or blue but remain neutral in color. The nucleus has several segmented lobes. This cell is a phagocyte that eats bacteria and cellular debris. [*see also*: complete blood count] F L S
nevus	Benign skin lesion that is present at birth and comes in a variety of colors and shapes. [*see also*: birthmark, dysplastic nevus, electrodesiccation, laser surgery] S
night blindness [386.xx]	Marked decrease in visual acuity at night or in dim light. This occurs with aging or when the diet does not contain enough vitamin A. [*see also*: blindness, presbyopia, retinitis pigmentosa]
nipple	Projecting point of the breast where the lactiferous ducts converge. It is surrounded by the pigmented areola.
nocturia [788.xx]	Increased frequency and urgency of urination during the night. It can be due to cystitis, an enlarged prostate gland, or decreased

A= Abbreviations Section   F= Figures Section   L= Laboratory Section   S= Synonyms Section
Sx(Symptoms)   Dx(Diagnosis)   Tx(Treatment)

	capacity of the bladder due to aging. [*see also*: nocturnal enuresis, urination]	
nocturnal enuresis [788.xx]	Involuntary urination during sleep. It is only considered a disease in older children or adults who should have voluntary bladder control. [*see also*: encopresis]	S
nondisplaced fracture	Broken bone ends remain in their normal anatomical alignment. [*see also*: fracture]	
non-Hodgkin's lymphoma [200.xx; 202.xx]	A group of more than 20 different types of lymphomas that occur in older adults and do not show Reed-Sternberg cells. [*see also*: Hodgkin's lymphoma]	
non-stress test	An external monitor on the mother's abdomen prints out the fetal heart rate. A normal test (reactive test) will show at least two fetal heart rate accelerations associated with fetal movement. A non-reactive test is abnormal. It is followed up by a biophysical profile that combines a non-stress test with an ultrasound to rate fetal movement, fetal heart rate, and amniotic fluid volume.	A
norepinephrine	Hormone secreted by the adrenal medulla in response to stimulation by nerves of the parasympathetic nervous system. It controls the daily involuntary processes of the body.	S
normal sinus rhythm	A heart rate of 70 to 80 beats per minute that is the normal resting rate set by the sinoatrial node. [*see also*: conduction system, dysrhythmia]	A
nosocomial disease	A new disease in a hospitalized patient because of exposure to the hospital environment. Example: Surgical wound infection.	
nuchal cord [762.xx]	Umbilical cord is wrapped around the neck of the fetus. A loose nuchal cord can be an incidental finding that causes no problems. A tight nuchal cord with one or more loops around the neck can impair blood flow to the brain, causing brain damage or fetal death. [*see also*: prolapsed cord]	S
nuclear medicine	Uses radioactive substances to create images of the internal structures of the body. [*see also*: Cardiolite stress test, myocardial perfusion scan, positron emission tomography, radioactive iodine uptake and thyroid scan, radionuclide ventriculography, renal scan, scintigraphy, SPECT scan, ventilation-perfusion scan]	
nucleolus	Round, central region within the nucleus. It makes RNA and ribosomes. [*see also*: nucleus]	
nucleus	Large, round, centralized intracellular body that contains chromosomes and their DNA. It controls all of the cell's activities. It is surrounded by a nuclear membrane. [*see also*: nucleolus]	
nutritional disease	Caused by lack of nutritious food, insufficient amounts of food, or an inability to utilize nutrients in the food. Examples: Malnutrition, pernicious anemia caused by lack of intrinsic factor production in the stomach.	
nystagmus [379.xx]	Involuntary rhythmic motions of the eye, particularly when looking to the side. Each back-and-forth motion is known as a "beat." Nystagmus can be caused by multiple sclerosis or Ménière's disease.	

O

oblique	On a slant or angle midway between anterior and lateral. [*see also*: coronal plane, midsagittal plane, projection]	
oblique fracture	Bone is broken on an oblique angle. [*see also*: fracture, oblique]	

A= Abbreviations Section   **F**= Figures Section   **L**= Laboratory Section   **S**= Synonyms Section
Sx(Symptoms)   **Dx**(Diagnosis)   **Tx**(Treatment)

obsessive-compulsive disorder [300.xx]	Constant, persistent, uncontrollable thoughts (obsessions) that occupy the mind, cause anxiety, and compel the patient to perform excessive, repetitive, meaningless activities (compulsions) for fear of what might happen if these are not done. These activities consume a significant portion of each day. [*see also*: Tourette's syndrome] **A**

> **Dx**   Utilization of the DSM-IV criteria. There is impairment in life, work, or social activities, or the patient spends more than one hour per day performing obsessive and/or compulsive activities.
>
> **Tx**   Psychological or psychiatric intervention may be warranted. [*see also*: cognitive-behavioral therapy, psychotherapy]

obsessive-compulsive personality [301.xx]	Inflexible and perfectionistic. Patients feel that everything must be accounted for and in its place, nothing can be left to chance, and they are unwilling to compromise. Patients feel that there is always one best way to do everything and they expect others to act accordingly. Patients keep lists and schedules and are concerned about productivity, but may be so consumed by minor details that they sometimes cannot get the job done. These patients do not have obsessive-compulsive disorder.
obstetrical history	Good prenatal care includes documentation of past pregnancies and deliveries. In the past, documentation of the number of pregnancies, deliveries, and abortions was done using the gravida (G), para (P), and abortion (A) system. Now, the G/TPAL is more commonly used to track each pregnancy and its outcome, because it also includes term (T) and living (L) births.
obstipation [564.xx]	Severe, unrelieved constipation. [*see also*: constipation, defecation, fecalith]
occipital lobe	Lobe of the cerebrum that receives and analyzes sensory information from the eyes. Contains the visual cortex for the sense of sight. [*see also*: visual cortex] **F**
oculomotor nerve	Cranial nerve III. Movement of the eyeball, upper eyelid, pupil, and lens. [*see also*: convergence, pupillary response] **S**
olfactory cortex	Area in the temporal lobe of the cerebrum that receives and analyzes nerve impulses from the nose. **S**
olfactory nerve	Cranial nerve I. Sense of smell. [*see also*: anosmia]
oligodendroglia	Cells that form the myelin sheath around axons of neurons in the brain and spinal cord. [*see also*: myelin, Schwann cell]
oligohydramnios [658.xx]	Decreased volume of amniotic fluid. The fetus swallows amniotic fluid but does not excrete a similar volume in its urine because of a congenital abnormality of the fetal kidneys. [*see also*: polyhydramnios] **S**
oligomenorrhea [626.xx]	Very light menstrual flow or infrequent menstrual cycles (longer than 35 days between the end of one cycle and the beginning of the next cycle) in a woman who previously had normal menstruation. It is caused by a hormone imbalance. [*see also*: menorrhagia, menstruation] **S**
oligospermia [606.xx]	Less than normal amount of spermatozoa produced by the testes. This results in male infertility. Caused by a hormone imbalance or an undescended testicle. [*see also*: cryptorchism, FSH assay and LH assay, varicocele]

oliguria [788.xx]
Decreased production of urine associated with kidney failure, although dehydration can be a temporary cause. [*see also*: renal failure, urination]

omentum
Broad, fatty pouch of peritoneum that supports the stomach and hangs down over the small intestine to protect and cushion it. [*see also*: peritoneum]

omphalocele [756.xx]
An umbilical hernia that is present at birth and only has a thin covering of peritoneum without any abdominal skin or subcutaneous fat. [*see also*: hernia, umbilical hernia] S

oncogene
Damaged and mutated genes that cause a cell to become cancerous. A virus can carry an oncogene in its RNA. Then when it enters a normal cell, the oncogene becomes incorporated into the cell's DNA and changes it into a cancerous cell.

OncoScint scan
Nuclear medicine procedure that uses scintigraphy and the radiopharmaceutical indium-111 as a tracer to create an image of metastases from cancer of the colon or ovary. The indium is attached to a monoclonal antibody that binds to receptors on the cancerous cells. The indium plus monoclonal antibody is the trade name drug OncoScint. [*see also*: colon]

onychomycosis [110.xx]
Fungal infection of the fingernails or toenails. A fungus infects the nail root and deforms the nail as it grows. The nail is discolored, misshapen, thickened, and raised up from the nail bed. [*see also*: herpes whitlow, paronychia]

oocyte
Immature egg in the fetal ovary. [*see also*: ovary, ovum]

oogenesis
Production of a mature ovum from an oocyte through the processes of mitosis and then meiosis. [*see also*: spermatogenesis]

oophorectomy
Surgical procedure to remove an ovary because of large ovarian cysts or ovarian cancer. A bilateral oophorectomy removes both ovaries. [*see also*: hysterectomy, salpingectomy]

open reduction and internal fixation
Surgical procedure to treat a complicated fracture. An incision is made at the fracture site, the fracture is realigned, and an internal fixation procedure is done using screws, nails, or plates to hold the fracture fragments in correct anatomical alignment. [*see also*: fracture] A

open-angle glaucoma [365.xx]
Increased intraocular pressure because aqueous humor cannot circulate freely. The angle where the edges of the iris and cornea touch is normal and open, but the trabecular meshwork is blocked. While painless, it destroys peripheral vision, leaving the patient with tunnel vision. Glaucoma can progress to blindness. [*see also*: glaucoma, gonioscopy, trabeculoplasty]

oppositional defiant disorder [313.xx]
Persistent, aggressive behavior (fighting, arguing, provoking, annoying), defiance of and refusal to obey rules, disrespect for authority figures, with anger, stubbornness, and touchiness. [*see also*: conduct disorder]

optic chiasm
Crossroads in the brain where parts of the right and left optic nerves cross and join the optic nerve on the opposite side.

optic disk
Bright yellow-white circle on the retina where the optic nerve and retinal arteries enter the posterior cavity. It cannot perceive visual images and is known as the blind spot. F

optic globe
The eyeball.

optic nerve
Cranial nerve II. A sensory nerve that carries nerve impulses of visual images from the rods and cones of the retina to the visual cortex in the brain. [*see also*: visual cortex] F S

A = Abbreviations Section   F = Figures Section   L = Laboratory Section   S = Synonyms Section
Sx (Symptoms)   Dx (Diagnosis)   Tx (Treatment)

oral cavity	Hollow area inside the mouth that contains the tongue, teeth, hard and soft palates, uvula, and salivary glands. It is lined with oral mucosa.	F S
oral cholecysto-graphy	Radiologic procedure that uses tablets of radiopaque contrast dye taken orally. The tablets dissolve in the intestine. The contrast dye is absorbed into the blood, travels to the liver, and is excreted with bile into the gallbladder. An x-ray is taken to identify stones in the gallbladder and biliary ducts or thickening of the gallbladder wall.	A
OraSure	Quick screening test done in a doctor's office or clinic that detects antibodies to HIV in the saliva. [*see also*: enzyme-linked immunosorbent assay, p24 antigen test, viral load test, Western blot]	
orbit	Bony socket in the cranium that surrounds all but the anterior part of the eyeball.	
orchiectomy	Surgical procedure to remove a testis because of testicular cancer. [*see also*: testes]	
orchiopexy	Surgical procedure to reposition an undescended testicle and fix it within the scrotum. [*see also*: cryptorchism]	
orchitis [604.xx]	Inflammation or infection of the testes. Usually caused by a bacterium, the mumps virus, or trauma. [*see also*: bacteriuria, testes]	S
organelles	Small structures in the cytoplasm of a cell that have various specialized functions. Organelles include mitochondria, ribosomes, the endoplasmic reticulum, the Golgi apparatus, and lysosomes. [*see also*: cytoplasm]	
origin	Where a muscle begins and is attached to a stationary or nearly stationary bone.	
oropharynx	Middle portion of the throat just behind the the oral cavity. It begins at the level of the soft palate and ends at the epiglottis. It contains the palatine tonsils. [*see also*: pharynx]	F
orthopnea [786.xx]	Lung disease that causes the patient to assume an upright or semi-upright position in order to breathe and sleep comfortably due to dyspnea and congestion in the lungs that occur when lying down. [*see also*: dyspnea]	
orthosis	Orthopedic device such as a brace, splint, or collar that is used to immobilize or correct an orthopedic problem. These are often custom made to fit the patient's specific measurements. [*see also*: brace, cast, prosthesis]	
orthostatic hypotension [458.xx]	The sudden, temporary, but self-correcting decrease in systolic blood pressure that occurs when the patient changes from a lying to a standing position and experiences lightheadedness.	
osseous tissue	Bone, which is a type of connective tissue.	
ossicles	Three tiny bones in the middle ear that function in the process of hearing: malleus, incus, and stapes. [*see also*: cholesteatoma, conductive hearing loss, sensorineural hearing loss]	S F
ossification	Process by which cartilaginous tissue is changed into bone from infancy through puberty.	
osteoblast	Osteocyte that forms new bone or rebuilds bone. [*see also*: fracture]	
osteoclast	Osteocyte that breaks down old or damaged areas of bone. [*see also*: fracture]	

A= Abbreviations Section   **F**= Figures Section   **L**= Laboratory Section   **S**= Synonyms Section
Sx(Symptoms)   **Dx**(Diagnosis)   **Tx**(Treatment)

osteocyte	Bone cell. There are two types: osteoclasts and osteoblasts. [*see also*: osteoblast, osteoclast]	
osteomalacia [268.xx]	Abnormal softening of the bones due to a deficiency of vitamin D or inadequate exposure to the sun. [*see also*: chrondomalacia patellae, rickets]	L S
osteomyelitis [730.xx]	Infection in the bone and the bone marrow. Bacteria enter the bone following an open fracture, crush injury, or surgical procedure. [*see also*: bone scintigraphy]	S
osteoporosis [733.xx]	Abnormal thinning of the bone structure. Occurs in postmenopausal women and elderly men. A lack of dietary calcium and a lack of exercise contribute to the process. [*see also*: bone density tests, densitometry, dual energy x-ray absorptiometry, pathological fracture, quantitative computerized tomography]	L
otitis externa [380.xx]	Bacterial infection of the external auditory canal. There is throbbing earache pain with a swollen, red canal and serous or purulent drainage. Caused by a foreign body in the ear or the patient scratching or probing inside the ear. [*see also*: otorrhea]	S
otitis media [381.xx]	Acute or chronic bacterial infection of the middle ear. Symptoms include myringitis and otalgia. There can be a collection of fluid behind the tympanic membrane that creates an air-fluid level. This fluid can be serous or suppurative. Otitis media is common in young children because the short eustachian tube is in a nearly horizontal position that allows bacteria to enter from the nasopharynx. If left untreated, the tympanic membrane can rupture or the bones of the middle ear can degenerate, resulting in permanent hearing loss. The mastoid process of the temporal bone also can become infected. [*see also*: cholesteatoma, otorrhea]	
otoplasty	Surgical procedure that uses plastic surgery to correct deformities of the external ear such as correcting a protruding ear, which is known as an ear pinning.	
otorrhea [388.xx]	Drainage of serous fluid or pus from the ear. It can be caused by otitis externa or otitis media (with a ruptured tympanic membrane). It can also be caused by a fracture of the temporal bone of the cranium with leakage of cerebrospinal fluid.	
otosclerosis [387.xx]	Abnormal formation of bone in the inner ear, particularly between the stapes and the oval window. The stapes becomes immoveable, causing conductive hearing loss. Certain families have a genetic predisposition to develop otosclerosis. [*see also*: conductive hearing loss, mixed hearing loss, ossicles]	
otoscopy	Medical procedure to examine the external auditory canals and tympanic membranes. The physician gently pulls the helix of the external ear back and up, to straighten the external auditory canal and better visualize the tympanic membrane. In infants younger than 3, the helix is pulled back and down. The otoscope provides light and magnification. Some otoscopes have a rubber bulb that forces air into the external auditory canal. A normal tympanic membrane moves in and out in response.	
ova and parasites	Diagnostic test to determine if there is a parasitic infection of the gastrointestinal tract. Ova are the eggs of parasitic worms. They can be seen in the stool or by examining a sample of stool under a microscope. [*see also*: wet mount]	A
oval window	Opening in the temporal bone between the middle ear and the vestibule of the inner ear. The opening is covered by the end of the stapes.	F

A= Abbreviations Section   **F**= Figures Section   **L**= Laboratory Section   **S**= Synonyms Section
Sx(Symptoms)   **Dx**(Diagnosis)   **Tx**(Treatment)

ovaries
Endocrine glands near the uterus. FSH from the anterior pituitary gland stimulates the ovary to develop follicles and stimulates the follicles to secrete estradiol. [*see also*: alpha fetoprotein, BRCA1 or BRCA2 gene, corpus luteum, culdoscopy, follicle, FSH assay and LH assay, Her2/neu, oocyte, oophorectomy, pelvic inflammatory disease, polycystic ovary syndrome, precocious puberty, tumor markers (CA 125)]

overactive bladder [596.xx]
Urinary urgency and frequency due to involuntary contractions of the bladder wall as the bladder fills with urine. This sometimes causes incontinence. [*see also*: cystometry, incontinence, urination]

ovulation
Day 14 of the menstrual cycle when LH from the anterior pituitary gland causes the ovarian follicle to rupture, releasing the mature ovum. The menstrual cycle consists of the menstrual phase, proliferative phase, secretory phase, ovulation, and ischemic phase. [*see also*: anovulation, dysfunctional uterine bleeding, follicle, infertility, luteinizing hormone, menstrual cycle, ovaries, ovum, precocious puberty]

ovum
An egg within a follicle in the ovary. A mature ovum is released during ovulation. An ovum is a gamete because it has only 23 chromosomes. [*see also*: anovulation, fertilization, fimbriae, gamete, human chorionic gonadotropin, hydatidiform mole, oogenesis, ovulation, polycystic ovary syndrome, pregnancy test, zygote]   S

oxygen
Inhaled gas that is transported to each cell and used to produce energy in the process of metabolism. [*see also*: anoxia, arterial blood gases, blood, carboxyhemoglobin, clubbing, cyanosis, deoxygenated, erythrocyte, hemoglobin, hypoxemia, metabolism, oxygenated, oxyhemoglobin, pulse oximetry, respiration, retrolental fibroplasia]   A

oxygen therapy
Medical procedure to provide supplemental oxygen to patients with pulmonary disease. Room air is 21% oxygen. Patients with respiratory conditions may require amounts of oxygen ranging from 22% to 100%. Oxygen can be delivered to a patient via a nasal cannula, face mask, or a respirator. Oxygen alone is very drying, so it is humidified. [*see also*: adult respiratory distress syndrome, arterial blood gases]

oxygenated
Blood that contains high levels of oxygen. [*see also*: cyanosis, deoxygenated, erythrocyte, hemoglobin, pulse oximetry]

oxyhemoglobin
Compound that transports oxygen in the blood and is formed by the combination of oxygen with the hemoglobin of red blood cells. [*see also*: hemoglobin]

oxytocin
Hormone released by the posterior pituitary gland. It stimulates the uterus to contract and begin labor. It also stimulates the let-down reflex to get milk flowing for breastfeeding. [*see also*: induction of labor, lactation, posterior pituitary gland, postpartum hemorrhage, uterine inertia]

P

p24 antigen test
Detects p24, a protein in HIV. The results are reported as a titer. This test is also used to screen donated blood for the presence of HIV. [*see also*: blood donation, blood transfusion, enzyme-linked immunosorbent assay, OraSure, viral load test, Western blot]

pacemaker insertion
Surgical procedure in which an automated device is implanted to control the heart rate and rhythm. Pacemakers use two or three wires (or leads) positioned to coordinate the heart beat with an electrical impulse. [*see also*: conduction system, dysrhythmia]

---

pain management	This subspecialty for treating chronic or severe pain is shared by both neurology and anesthesiology. Pain management procedures include a dorsal nerve root injection into an area where a nerve is compressed. Surgical treatment includes a rhizotomy, an incision to cut spinal nerve roots. The dorsal (sensory) nerve roots can be cut to relieve severe pain. The ventral (motor) nerve roots can be cut to relieve severe muscle spasticity and spasm. [see also: causalgia, complex regional pain syndrome, corticosteroid injection, muscle spasm, myalgia, neuralgia, sciatica, tenosynovitis, torticollis, transcutaneous electrical nerve stimulation, tic douloureux, trigger point injections]	
palate	The hard bone and posterior soft, fleshy area that form the roof of the mouth. [see also: oral cavity]	S F
palatine tonsils	Lymphoid tissue on either side of the throat where the soft palate arches downward in the oropharynx. [see also: tonsillitis]	F
pallor [782.xx]	Unnatural paleness due to a lack of blood supply to the tissue. [see also: cyanosis]	S
palpitation [785.xx]	An uncomfortable sensation felt in the chest during a premature contraction of the heart. It is often described as a "thump." [see also: conduction system, premature contraction]	S
pancreas	Triangular endocrine gland located in the abdominal cavity, posterior to the stomach. It contains the islets of Langerhans (alpha, beta, and delta cells) that produce and secrete the hormones glucagon, insulin, and somatostatin. It also produces digestive enzymes (amylase, lipase, protease, peptidase) and releases them into the duodenum. [see also: diabetes mellitus, fasting blood sugar, glucose tolerance test, hyperinsulinism, pancreatitis, tumor markers (CA 19-9)]	F L
pancreatitis [577.xx]	Inflammation or infection of the pancreas. [see also: pancreas]	
pancytopenia [284.xx]	Decreased numbers of all types of blood cells due to failure of the bone marrow to produce stem cells. [see also: anemia, aplastic anemia, leukemia]	
panhypopituitarism [253.xx]	Condition in which there is hyposecretion of all of the hormones of the anterior pituitary gland. [see also: anterior pituitary gland, hypopituitarism]	S
panic disorder [300.xx]	Sudden attacks of severe, overwhelming anxiety without an identifiable cause. Patients often feel that they are choking or dying of a heart attack. [see also: anxiety disorder, borderline personality, cognitive-behavioral therapy]	
pansinusitis [461.xx; 473.xx]	Acute or chronic bacterial infection in all of the sinus cavities, or all the sinuses on one side of the face. Symptoms include headache, pain in the face over the sinus, postnasal drainage, fatigue, and fever. [see also: ethmoid sinuses, frontal sinuses, maxillary sinuses, sinusitis, sphenoid sinuses]	
Papanicolaou smear	Cytology test used as a screening test to detect abnormal cells or carcinoma in situ in the cervix. A small plastic or wooden spatula is used to obtain ectocervical cells. Then a cytobrush is inserted into the cervical os to obtain endocervical cells. A cervical broom can obtain both types of cells at the same time and also test for HPV. The cell specimen is transferred to a glass slide and sprayed with a fixative. The slides are sent to the laboratory where the cells are examined under the microscope for abnormalities. The Bethesda system is used to report Pap smear results.	A S

[*see also*: cervical dysplasia, colposcopy, conization, dysplasia, exfoliative cytology, genital warts]

papilledema
[377.xx]

Inflammation and edema of the optic disk. Caused by increased intracranial pressure from a brain tumor or head trauma. [*see also*: diplopia, photophobia]   S

papilloma

Small, soft, flesh-colored growth of epidermis and dermis that protrudes outwardly. [*see also*: electrodesiccation]   S

paraplegia
[344.xx]

An injury to the lower spinal cord causing an inability to voluntarily move the muscles of the legs. [*see also*: flaccid paralysis, quadriplegia, spastic paralysis, spinal cord injury]

**parasympathetic
nervous system**

Division of the autonomic nervous system that uses the neurotransmitter norepinephrine and carries nerve impulses to the heart, involuntary smooth muscles, and glands while the body is at rest. [*see also*: norepinephrine]

**parathyroid
glands**

Four endocrine glands on the posterior lobes of the thyroid gland. They produce and secrete parathyroid hormone. [*see also*: parathyroidectomy, parathyroid hormone]

**parathyroid
hormone**

Hormone secreted by the parathyroid glands. Along with calcitonin from the thyroid gland, it regulates the amount of calcium in the blood. If the calcium level is too low, parathyroid hormone moves calcium from the bones to the blood. [*see also*: calcitonin, hyperparathyroidism, hypoparathyroidism]   S

**parathy-
roidectomy**

Surgical procedure to remove one or more of the parathyroid glands to control hyperparathyoidism. Also, a parathyroidectomy can occur accidentally when the thyroid gland is surgically removed.

parenchyma

The functional area or unit of an organ.

paresthesia
[782.xx]

Condition in which abnormal sensations such as tingling, burning, or pinpricks are felt on the skin. Often the result of chronic nerve damage from pinched nerves or diabetic neuropathy. [*see also*: carpal tunnel syndrome, causalgia, diabetic neuropathy, hypothyroidism]

parietal lobe

Lobe of the cerebrum that receives and analyzes sensory information about temperature, touch, pressure, vibration, and pain from the skin and internal organs. [*see also*: Babinski's sign]   F

**parietal
pericardium**

Part of the pericardium that forms the outer wall of the pericardial sac. This sac is filled with pericardial fluid. [*see also*: cardiac tamponade]   S

parietal pleura

One of the two membranes of the pleura. It lines the thoracic cavity. [*see also*: thoracic cavity]

**Parkinson's
disease** [332.xx]

Chronic, degenerative disease due to an imbalance in the levels of the neurotransmitters dopamine and acetylcholine in the brain. [*see also*: acetylcholine, dopamine]   S

> **Dx** Definitive diagnosis is difficult and time consuming, as no distinctive diagnostic tests are available. Diagnosis is based on history and physical examinations repeated over time. [*see also*: bradykinesia, neurogenic bladder, positron emission tomography scan]
>
> **Tx** Presently there is no cure. Medications are provided to treat the underlying symptoms and provide comfort.

paronychia
[681.xx]

Inflammation and infection of the skin along the cuticle. [*see also*: herpes whitlow, onychomycosis]

paroxysmal nocturnal dyspnea

Shortness of breath that occurs at night. It is caused by fluid in the lungs because the patient is lying down. [*see also*: congestive heart failure, dyspnea] A

paroxysmal tachycardia [427.xx]

An episode of tachycardia, an arrhythmia in which there is a fast but regular rhythm (up to 200 beats/minute), that goes away without treatment. [*see also*: dysrhythmia]

partial thromboplastin time

Blood test to monitor the effectiveness of the anticoagulant drug heparin when it is given in regular dosages. A prolonged (rather than normal) PTT would be expected. [*see also*: activated clotting time, prothrombin time, thromboplastin] A

parturition

The process of labor and delivery. There are three stages: dilation and effacement of the cervix, delivery of the newborn, delivery of the placenta.

passive immunity

Immune response and defense against pathogens conveyed by the mother's antibodies to the fetus via the placenta or to the breastfeeding baby. These maternal antibodies provide protection from all the diseases the mother has had. [*see also*: active immunity, immunoglobulin A]

patent ductus arteriosus [747.xx]

Condition that occurs when the ductus arteriosus fails to close within 24 hours after birth. The ductus arteriosus is a normal fetal structure that allows the oxygenated blood to bypass the not-yet functioning fetal lungs. A

pathogen

Microorganism that causes a disease. Pathogens include bacteria, viruses, protozoa, and other microorganisms, as well as plant cells such as fungi or yeast. [*see also*: active immunity, antigen, complement proteins, culture and sensitivity, immunoglobulin G, immunoglobulin M, lysosome, microglia, natural killer cells, passive immunity, vaccination]

pathologic fracture [829.xx]

A fracture that is caused by a disease process such as osteoporosis, bone cancer, or metastases to the bone. [*see also*: fracture]

pectus excavatum [754.xx]

Congenital deformity in which the inferior tip of the sternum, particularly the xiphoid process, is bent inwards, creating a hollow depression in the anterior chest wall.

pediculosis [132.xx]

Infestation of lice and their eggs in the scalp, hair, eyelashes, or pubic hair. Lice are easily transmitted from one person to another by means of combs or hats. S

pedophilia [302.xx]

Obtaining power, control, and sexual arousal through contact or sexual acts with preadolescent children.

pelvic cavity

Cavity that is the inferior continuation of the abdominal cavity. It is surrounded by the pelvic bones and the base of the spinal column.

pelvic inflammatory disease [614.xx]

Infection of the cervix that ascends to the uterus, fallopian tubes, and ovaries. Often caused by a sexually transmitted disease. If untreated, it can cause scars in the fallopian tubes and infertility. [*see also*: dysmenorrhea, dyspareunia, infertility, myometritis, salpingitis, sexually transmitted diseases] A

pelvimetry

Medical procedure to determine the dimensions of the maternal bony pelvis to see if its size is adequate for a vaginal delivery. The measurement can be estimated by feel during a bimanual examination or measured on an x-ray of the pelvis. [*see also*: cephalopelvic disproportion, cesarean section, failure to progress]

penile implant	Surgical procedure to implant an inflatable penile prosthesis for patients with erectile dysfunction. [*see also*: impotence]
penis	Organ of erectile tissue that fills with blood during male sexual arousal. The corpora cavernosa are two columns of tissue that fill with blood along the upper surface of the penis. The corpus spongiosum is a column of tissue that fills with blood on the underside of the penis. The urethra travels through the corpus spongiosum. During sexual arousal, the penis becomes firm and erect (an erection). [*see also*: adrenogenital syndrome, balanitis, chordee, circumcision, dyspareunia, epispadias, hypospadias, impotence, phimosis, premature ejaculation, priapism, semen]
pepsin	Digestive enzyme from the stomach. It breaks down protein foods into large protein molecules. [*see also*: hydrochloric acid, pepsinogen]
pepsinogen	Substance produced by the stomach. It is converted by hydrochloric acid to the digestive enzyme pepsin. [*see also*: gastrin]
peptic ulcer disease [533.xx]	Chronic irritation, burning pain, and erosion of the mucosa of the esophagus, stomach, or duodenum to the point of forming an ulcer. [*see also*: *Campylobacter*-like organism test]
percutaneous endoscopic gastrostomy	A tube is inserted through the abdominal wall. Then, under visual guidance from an endoscope that was previously passed through the mouth into the stomach, the PEG tube is positioned in the stomach. [*see also*: gastrostomy]
percutaneous radiofrequency ablation	Surgical procedure in which a needle electrode or metal prong electrodes are placed through the skin and into a cancerous tumor less than 2 inches in diameter. High-frequency radiowaves (similar to microwaves) heat and kill the cancerous cells.
percutaneous transhepatic cholangiography	Radiologic procedure that uses a contrast dye to outline the bile ducts. A needle is passed through the abdominal wall, and the contrast dye is injected into the liver. An x-ray is taken to identify stones in the gallbladder and biliary ducts or thickening of the gallbladder wall. [*see also*: bile ducts, cholangiography]
percutaneous transluminal coronary angioplasty	Surgical procedure to reconstruct an artery that is narrowed because of atherosclerosis. A catheter is inserted into the femoral artery and threaded to the site of the stenosis. In a balloon angioplasty, a balloon within the catheter is inflated, compressing the atheromatous plaque and widening the lumen of the artery. The catheter and balloon are then removed. Alternatively, an intravascular stainless steel mesh stent can be inserted on the catheter. The catheter is removed, but the expanded stent remains in the artery. [*see also*: coronary artery disease, myocardial infarction]
percutaneous ultrasonic lithotripsy	An endoscope is inserted through the flank skin and into the kidney. A lithotriptor probe is inserted through the endoscope and into the kidney to break up large stones. Sometimes a holmium laser that generates a laser beam is used to break up very hard kidney stones. [*see also*: extracorporeal shock wave lithotripsy]
pericardiocentesis	Surgical procedure that uses a needle to puncture the pericardium and withdraw inflammatory fluid accumulated in the pericardial sac. Used to treat pericarditis and cardiac tamponade. [*see also*: cardiac tamponade]

(marginal section markers, top to bottom: F S *beside "penis";* S *beside "pepsinogen";* A *beside "peptic ulcer disease";* A *beside "percutaneous endoscopic gastrostomy";* A *beside "percutaneous transhepatic cholangiography";* A *beside "percutaneous transluminal coronary angioplasty")*

pericarditis [391.xx; 420.xx]	Inflammation or infection of the pericardial sac with an accumulation of pericardial fluid. [*see also*: cardiac tamponade, echocardiography]	
perimenopausal period	The time around menopause when menstrual periods first become irregular and menstrual flow is light. [*see also*: menopause]	
perineum	♀: The area between the edge of the vulva and the anus. [*see also*: episiotomy]	F
	♂: Area of skin between the anus and where the scrotum attaches to the body.	
periosteum	Thick, fibrous membrane that covers the outside surface of a bone.	
peripheral artery disease [443.xx]	Arteriosclerosis of the arteries of the legs. Blood flow to the extremities is poor, and there is ischemia of the tissues. While walking, the patient experiences pain in the calf. In severe PAD, the feet and toes remain cool and cyanotic and may become necrotic as the tissues die. [*see also*: arteriosclerosis, peripheral vascular disease]	A
peripheral nervous system	Division of the nervous system that includes the cranial nerves and the spinal nerves. [*see also*: diabetic neuropathy, Guillain-Barré syndrome, neurofibromatosis]	
peripheral vascular disease [459.xx]	Any disease of the arteries of the extremities. It includes peripheral artery disease as well as Raynaud's disease. [*see also*: peripheral artery disease, Raynaud's disease]	A
peripheral vision	Medical procedure to test the visual acuity at the edges of the visual field. The patient looks straight ahead while the physician moves an object from behind the patient's head toward the edge of the visual field. The patient indicates when the object is first seen. [*see also*: hemianopia, open-angle glaucoma, retinitis pigmentosa]	
peristalsis	Contractions of the smooth muscle that move substances through an organ or structure. [*see also*: ileus]	S
peritoneal dialysis	Medical procedure to remove waste products from the blood of patients in renal failure. A permanent catheter is inserted through the abdominal wall. Dialysate fluid flows through the catheter and remains in the abdominal cavity for several hours. During that time, the fluid pulls body wastes from the blood. Then the fluid is removed, carrying waste products with it. [*see also*: continuous ambulatory peritoneal dialysis, continuous cycling peritoneal dialysis, dialysis, hemodialysis]	
peritoneum	Membrane that lines the abdominopelvic cavity and secretes peritoneal fluid to fill the spaces between the organs. [*see also*: mesentery, omentum, peritonitis]	
peritonitis [567.xx]	Inflammation and infection of the peritoneum. [*see also*: peritoneum]	
pernicious anemia [281.xx]	Caused by a lack of vitamin B_{12} in the diet (from animal foods) or a lack of intrinsic factor in the stomach. Can be seen in vegetarians or the elderly. Untreated, it can cause permanent damage to the nerves. The erythrocytes are abnormally large and very immature. [*see also*: anemia, anisocytosis, Schilling test]	L S
perspiration	Process of sweating and the sweat itself. Sweat is produced by sudoriferous glands. It contains sodium and waste products. As its water content evaporates from the skin, it cools the body. [*see also*: anhidrosis, diaphoresis, sudoriferous gland]	S

A = Abbreviations Section   F = Figures Section   L = Laboratory Section   S = Synonyms Section
Sx (Symptoms)   Dx (Diagnosis)   Tx (Treatment)

petechiae [782.xx]	Pinpoint hemorrhages in the skin from ruptured capillaries. [see also: ecchymosis, hemorrhage]
petit mal seizure [345.xx]	Impaired consciousness with slight or no muscle activity. Muscle **S** tone is retained and the patient does not fall down, but is unable to respond to external stimuli. After an episode, the patient resumes activities and is unaware of the seizure. [see also: epilepsy, seizures]
phacoemul- sification	A small, self-sealing (stitchless) incision is made in the cornea. An ultrasonic probe is inserted and sound waves are used to break up the lens. The pieces are removed with irrigation and aspiration. The central part of the lens is removed and replaced with an artificial intraocular lens implant. The implant folds to pass through the incision and then unfolds. [see also: aphakia, astigmatism, cataract extraction, extracapsular cataract extraction]
phagocyte	Category of leukocytes that engulfs foreign cells and cellular **S** debris and destroys them with digestive enzymes. Phagocytes include neutrophils, eosinophils, and monocytes.
phagocytosis	The process by which a phagocyte destroys a foreign cell or cellular debris. [see also: phagocyte]
pharmacologic stress test	Performed in patients who cannot exercise vigorously. A vasodilator drug is given to cause normal coronary arteries to dilate. Occluded arteries cannot dilate, and this stresses the heart in a way that is similar to exercise and provokes angina. [see also: angina pectoris, stress test]
pharyngeal tonsils	Lymphoid tissue in the superior part of the nasopharynx. Also known as adenoids. [see also: tonsils] **S**
pharyngitis [462.xx; 472.xx]	Bacterial or viral infection of the throat. [see also: heterophil **S** antibody test, strep throat]
pharynx	The throat, a shared passageway for both air and food. It is **F** composed of the nasopharynx, oropharynx, and hypopharynx. **S**
pheochromo- cytoma [255.xx]	Hypersecretion of epinephrine and norepinephrine. Caused by **L** an adenoma in the adrenal medulla. There are headaches and severe hypertension that can cause a stroke. [see also: adrenal medulla, epinephrine]
	Dx H&P. The classic triad of symptoms is present: headache, heart palpitations, and sweating. Lab studies are done to measure hormone levels. Imaging studies to visualize the gland and tumor. [see also: cephalalgia, diaphoresis, palpitation]
	Tx Surgical removal of the tumor is paramount, but treating the cardiovascular symptoms associated with hypersecretion is also important. Medications may be given to block the hormone formation.
philtrum	Area with vertical grooves in the skin of the upper lip. [see also: cleft palate]
phimosis [605.xx]	Congenital condition in which the opening of the foreskin is too small to allow the foreskin to pull back over the glans penis. This traps smegma (a white, cheesy, discharge of skin cells and oil) and can cause an infection. [see also: balanitis, circumcision, dyspareunia]
phlebitis [451.xx]	Inflammation of a vein, usually accompanied by infection. The area around the vein is painful, and the skin may show a red streak that follows the course of the vein. A severe inflammation can

partially occlude the vein and slow the flow of blood. [see also: thrombophlebitis]

phlebotomy

Medical procedure for drawing a sample of venous blood into a vacuum tube. The vacuum tubes have different colored rubber stoppers that indicate what additive or anticoagulant is in the tube; this determines what blood test can be performed on the blood in that tube.

S

phobia [300.xx]

Intense, unreasonable fear of a specific thing or situation or even the thought of it. Phobias occur when the unconscious mind avoids a real, ongoing conflict by projecting the anxiety onto an unrelated situation or object. Avoidance of the phobia can severely restrict the normal activities of daily life. [see also: cognitive-behavioral therapy, hypnosis]

phorometry

Medical procedure to select the strength of lens that corrects the patient's refractive error and gives 20/20 vision. The specifications of that lens are written as a prescription that is duplicated in eyeglasses or contact lenses. [see also: accommodation, astigmatism]

photophobia [368.xx]

Abnormal sensitivity to bright light. Can be associated with inflammation and external or internal diseases of the eye, increased intracranial pressure, or migraine headache. [see also: closed-angle glaucoma, migraine headache, papilledema]

S

phrenic nerve

Nerve, that when stimulated, causes the diaphragm to contract and initiate respiration. [see also: respiration, vagus nerve]

physical therapy

Medical procedure that uses active or passive exercises to improve a patient's range of motion, joint mobility, and balance while walking. [see also: muscle strength test, rehabilitation exercises]

A

pia mater

Thin, delicate, innermost layer of the meninges. It covers the surface of the brain and contains many small blood vessels. [see also: meninges]

F

piloerection

Process in which erector muscles contract (to form a goose bump) and the body hair becomes erect when the skin is cold. This generates heat that is trapped as a layer of warm air near the surface of the skin.

pilonidal sinus [685.xx]

Abnormal passageway that begins as an enlarged, abnormal hair follicle that contains a hair that is never shed. Irritation causes the hair follicle to become infected, eventually creating a sinus into the subcutaneous tissue. [see also: boil, folliculitis]

pineal gland

Endocrine gland in the brain that lies posterior to the pituitary gland. It secretes the hormone melatonin, which controls the body's circadian rhythm. [see also: melatonin, seasonal affective disorder]

S

pink eye [372.xx]

Inflamed, reddened, and swollen conjunctiva with dilated blood vessels on the sclera. Caused by an acute contagious bacterial conjunctivitis. Patients have a mucus discharge from the eye. [see also: conjunctivitis]

S

pituitary gland

Endocrine gland in the brain that is connected by a stalk of tissue to the hypothalamus. It sits in the bony sella turcica of the sphenoid bone. It is known as the master gland of the body. It consists of the anterior pituitary gland and the posterior pituitary gland. [see also: anterior pituitary gland, posterior pituitary gland, transphenoidal hypophysectomy]

S

placenta

Large, pancake-like organ that develops from the chorion. It provides nutrients and oxygen to the developing fetus and

S

removes carbon dioxide and waste products. It assumes the job of the corpus luteum and secretes estradiol and progesterone to maintain the endometrium during pregnancy. [*see also*: abruptio placentae, chorion, corpus luteum, estradiol, fetal distress, immunoglobulin G, miscarriage, placenta previa, postpartum hemorrhage, progesterone, umbilical cord]

placenta previa
[641.xx]
Incorrect placement of the placenta with its edge partially or completely covering the cervical canal. During labor when the cervix dilates, the connection between the placenta and uterus is disrupted. This causes moderate-to-severe bleeding in the mother and disrupts the flow of blood to the fetus. [*see also*: dystocia]

plain film
Radiograph obtained without the use of a contrast dye. [*see also*: x-ray]

plane
An imaginary flat surface, like a plate of glass, that divides the body into parts. There are three planes: the coronal plane, midsagittal plane, and transverse plane. [*see also*: oblique]

plasma
Clear, straw-colored fluid portion of the blood that carries blood cells and contains dissolved substances such as proteins, glucose, minerals, electrolytes, clotting factors, complement proteins, hormones, bilirubin, urea, and creatinine. [*see also*: ABO blood group, blood, complement proteins, plasmapheresis, polycythemia vera, serum, type and crossmatch]

plasma proteins
Protein molecules in the blood. The most important one is albumin. [*see also*: albumin, complement proteins]

plasmapheresis
Medical procedure in which plasma is separated from the blood cells. A donor gives a unit of blood, which is rapidly spun in a centrifuge. Centrifugal force pulls the blood cells to the bottom of the bag. The plasma portion at the top is siphoned off and pooled with plasma from other donors to make fresh frozen plasma, albumin, or clotting factors. The blood cells are then given back to the donor. [*see also*: albumin, Guillain-Barré syndrome, myasthenia gravis, plasma]

play therapy
Uses toys and other objects (often dolls) to help young children express emotions and reenact traumatic or abusive events (on a small scale they can control). Used to treat social withdrawal, anxiety, depression, aggression, and ADHD.

pleura
Serous membrane that lines the thoracic cavity (parietal pleura) and folds back on itself (visceral pleura) to cover the surface of the lung. It secretes pleural fluid into the pleural space (space between the two layers). [*see also*: hemothorax, pleural effusion, pleurisy, pneumothorax]

pleural effusion
[511.xx]
Accumulation of fluid within the pleural space due to inflammation or infection of the pleura and lungs. [*see also*: pleura, thoracentesis]

pleurisy [511.xx]
Inflammation of the pleura as a result of pneumonia or other infection, trauma, or tumor. The inflamed parietal pleura and visceral pleura rub against each other, causing pain, particularly when the patient takes a deep breath. The sound heard through the stethoscope is known as a pleural friction rub. [*see also*: pneumonia, pyothorax]   S

pneumoconiosis
[500.xx–508.xx]
Constant exposure to inhaled particles causes pulmonary fibrosis, in which the alveoli lose their elasticity. Pneumoconiosis is a general word for any occupational lung disease caused by   S

chronically inhaling some type of dust or particle. [*see also*: anthracosis, asbestosis]

***Pneumocystis carinii* pneumonia**
[136.xx]

Severe form of pneumonia caused by the amoeba *Pneumocystis carinii*. Most people are infected with this microorganism in childhood. It causes a mild infection, and then lies dormant in the body within small cyst-like structures. In debilitated patients, particularly those with AIDS, it emerges from the cyst and causes disease. [*see also*: acquired immunodeficiency syndrome]   A

pneumonia
[480.xx–486.xx]

Inflammation or infection of some or all of the lobes of the lungs   L
and the bronchi. The pneumonia is named according to its cause or its location in the lungs. Fluid from inflamed tissues, plus microorganisms and white blood cells, fill the alveoli and air passages. [*see also*: adult respiratory distress syndrome, aspiration pneumonia, incentive spirometry, *Pneumocystis carinii* pneumonia, walking pneumonia]

pneumothorax
[512.xx]

Large volume of air that forms in the pleural space and progressively   S
separates the two pleural membranes. This compresses or even collapses the lung. Can be caused by a penetrating injury that allows outside air to flow into the thoracic cavity. It can also occur when alveoli rupture from lung disease and release air into the thoracic cavity. [*see also*: chest tube insertion, hemothorax, pleura]

poikilocytosis
[790.xx]

Erythrocytes that vary in shape. [*see also*: sickle cell anemia]

polycystic kidney disease [753.xx]

Congenital disease characterized by cysts in the kidney that   A
eventually obliterate the nephrons, causing kidney failure.

polycystic ovary syndrome [256.xx]

A follicle matures and enlarges, but fails to rupture to release an ovum and then becomes a cyst. This occurs month after month until the ovaries are filled with multiple cysts. The cysts enlarge each month in response to LH, causing pain.

polycythemia vera [268.xx]

Increased number of erythrocytes due to uncontrolled production   L
by the red bone marrow. The cause is unknown. The viscosity of   S
the blood increases and the total blood volume is increased. [*see also*: blood, plasma, splenomegaly]

polydactyly
[755.xx]

Congenital abnormality in which there are extra fingers or toes.   S
[*see also*: syndactyly]

polyhydramnios
[761.xx]

Increased volume of amniotic fluid. Caused by maternal diabetes mellitus, twin gestation, and different types of fetal abnormalities. [*see also*: gestational diabetes, oligohydramnios]

polymyalgia
[725.xx]

Pain in several muscle groups due to injury or muscle disease. [*see also*: hypokalemia, myalgia]

polymyositis
[710.xx]

A chronic, progressive disease that causes widespread inflammation of muscles with weakness and fatigue. The cause is unknown, although it may be an autoimmune disease. [*see also*: autoimmune disease, C-reactive protein, myositis, muscle biopsy]

polyneuritis
[729.xx]

Generalized inflammation of many nerves, in one part of the body or all the nerves in the body. [*see also*: neuritis]

polypectomy

Surgical excision of polyps using forceps or a snare. [*see also*: polyps]

polyphagia
[783.xx]

Excessive overeating. [*see also*: bulimia, cognitive-behavioral therapy, diabetes mellitus]

polyps
colon [211.xx]
nasal [471.xx]

Small, fleshy, benign or precancerous growths that arise from the mucosa of the nose, sinuses, vocal cords or colon. [*see also*: barium enema, colon, mucosa, nasal polyp, polypectomy]

polysomnography	Multifaceted test to diagnose the underlying conditions that can cause insomnia, sleep disruption, sleep apnea, or narcolepsy. Electrodes on the face and head and various other monitors are applied to the patient. During sleep, the patient's EEG, eye movements, muscle activity, heartbeat, and respirations are monitored. [*see also*: electroencephalography, narcolepsy, sleep apnea]	S
polyuria [788.xx]	Excessive production of urine associated with diabetes mellitus and diabetes insipidus. [*see also*: diabetes mellitus, diabetes insipidus, urination]	
pons	Area of the brainstem that relays nerve impulses from the body to the cerebellum and back to the body. Area where nerve tracts cross from one side of the body and relay nerve impulses to the opposite side of the cerebrum. Cranial nerves V through VIII originate there. [*see also*: brainstem, cranial nerves, hypothalamus]	
popliteal space	Area at the back of the knee that is bordered by muscles and contains blood vessels and nerves.	S
portal hypertension [572.xx]	An increase in blood pressure in the portal vein. [*see also*: ascites, hypertension, splenomegaly, varices]	
positron emission tomography (PET) scan	Nuclear medicine procedure that uses the radiopharmaceutical fluorine-18 combined with glucose molecules. As the glucose is metabolized, the radioactive substance emits positrons, which form gamma rays that are detected by a gamma camera. A circular gamma scintillation camera detects the gamma rays and creates an image that shows cellular metabolism. Shows areas of increased or decreased metabolism due to cancerous tumors and some diseases. [*see also*: Alzheimer's disease, epilepsy, Parkinson's disease, schizophrenia, seizure]	A
posterior	Pertaining to the back of the body or the back part of an organ or structure. Posteroanterior means moving from the back to the front. Opposite of anterior. [*see also*: coronal plane]	
posterior cavity	Large space in the posterior aspect of the eye. It contains vitreous humor. [*see also*: dilated funduscopy]	F
posterior chamber	Thin space behind the iris of the eye. Aqueous humor circulates through it. [*see also*: aqueous humor]	
posterior pituitary gland	Part of the pituitary gland that stores and releases antidiuretic hormone (ADH) and oxytocin produced by the hypothalamus. [*see also*: anterior pituitary gland, antidiuretic hormone, oxytocin, pituitary gland]	S
posteroanterior	Pertaining to going from the back to the front.	A
postictal state	Occuring after a tonic-clonic seizure, the patient experiences sleepiness and confusion. [*see also*: epilepsy, seizure, status epilepticus]	
postnatal period	From the newborn's standpoint, the period of time after birth.	
postpartum	From the mother's standpoint, the period of time after delivery. [*see also*: antepartum, postpartum depression]	
postpartum depression [648.xx]	A mood disorder with symptoms of mild-to-moderate depression, anxiousness, irritability, tearfulness, and fatigue. It is caused by hormonal changes after birth and by feelings of overwhelming responsibility and fatigue. Formerly known as involutional melancholia because it occurs at the time of involution of the uterus. [*see also*: Beck Depression Inventory, dysthymia, involution]	S

A= Abbreviations Section   **F**= Figures Section   **L**= Laboratory Section   **S**= Synonyms Section
Sx(Symptoms)   **Dx**(Diagnosis)   **Tx**(Treatment)

postpartum hemorrhage [666.xx]	Continual bleeding from the uterus at the site where the placenta separated after a normal birth. The empty uterus is boggy and does not become firm. Caused by hyposecretion of oxytocin from the posterior pituitary gland in the brain. [see also: disseminated intravascular coagulation, oxytocin, placenta]

posttraumatic stress disorder [309.xx]

Continuing, disabling reaction to an excessively traumatic situation or event. The patient feels helpless, has a numbed emotional response with disinterest in people and current events, and relives the trauma of the event over and over. Other symptoms include chronic anxiety, insomnia, irritability, and occasional violent outbursts. Previously known as combat fatigue or shell shock.

A
S

> **Dx** Following a trauma, there are three subdivisions in the DSM-IV, with varying numbers of criteria for each subdivision.
>
> **Tx** Psychotherapy. Pharmacological treatment usually isn't warranted.

potassium

Ion (K^+) that plays a role in the contraction of the myocardium. [see also: metabolic panel]

L

precocious puberty [259.xx]

Early onset of puberty along with the premature development of the physical characteristics and hormonal changes associated with puberty. (It can also be caused by hypersecretion of FSH and LH from an adenoma in the anterior pituitary gland.) [see also: androgenital syndrome, estradiol, FSH assay and LH assay, luteinizing hormone, puberty]

> ♀: Hypersecretion of estradiol. Caused by an adenoma in the ovary. There is premature development of the breasts, menstruation, and ovulation in a child. [see also: ovulation]
>
> ♂: Hypersecretion of testosterone. Caused by an adenoma in the testis. There is premature development of a beard, deepening of the voice, and sperm production in a child.

preeclampsia [642.xx]

Hypertensive disorder of pregnancy with increased blood pressure, edema, weight gain, and protein in the urine. The nephrons of the kidneys allow large protein molecules from the blood to be lost in the urine. A low level of protein changes the osmotic pressure of the blood and allows fluid to move into the tissues, where it collects as edema. Preeclampsia can progress to eclampsia. [see also: albuminuria, dystocia, eclampsia, hypertension]

L

pregnancy

State of being with child. It begins at the moment of conception and ends with delivery of the newborn. [see also: chloasma, dystocia, gestational diabetes, hydatidiform mole, hyperemesis gravidarum, lecithin/sphingomyelin ratio, linea nigra, morning sickness, obstetrical history, tubal ligation, vasectomy]

L

pregnancy test

Blood test to detect human chorionic gonadotropin (HCG) secreted by the fertilized ovum. Serum HCG is positive just nine days after conception. Home pregnancy tests that detect HCG in the urine are easy to use but are not always accurate. Only a positive blood test (serum beta HCG) is diagnostic of pregnancy. The presence of HCG does not indicate that the pregnancy is normal because HCG is also produced in an ectopic pregnancy and hydatidiform mole. [see also: dystocia, ectopic pregnancy, hydatidiform mole, pregnancy]

premalignant skin lesions

Abnormal but not yet clearly cancerous lesions. Over time and with continued exposure to sunlight or irritation, these lesions can become cancerous. [see also: basal cell carcinoma]

---

premature atrial contractions [427.xx]	Arrhythmia in which there are one or more extra contractions of the atrium within a cardiac cycle. [*see also*: cardiac cycle, dysrhythmia, premature contraction]	A
premature contraction [427.xx]	Arrhythmia in which there are one or more extra contractions within a cardiac cycle. There are two types of premature contractions: premature atrial contractions (PACs) and premature ventricular contractions (PVCs). [*see also*: cardiac cycle, dysrhythmia, palpitation]	S
premature ejaculation [302.xx]	Ejaculation of semen that often occurs with minimal stimulation and before the penis becomes fully erect to penetrate the vagina. This lessens the enjoyment of sexual intercourse and decreases the chance of conception. Can be caused by a hormonal imbalance but more often by stress or a psychological reason.	
premature labor [644.xx]	Regular uterine contractions that occur before the fetus is mature (before full-term gestation of 38 to 42 weeks). The cervix may dilate and small amounts of blood or amniotic fluid may leak out. [*see also*: Braxton Hicks contractions]	
premature rupture of membranes [658.xx]	Spontaneous rupture of the amniotic sac and loss of amniotic fluid before labor begins. The mother must deliver or risk the development of infection within 24 hours. [*see also*: cesarean section, dystocia]	A
premature ventricular contractions [427.xx]	Arrhythmia in which there are one or more extra contractions of the ventricle within a cardiac cycle. [*see also*: cardiac cycle, dysrhythmia, palpitation]	A
premenstrual dysphoric disorder [625.xx]	Occurs before the onset of the menstrual cycle and combines the symptoms of premenstrual syndrome with depression, anxiety, tearfulness, difficulty concentrating, and sleep and eating disturbances. It is a psychiatric mood disorder caused by an alteration in the level of neurotransmitters in the brain. [*see also*: Beck Depression Inventory, premenstrual syndrome]	A
premenstrual syndrome [625.xx]	Occurring a few days before the onset of menstruation: breast tenderness, fluid retention, bloating, and mild mood changes. Caused by the high levels of estradiol and progesterone just prior to menstruation, which affect the levels of serotonin and norepinephrine in the brain. [*see also*: menstruation, premenstrual dysphoric disorder]	A
prenatal period	From the fetus' standpoint, the period of time from conception to birth.	
presbyacusis [388.xx]	Bilateral hearing loss due to aging. [*see also*: audiometry, conductive hearing loss, mixed hearing loss, sensorineural hearing loss]	
presbyopia [367.xx]	Loss of flexibility of the lens with blurry near vision and loss of accommodation caused by aging. [*see also*: accommodation]	
presenile dementia [290.xx]	Alzheimer's disease that occurs in early middle age. [*see also*: Alzheimer's disease, dementia]	
priapism [607.xx]	Continuing erection of the penis with pain and tenderness. Caused by spinal cord injury or a side effect of drugs to treat erectile dysfunction. [*see also*: impotence, spinal cord injury]	
primary site	Area where the cancerous cell first formed and grew into a cancerous tumor. There is just one primary site. [*see also*: in situ, secondary site]	S
products of conception	The fetus, placenta, and all fluids and tissue in the pregnant uterus. [*see also*: lochia]	

progesterone	Female sex hormone produced and secreted by the corpus luteum of the ovary, after ovulation, when stimulated by LH from the anterior pituitary gland. It causes the uterine lining to thicken to prepare for a possible fertilized ovum. During pregnancy, it is secreted by the placenta. [*see also*: corpus luteum, gestational diabetes mellitus, human chorionic gonadotropin, hyperemesis gravidarum, morning sickness, premenstrual syndrome]
projection	Direction in which the x-ray beam travels through the patient. [*see also*: plane, x-ray]
prolactin	Hormone secreted by the anterior pituitary gland. It stimulates lactiferous glands of the breasts to develop during puberty and to produce milk during pregnancy. [*see also*: failure of lactation, galactorrhea]
prolapsed cord [762.xx]	A loop of umbilical cord becomes caught between the presenting part of the fetus and the birth canal. This occurs if the membranes rupture before the fetal head (or other presenting part) is fully engaged in the mother's pelvis. With each uterine contraction, the umbilical cord is compressed, causing decreased blood flow to the fetus and fetal distress. [*see also*: fetal distress, nuchal cord]
proliferative phase	Days 7–13 of the menstrual cycle when a follicle matures in the ovary and the thickness of the endometrium increases. The menstrual cycle consists of the menstrual phase, proliferative phase, secretory phase, ovulation, and ischemic phase. [*see also*: menstruation]
pronation	Turning the palm of the hand down. Opposite of supination. [*see also*: prone]
pronator	Muscle that produces pronation when it contracts.
prone	Position of lying on the anterior surface of the body. Opposite of supine. [*see also*: pronation, supination]
prophylactic mastectomy	Surgical resection of all or part of the breast in women who have a strong family history of breast cancer to prevent breast cancer from occurring. [*see also*: mastectomy]
ProstaScint scan	Nuclear medicine procedure that uses ProstaScint to detect areas of metastasis from a primary site of prostate cancer. ProstaScint is a combination of a radioactive tracer (indium-111) and a monoclonal antibody that binds to receptors on cancer cells in the prostate gland and elsewhere in the body. The radioactive tracer emits gamma rays that are detected by a gamma scintillation camera and made into an image. [*see also*: scintigraphy]
prostate gland	Round gland at the base of the bladder in a male. It surrounds the first part of the urethra and produces prostatic fluid that contributes to the volume of semen. [*see also*: acid phosphatase, benign prostatic hypertrophy, digital rectal examination, ProstaScint scan, prostate-specific antigen, prostatectomy, prostatitis, transurethral resection of the prostate]
prostatectomy	Surgical procedure to remove the entire prostate gland, lymph nodes, seminal vesicles, and vas deferens because of prostate cancer. A retropubic or a suprapubic surgical approach can be used. [*see also*: prostate gland]
prostate-specific antigen	Blood test that detects a glycoprotein in cells of the prostate gland. PSA is increased in men with prostate cancer. The higher the level, the more advanced the cancer. PSA levels fall after successful treatment of the cancer. [*see also*: acid phosphatase]

S

S

F

A

prostatitis [601.xx]	Acute or chronic bacterial infection of the prostate gland. Usually caused by a urinary tract infection or a sexually transmitted disease. [*see also*: prostate gland, sexually transmitted disease, urinary tract infection]
prosthesis	Orthopedic device, such as an artificial leg, that is used by a patient who has had an amputation of a limb. [*see also*: amputation, augmentation mammaplasty, joint replacement surgery, orthosis, penile implant, reconstructive mammaplasty] S
protease	Digestive enzyme from the pancreas. It breaks down large protein molecules in the duodenum into smaller ones.
prothrombin	Blood clotting factor II. It is activated just before the thrombus is formed. (*see also*: thrombus) S
prothrombin time	Blood test to evaluate the effectiveness of the anticoagulant drug Coumadin. A prolonged (rather than normal) PT would be expected. The international normalized ratio (INR) reports the PT value in a standardized way, regardless of what laboratory performed the PT test. [*see also*: partial thromboplastin time] A
proximal	Pertaining to near the point of origin, particularly of an arm or leg. Opposite of distal.
proximal convoluted tubule	Tubule of the nephron that begins at Bowman's capsule and ends at the loop of Henle in the nephron. Reabsorption takes place there. [*see also*: distal convoluted tubule]
pruritus [698.xx]	Itching. Pruritus is associated with many skin diseases. It is also present during an allergic reaction because of the release of histamine. [*see also*: allergic reaction, histamine] S
psoriasis [696.xx]	Autoimmune disorder characterized by the production of excessive amounts of epidermal cells. Skin lesions are itchy and show erythema covered with silvery scales and plaques, particularly on the scalp, elbows, hands, and knees. [*see also*: autoimmune disease]
psychiatric diagnosis	Stated in a specific way that involves five axes or aspects, as required by the American Psychiatric Association's publication *Diagnostic and Statistical Manual of Mental Disorders*, (DSM-IV). [*see also*: anxiety disorder, bipolar disorder, obsessive-compulsive disorder, posttraumatic stress disorder, psychopath, schizophrenia]
psychiatry	Medical specialty that deals with the mind, mental health, and mental illness. [*see also*: psychiatric diagnosis, psychotherapy] A
psychoanalysis	Based on the ideas of conscious and subconscious as developed by Sigmund Freud to analyze a patient's thoughts and behavior. It includes interpretation of dreams and hypnosis.
psychopath [301.xx]	Disregard for the written and unwritten rules and standards of conduct (laws, morals, ethics) of society. Patients lie, steal, and manipulate, showing no empathy for others or guilt or remorse for their actions. There is also fighting, failure to attend school (truancy), vandalism, sexual promiscuity, excessive drinking, the use of illegal drugs, and criminal acts. Also known as sociopath. [*see also*: psychotherapy] S
	Dx Symptoms not due to another mental disorder and all medical conditions have been ruled out. The patient is at least 18 years of age, but has had evidence of a conduct disorder before the age of 15. A disregard for the law and the rights of others, society, or culture, evidencing three of the seven criteria listed in the DSM-IV.
	Tx Psychological or psychiatric intervention is warranted.

psychotherapy	Any therapy (except drug therapy and electroconvulsive therapy) that uses verbal or nonverbal communication between a patient or a group of patients and a psychologist or psychiatrist to treat a mental disorder. [*see also*: psychoanalysis]	
puberty	Period of time when FSH and LH from the anterior pituitary gland first begin to stimulate the sex organs. The sexual characteristics develop, and there is a growth spurt. [*see also*: acne vulgaris, comedo, dwarfism, estradiol, follicle-stimulating hormone, gigantism, gynecomastia, mammary glands, menarche, prolactin, precocious puberty, Tanner staging]	**S**
pulmonary artery	Artery that carries blood from the heart to the lungs. The pulmonary artery is the only artery in the body that carries oxygen-poor blood. [*see also*: ductus arteriosus, pulmonary embolism]	**F**
pulmonary circulation	The blood vessels (arteries, capillaries, and veins) that go in and out of the lungs, but not to the rest of the body. [*see also*: systemic circulation]	
pulmonary edema [514.xx]	Fluid in the alveoli because of failure of the left side of the heart to adequately pump blood. There is a backup of blood in the pulmonary circulation. [*see also*: congestive heart failure]	**L**
pulmonary embolism [415.xx]	Blockage of one of the pulmonary arteries by an embolus. A blood clot can develop in the legs of a patient on prolonged bed rest, or it can be a fat globule that is released from yellow marrow when a long bone is fractured. The embolus travels to the heart and into the pulmonary artery. As the pulmonary artery divides into smaller branches, the embolus becomes trapped and blocks the arterial blood flow going to that part of the lung. [*see also*: deep vein thrombosis] **Dx** H&P. ABGs to assess blood oxygen levels. An angiogram may be performed to locate the clots. A V/Q scan is used to visualize the lung vasculature that may be blocked. [*see also*: ventilation-perfusion scan] **Tx** Anticoagulants to thin the blood and prevent more clots from forming. Sometimes localized thrombolytics may be given to dissolve the clot. A surgically inserted venous filter (Greenfield filter) may be inserted to catch the clots before they get to the heart and lungs.	**A** **L**
pulmonary function tests	Diagnostic procedure to measure the capacity of the lungs and the volume of air during inhalation and exhalation. The FVC (forced vital capacity) measures the amount of air that can be forcefully exhaled from the lungs after the deepest inhalation. The FEV_1 (forced expiratory volume in one second) measures the volume of air that can be forcefully exhaled during the first second of measuring the FVC. [*see also*: adult respiratory distress syndrome, bronchitis, chronic obstructive pulmonary disease, cystic fibrosis]	**A**
pulmonary valve	Heart valve located between the right ventricle and the pulmonary artery. [*see also*: tetralogy of Fallot]	**F**
pulmonary vein	Vein that carries blood from the lungs to the heart. The pulmonary vein is the only vein in the body that carries oxygen-rich blood.	
pulse	The bulging of an artery wall from blood pumped by the heart.	**A**
pulse oximetry	Diagnostic procedure in which a pulse oximeter, a small, noninvasive clip device, is placed on the patient's index finger or earlobe to measure the degree of oxygen saturation of the blood. It emits light waves that penetrate the skin and are absorbed or reflected	

by saturated hemoglobin bound to oxygen versus unsaturated hemoglobin. The oximeter then calculates the oxygen saturation. The oximeter does not measure CO_2 levels. [*see also*: anoxia]

punch biopsy Special forceps are used to grasp part of a tumor. As the forceps closes, it punches out a small, cylindrical tissue specimen. Multiple punch biopsies can be taken at one time. [*see also*: biopsy]

pupil Dark, round, central opening in the iris that allows light rays to enter the internal eye. [*see also*: anisocoria, iris] F

pupillary response Medical procedure to test if the pupils will constrict briskly and equally in response to a bright light. This is documented in the patient's record as PERRL (pupils equal, round, and reactive to light). [*see also*: anisocoria, miosis, mydriasis, oculomotor nerve]

Purkinje fibers Network of interlacing fibers of the conduction system of the heart. They arise from the bundle branches and spread throughout the ventricles. [*see also*: conduction system, dysrhythmia] F

pyelography Radiologic procedure that uses x-rays and radiopaque contrast dye. The dye is injected intravenously and flows through the blood and into the kidneys. It outlines the renal pelves, ureters, bladder, and urethra. It shows any obstruction, blockage, kidney stone, or abnormal anatomy in the urinary tract. [*see also*: nephrolithiasis, retrograde pyelography] S

pyelonephritis
[590.xx] Inflammation and infection of the pelves of the kidneys. Caused by a bacterial infection of the bladder that ascends up the ureters to the kidneys. [*see also*: urinary tract infection]

pylorus Narrowing channel of the stomach just before it joins the duodenum. It contains the pyloric sphincter.

pyometritis
[615.xx] Infection and inflammation of the myometrium that creates pus in the intrauterine cavity. [*see also*: myometritis]

pyosalpinx
[614.xx] Infection of the fallopian tube, where the infection fills the tube with pus. [*see also*: fallopian tube]

pyothorax
[510.xx] Localized collection of purulent material (pus) in the thoracic cavity from an infection in the lungs. [*see also*: atelectasis, chest tube insertion, thoracentesis] S

pyromania
[312.xx] Deliberately setting fires for the pleasure of watching the fire and the people sent to fight the fire. Fires are not set to take revenge, conceal a crime, or collect insurance money.

pyuria White blood cells in the urine, indicating a urinary tract infection. Can be seen with the naked eye when the urine is cloudy or milky, or the number of white blood cells may be so few that only microscopic examination during urinalysis reveals them. [*see also*: leukocyte esterase, urinalysis]

Q

quadrant One-quarter of an area that has been divided into four parts by an imaginary grid. The four quadrants of the surface of the abdominopelvic area are the right upper quadrant (RUQ), the left upper quadrant (LUQ), the left lower quadrant (LLQ), and the right lower quadrant (RLQ). [*see also*: epigastric region, hypochondriac region, hypogastric region, inguinal region, lumbar region, umbilical region]

quadriplegia
[344.xx] An injury to the upper spinal cord causing an inability to voluntarily move all four extremities. [*see also*: flaccid paralysis, paraplegia, spastic paralysis]

quantitative
computerized Radiologic procedure that uses an x-ray beam and a CT scanner to create a three-dimensional image to measure the bone mineral A

tomography	density (BMD) to determine if demineralization from osteoporosis has occurred. QCT is able to take separate measurements for cancellous and cortical bone. Cancellous bone is the first to be affected by osteoporosis and the first to respond to therapy. [see also: densitometry]

R

radiation	The process of sending out some type of invisible ray, like x-rays or gamma rays. [see also: dosimetry, film badge, gamma ray, lead apron, radiation therapy]
radiation cystitis [990.xx]	Inflammation of the bladder caused by the irritating effects of radiation therapy given to treat bladder cancer. [see also: radiation therapy]
radiation therapy	Treatment that uses one of several types of radiation to disrupt the atoms in the DNA in cancer cells to keep them from dividing. The radiation is in the form of waves or particles. Radiotherapy destroys both cancerous and normal cells, but enough normal cells remain to divide and repair the damaged tissue. [see also: alopecia, aplastic anemia, burns, debulking, fractionation, nausea, radiation cystitis]
radical mastectomy	Surgical resection of all or part of the breast to excise a malignant tumor. The pectoralis major and minor muscles of the chest wall are removed along with an axillary lymph node dissection or removal. This procedure is performed infrequently. [see also: mastectomy, modified radical mastectomy]
radical neck dissection	Surgical procedure to treat extensive cancer of the mouth and neck. Parts of the jaw bone, tongue, lymph nodes, and muscles of the neck may be removed. The larynx can also be removed.
radical resection	Surgical procedure to excise the tumor as well as nearby lymph nodes, soft tissues, muscles, and even bones. [see also: cancer, metastases]
radioactive iodine uptake and thyroid scan	Nuclear medicine procedure that combines a radioactive iodine uptake procedure and a thyroid scan. The radioactive iodine uptake demonstrates how well the thyroid gland is able to absorb iodine from the blood. The thyroid scan shows the size and shape of the thyroid gland. Two radioactive tracers are given, orally and intravenously. A normal scan will show uniform distribution of the radioactive tracer throughout the thyroid gland. An adenoma appears as a bright ("hot") spot because of its increased uptake of radioactive iodine compared to the rest of the gland. A darker area (a "cold" spot) can either be a cyst or a cancerous tumor of the thyroid gland (neither of which take up iodine). [see also: Graves' disease, nuclear medicine, thyroid gland] A
radioactive substance	Substance that produces gamma rays or positrons as it decays and its atoms change from an unstable to a stable state. Used to create images in nuclear medicine. [see also: nuclear medicine]
radioallergosorbent test	Blood test that measures the amount of IgE produced each time the blood is mixed with a specific allergen. It shows which of many allergens the patient is allergic to and how severe the allergy is. [see also: allergen, immunoglobulin E] A
radiofrequency catheter ablation	Medical procedure to destroy ectopic areas in the heart that are emitting electrical impulses and producing arrhythmias. A catheter is inserted into the heart. Electromagnetic energy produced by a generator produces enough heat at the site to kill the cells causing the arrhythmia. Radiofrequency catheter occlusion uses A

heat to collapse and seal large varicose veins. [*see also*: dysrhythmia]

radiolucent
Areas of low density in the body (such as air-filled cavities) that allow x-rays to pass through and create a black area on a radiograph. Areas of high-density tissue (such as bone) are radiopaque, do not let x-rays pass through, and appear white on a radiograph. [*see also*: x-ray]

radionuclide
Radioactive form of a chemical element in which too many protons in the nucleus make the atom unstable.

radionuclide ventriculography
Nuclear medicine procedure that uses the radioactive tracer technetium-99m. A gamma camera records gamma rays emitted by a radioactive tracer that is bound to red blood cells. The camera is coordinated (gated) with the patient's EKG so that images of the heart chambers are taken at various times during the cardiac cycle. It calculates the ejection fraction. [*see also*: single-photon emission computed tomography scan] **A** **S**

radiopharma-ceutical
Naturally occurring or man-made radioactive radionuclide that has been processed and measured so that it can be given as a drug in nuclear medicine. Radiopharmaceuticals include gallium-67, indium-111, iodine-123, krypton-81m, technetium-99m, thallium-201, and xenon-133. [*see also*: tracer] **S**

rales [786.xx]
Irregular crackling or bubbling sounds during inspiration. [*see also*: rhonchi]

rapid strep test
Test kit for strep throat. It detects beta-hemolytic group A streptococcus. A color change means the test result is positive. Unlike a standard culture and sensitivity test, the result of a rapid strep test is available within the hour so that the physician can immediately prescribe an antibiotic drug. [*see also*: strep throat]

rash
Any type of skin lesion that is pink to red, flat or raised, pruritic or nonpruritic. Certain systemic diseases (chickenpox, measles) have distinctive, characteristic rashes. **S**

Raynaud's disease [443.xx]
Sudden, severe vasoconstriction and spasm of the arterioles in the fingers and toes, often triggered by cold or emotional upset. [*see also*: peripheral vascular disease]

reabsorption
Process by which water and substances in the filtrate move out of the renal tubule and into the blood in a nearby capillary. [*see also*: filtration]

reactive attachment disorder [313.xx]
Inability to bond emotionally and form intimate relationships with others because of severe abuse or neglect of the patient's basic needs before age 2, when trust is established. There is a lack of trust, watchful wariness, poor eye contact, lack of empathy, inability to show genuine affection, and a lack of a conscience. The patient is difficult to comfort and resists physical contact such as being held or cuddled, but sometimes exhibits inappropriate friendliness to strangers.

receptive aphasia [315.xx]
Loss of the ability to understand the spoken or written word caused by injury to the areas of the brain that deal with language and the interpretation of sounds and symbols. [*see also*: aphasia]

receptor
Structure on the cell membrane of a muscle fiber. It interacts with a neurotransmitter from a nerve. [*see also*: neurotransmitter]

receptor assays
Cytology test that measures the number of estrogen receptors (ER) or progesterone receptors (PR) in the cell to determine the prognosis and treatment options for breast cancer. A tumor with increased numbers of ER or PR receptors (ER-positive or PR-

positive) is dependent on those hormones and is most sensitive to treatment with male hormone therapy that creates the opposite hormonal environment. [*see also*: BRCA1 or BRCA2]

reconstructive mammaplasty

Surgical procedure to rebuild a breast after a mastectomy. This can be performed at the same time as a mastectomy or in a later, separate operation. A breast prosthesis or a TRAM flap is used to recreate the fullness of the breast. With a breast prosthesis procedure, a tissue expander (a saline-filled silicone bag) is first inserted to stretch the skin to accommodate a breast prosthesis, which is later inserted. A TRAM flap reconstructs the breast by using the transverse rectus abdominis muscle as a flap. [*see also*: augmentation mammaplasty, mammaplasty, mastectomy, reduction mammaplasty, transverse rectus abdominis muscle flap]

rectocele [618.xx]

Herniation of the rectum into the adjacent wall of the vagina.   **S**
The vaginal canal can become blocked, and there can be interference with the passage of stool through the rectum. It is caused by childbirth or age. [*see also*: colporrhaphy]

rectum

Final part of the large intestine. It is a short, straight segment that   **F**
lies between the sigmoid colon and the outside of the body.
[*see also*: anus, barium enema, digital rectal examination, double contrast enema, episiotomy, hemorrhoids, rectocele, ulcerative colitis, vesicocele]

reduction mammaplasty

Surgical procedure to reduce the size of a large, pendulous breast. The procedure can be performed in conjunction with a mastopexy or breast lift to reposition a sagging breast. [*see also*: augmentation mammaplasty, mammaplasty, reconstructive mammaplasty]

reflex

Involuntary muscle reaction that is controlled by the spinal cord. In response to pain, the spinal cord immediately sends a command to the muscles of the body to move. All of this takes place without conscious thought or processing by the brain. The entire circuit is also known as a reflex arc. [*see also*: Babinski's sign, deep tendon reflexes, lactation, spastic paralysis, uvula]

refractory period

Short period of time when the myocardium is resting and unresponsive to electrical impulses. [*see also*: diastole, myocardium, systole]

regurgitation [394.xx; 424.xx; 746.xx] [530.xx]

Cardiac: When blood flows backward into the atrium with each contraction because of valve problems. [*see also*: mitral valve prolapse]
Digestive: The reflux of small amounts of food and acid back into the mouth. [*see also*: emesis]

rehabilitation exercises

Physical therapy procedure that includes exercises to increase muscle strength and improve coordination and balance, prescribed as part of a rehabilitation plan. In active exercise, the patient exercises without assistance. In passive exercise, the physical therapist or nurse performs range of motion (ROM) exercises for a patient who is unable to move. This does not build muscle strength, but it decreases stiffness and spasticity and prevents contractures. [*see also*: physical therapy]

relapse

Return of the signs or symptoms of cancer after a period of improvement or even remission. [*see also*: remission]

remission

Period of time during which there are no signs or symptoms of cancer. Occurs after the successful treatment of cancer. [*see also*: relapse]

A = Abbreviations Section   **F** = Figures Section   **L** = Laboratory Section   **S** = Synonyms Section
Sx (Symptoms)   **Dx** (Diagnosis)   **Tx** (Treatment)

renal colic
[788.xx]

Spasm of the smooth muscle of the ureters or bladder, as a kidney stone's jagged edges scrape the mucosa and cause pain. [*see also*: lithogenesis, nephrolithiasis]

renal failure
[584.xx–585.xx]

Disease in which the kidney's urine production progressively decreases and then stops altogether. Symptoms do not appear until 80% of kidney function has been lost. [*see also*: acute renal failure, acute tubular necrosis, blood urea nitrogen, chronic renal failure, creatinine, dialysis, end-stage renal disease, nephrectomy]   L

renal pelvis

Large, funnel-shaped cavity within each kidney that collects urine from the major calices and sends it to the ureter. [*see also*: pyelonephritis]   F

renal pyramids

Triangular-shaped areas of tissue in the medulla of the kidney.   F

renal scan

Nuclear medicine procedure that uses a radioactive isotope injected intravenously. It is taken up by the kidney and emits radioactive particles that are captured by a scanner and made into an image. Used after a kidney transplant to look for signs of organ rejection.

renin

Enzyme secreted by special cells near the nephron when the blood pressure decreases. Renin stimulates the production of angiotensin, a powerful vasoconstrictor.   S

repolarization

The opposite of depolarization. Pumps in the cell move calcium and sodium ions out of the cell, causing potassium ions to come back into the cell. This restores the normal electrical state of the cell and puts it in a resting state.

reproductive

The other role of the female genital system in conceiving, carrying, and giving birth to a child.

reproductive system

♀: Body system that includes the breasts, ovaries, fallopian tubes, uterus, vagina, and external genitalia for the female. It produces eggs and sex hormones in the female and regulates menstruation, pregnancy, and milk production from the breasts.

♂: Body system that includes the scrotum, testes, epididymides, vas deferens, seminal vesicles, prostate gland, urethra, and penis for the male. It produces sperm and sex hormones in the male.

respiration

The movement of air through the respiratory system and into the lungs during inhalation (or inspiration) and out of the lungs with exhalation (or expiration). Oxygen and carbon dioxide are exchanged in the alveoli during external respiration, and at the cellular level during internal respiration. [*see also*: phrenic nerve]

respiratory system

Body system that includes the nose, nasal cavity, pharynx, larynx, trachea, bronchi, bronchioles, lungs, and alveoli. Its purpose is to bring oxygen into the body and expel carbon dioxide.

restless leg syndrome [333.xx]

Uncomfortable restlessness and twitching of the muscles of the legs, particularly the calf muscles, along with an indescribable tingling, aching, or crawling-insect sensation, the exact cause of which is unknown.

reticulocyte

Immature erythrocyte that is released into the blood. It has no nucleus, but contains a network of ribosomes in its cytoplasm. [*see also*: erythrocyte]   F

retina

Membrane lining the posterior cavity of the eye. It contains rods and cones. Landmarks on the retina include the optic disk and the macula. [*see also*: cones, diabetic retinopathy, dilated funduscopy, flashers and floaters, macula, retinal detachment, retinitis pigmentosa, retinoblastoma, retrolental fibroplasia, rods]   F

A = Abbreviations Section   F = Figures Section   L = Laboratory Section   S = Synonyms Section
Sx (Symptoms)   Dx (Diagnosis)   Tx (Treatment)

retinaculum	Thin, nearly translucent band of fibrous tissue and fascia that holds down extensor and flexor tendons that go across the wrist and ankle joints. [*see also*: carpal tunnel syndrome]	
retinal detachment [361.xx]	Separation of the retina from the choroid layer beneath it. This can be caused by head trauma. It can occur gradually during aging as the vitreous humor changes from a gel to a watery consistency that flows into a tear in the retina and separates the two layers. In diabetic patients, hemorrhage of the fragile retinal blood vessels can separate the layers. [*see also*: choroid, flashers and floaters, laser photocoagulation, retina, retinopexy]	S
retinitis pigmentosa [362.xx]	Inherited abnormality linked to 70 different genes. The retina has abnormal deposits of pigmentation behind the rods and cones, causing loss of color vision or night vision and loss of central or peripheral vision. It can progress to blindness. [*see also*: color blindness, night blindness, peripheral vision]	A
retinoblastoma [190.xx]	Cancerous tumor of the retina in children, arising from abnormal embryonic retinal cells.	
retinopexy	Surgical procedure to reattach a detached retina. Cryotherapy is used to freeze the tissue and fix all three layers (sclera, choroid, retina) together. Alternatively, laser photocoagulation can be done to heat spots on the retina to coagulate and seal them to the layers beneath. [*see also*: choroid, laser photocoagulation, retinal detachment]	
retrograde amnesia [780.xx]	Partial or total loss of long-term memory due to trauma or disease of the hippocampus. No events before the onset of the amnesia can be recalled. [*see also*: anterograde amnesia, global amnesia]	
retrograde pyelography	Radiologic procedure that uses x-rays and radiopaque contrast dye. A cystoscopy is performed first, and then a catheter is advanced into the ureter and dye is injected. It outlines the ureter, as well as the renal pelvis and calices of the kidney. It shows any obstruction, blockage, kidney stone, or abnormal anatomy in the urinary tract. [*see also*: intravenous pyelography]	
retrolental fibroplasia [362.xx]	Developing retinal tissue is replaced with fibrous tissue because of using high levels of oxygen therapy in premature babies with immature lungs.	S
retroperitoneal space	Area behind the peritoneum that lines the abdominal cavity. The retroperitoneal space contains the kidneys, adrenal glands, and fatty tissue. [*see also*: kidney]	
retroversion of the uterus [621.xx]	Abnormal position in which the entire uterus is bent backward while the cervix is in a normal position. [*see also*: anteflexion, dyspareunia, endometriosis]	S
reversible ischemic neurologic deficit	A temporary lack of oxygenated blood to an area of brain. It is like a TIA but its effects last for several days. [*see also*: cerebrovascular accident, transient ischemic attack]	A
Reye's syndrome [331.xx]	The use of aspirin to relieve the symptoms of the flu can cause Reye's syndrome. The reason for this is not known. Symptoms include very high levels of ammonia in the blood and brain, vomiting, seizures, and liver failure. These symptoms are acute and occasionally fatal.	L
Rh blood group	Category of blood type. When the Rh factor is present, the blood is Rh positive. Without the Rh factor, the blood is Rh negative. [*see also*: ABO blood group]	

A = Abbreviations Section   **F** = Figures Section   **L** = Laboratory Section   **S** = Synonyms Section
Sx (Symptoms)   **Dx** (Diagnosis)   **Tx** (Treatment)

rheumatic heart disease [390.xx–398.xx]	Autoimmune response to a previous streptococcal infection, such as a strep throat. It occurs most often in children. The body makes antibodies to fight the bacteria, but after the infection is gone the antibodies attack the connective tissue in the body, particularly the joints and/or the heart. The joints become swollen with fluid and inflamed. The mitral and aortic valves of the heart become inflamed and damaged. Vegetations form on the valves of the heart, which become scarred and narrowed, a condition known as stenosis. [*see also*: autoimmune disease, strep throat, valve]	L S
rheumatoid arthritis [714.xx]	An autoimmune disease in which the patient's own antibodies attack the cartilage and connective tissues, causing inflammatory disease, particularly of the joints. [*see also*: autoimmune disease, bone scintigraphy, C-reactive protein]	A L S
rhinophyma [695.xx]	Redness and hypertrophy of the nose with small-to-large, irregular lumps in the skin. It is caused by an increased number of sebaceous glands and acne rosacea.	S
rhinoplasty	Surgical procedure that uses plastic surgery to change the size or shape of the nose. [*see also*: body dysmorphic disorder, rhytidectomy]	
rhonchi	Humming, whistling, or snoring sounds during inspiration or expiration. [*see also*: rales]	
rhytidectomy	Surgical procedure to remove wrinkles and tighten loose, aging skin on the face and neck. A blepharoplasty may be performed at the same time. [*see also*: blepharoplasty, blepharoptosis, body dysmorphic disorder, rhinoplasty]	S
ribosome	Granular organelle located throughout the cytoplasm and on the endoplasmic reticulum. Ribosomes contain RNA and proteins and are the site of protein synthesis within each cell.	
right bundle branch block [426.xx]	Arrhythmia in which the electrical impulses from the AV node do not travel down the right bundle of His. [*see also*: dysrhythmia]	A
right-sided congestive heart failure [428.xx]	In right-sided congestive heart failure, the right ventricle is unable to pump blood adequately. Blood backs up in the superior vena cava, causing jugular venous distention. Blood also backs up in the inferior vena cava, causing hepatomegaly and peripheral edema in the legs, ankles, and feet. [*see also*: congestive heart failure]	
rigor mortis	A normal condition of the muscles that occurs several hours after death. As the muscle fibers die, the permeability of the cell membrane changes and calcium ions enter the cells. This causes all the muscles of the body to contract. Because the cells are dead, they can no longer pump out calcium ions and so the muscles remain contracted for about 72 hours until the cells begin to decompose.	S
ringworm [110.xx]	Skin infection caused by a microscopic fungus that feeds on epidermal cells. Occurring on any part of the body, the round lesions led to the erroneous conclusion that the disease was caused by a worm. [*see also*: tinea]	S
Rinne and Weber hearing tests	The Rinne tuning fork test evaluates bone conduction versus air conduction of sound in one ear at a time. A vibrating tuning fork is placed against the mastoid process behind the ear to test bone conduction of sound. Then it is placed next to (but not touching) the same ear. The Weber tuning fork test evaluates bone	

A = Abbreviations Section   **F** = Figures Section   **L** = Laboratory Section   **S** = Synonyms Section
Sx (Symptoms)   **Dx** (Diagnosis)   **Tx** (Treatment)

	conduction of sound in both ears at the same time. The vibrating tuning fork is placed against the center of the forehead or on the top of the head. The sound should be heard equally in both ears. [see also: audiometry, conductive hearing loss, mixed hearing loss, sensorineural hearing loss]
rods	Light-sensitive cells in the retina that detect black and white and function in daytime and nighttime vision. [see also: retina]
Romberg's sign	Medical procedure to assess equilibrium. The patient stands with the feet together and the eyes closed. Swaying or falling to one side indicates a loss of balance and inner ear dysfunction. [see also: vertigo]
Rorschach test	Uses cards with abstract shapes on them. Patients are asked to describe what the shape of the inkblot represents to them. **S**
rotation	Moving a body part around its axis.
rotational angiography	The x-ray machine moves around the area to be examined and multiple x-rays are taken after contrast dye is injected. Over 100 separate images can be taken in about one minute. The computer creates a three-dimensional image that can be rotated and viewed from all angles. This technique is particularly helpful in documenting tortuous arteries or areas where the normal anatomy is distorted. [see also: angiography, aortography, arteriography, coronary angiography, venography]
rotator	Muscle that produces rotation when it contracts. [see also: rotation]
rotator cuff tear	Tear in the rotator muscles of the shoulder that surround the head of the humerus. These muscles help to abduct the arm.
round window	Opening in the temporal bone between the middle ear and the vestibule of the inner ear. The opening is covered with a membrane. **F**
rugae	Digestive: Deep folds in the gastric mucosa that expand or contract to accomodate varying amounts of food.
	Urinary: Folds in the mucosa of the bladder that disappear as the bladder fills with urine
ruptured tympanic membrane [384.xx]	Tear in the tympanic membrane due to excessive pressure or infection. In pilots and deep sea divers, unequal air pressure in the middle ear compared to the surrounding air or water pressure can rupture the tympanic membrane.

S	
sadism [302.xx]	Obtaining power, control, and sexual arousal by deliberately causing abuse, pain, humiliation, or bondage to another person. [see also: masochism]
sagittal suture	Midline suture between the two parietal bones on the right and left sides of the cranium.
saliva	Watery substance secreted by the salivary glands. It contains amylase, a digestive enzyme that begins the process of chemical digestion in the mouth. [see also: amylase, immunoglobulin A, mononucleosis, OraSure, salivary gland] **S**
salivary gland	Three pairs of glands (parotid, submandibular, and sublingual) that produce and release saliva. [see also: saliva, sialolithiasis]
salpingectomy	Surgical procedure to remove a fallopian tube because of ovarian cancer or an ectopic pregnancy in the tube. A bilateral salpingectomy removes both fallopian tubes. A bilateral salpingo-

	oophorectomy removes both fallopian tubes and both ovaries. [see also: hysterectomy, oophorectomy]
salpingitis [614.xx]	Inflammation or infection of the fallopian tube. Caused by endometriosis or pelvic inflammatory disease that can narrow or block the lumen of the tube. [see also: endometriosis, pelvic inflammatory disease]
scabies [133.xx]	Infestation of parasitic mites that tunnel under the skin and produce vesicles. These lesions are pruritic.
Schilling test	Urine test used to diagnose pernicious anemia. It measures the amount of radioactive vitamin B_{12} excreted in the urine. The patient swallows a capsule that contains intrinsic factor and vitamin B_{12} labeled with a radioactive tracer. The patient swallows a second capsule that contains vitamin B_{12} labeled with a different radioactive tracer but no intrinsic factor. If the patient has pernicious anemia, only the capsule that contained vitamin B_{12} and intrinsic factor will be absorbed into the blood and then excreted in the urine. [see also: pernicious anemia]
schizophrenia [295.xx]	Chronic loss of touch with reality in most or all aspects of life with bizarre behavior and breakdown of thought processes. Many patients have their first episode as young adults.
	Dx Due to the different types and degrees of schizophrenia, diagnosis can be difficult. The DSM-IV is consulted for diagnostic criteria. [see also: positron emission tomography scan]
	Tx Psychological or psychiatric intervention is warranted. [see also: electroshock therapy, psychotherapy]
schizotrichia	Split ends on hairs.
Schwann cell	Cell that forms the myelin sheaths around axons of the cranial and spinal nerves. [see also: myelin]
sciatica [724.xx]	Acute or chronic condition that occurs when the herniated nucleus pulposus (HNP) of an intervertebral disk is forced out through a weak area in the disk wall and presses on adjacent spinal nerve roots. Usually involves a lumbar disk that causes pain from compression of several branches of the sciatic nerve. [see also: diskectomy, intervertebral disk, laminectomy, myelography, pain management, radiculopathy]
scintigraphy	Nuclear medicine procedure that uses a radioactive radiopharmaceutical as a tracer that collects in particular organs or tissues. It emits gamma rays that produce a flash of light. A gamma camera scans and counts the radioactivity (gamma rays) and creates an image. Areas of increased uptake are abnormal and can be an infection, cancer, or metastases. [see also: bone scintigraphy, hydroxyiminodiacetic acid scan, OncoScint scan, positron emission tomography scan, ProstaScint scan, single-photon emission computed tomography scan]
sclera	White, tough, fibrous connective tissue that forms the outer layer around most of the eye. [see also: scleral icterus]
scleral icterus [379.xx]	Yellow coloration of the conjunctivae which makes the sclerae also appear yellow. Caused by jaundice due to liver disease. [see also: conjunctiva, hepatitis, jaundice]
scleroderma [710.xx]	Autoimmune disorder that causes the skin and internal organs to become progressively hardened due to deposits of collagen. [see also: autoimmune disease]
sclerotherapy	Medical procedure in which a sclerosing drug (liquid or foam) is injected into a varicose vein. The drug causes irritation and

The following single-letter markers appear in the right margin: S (scabies), S (schizophrenia), S (schizotrichia), S (Schwann cell), S (sciatica), S (sclera), F (scleral icterus)

inflammation that later hardens as fibrosis that occludes the vein. [*see also*: varicose veins]

scoliosis [737.xx]
Abnormal, excessive, C-shaped or S-shaped lateral curvature of the spine. The back is said to have a scoliotic curvature. Scoliosis can be congenital but most often the cause is unknown. [*see also*: dextroscoliosis, kyphosis, kyphoscoliosis, levoscoliosis, lordosis]

scotoma [368.xx]
Temporary or permanent visual field defect in one or both eyes. These vary in size and can be patchy or solid, stationary or moving. Caused by glaucoma, diabetic retinopathy, or macular degeneration when various parts of the retina or optic nerve branches are destroyed. Also, a hemorrhage (stroke), tumor, or trauma on one side of the brain can cause a scotoma in the opposite visual field. Prior to a migraine headache, a patient may see a scintillating scotoma, a moving line of brilliantly flashing bars of light. [*see also*: cerebrovascular accident, diabetic neuropathy, diplopia, glaucoma, gonioscopy, hemianopia, macular degeneration, migraine headache]

scout film
Radiograph obtained to provide a preliminary view of an area before radiopaque contrast dye is administered.

scratch test
Solutions of various antigens are scratched into the skin. If the patient is allergic to a particular antigen, a wheal will form at the site of the scratch. [*see also*: allergen] S

scrotum
Pouch of skin that holds the two testes. [*see also*: cryptorchism, inguinal hernia, orchiopexy, perineum] F

seasonal affective disorder
Hypersecretion of melatonin. Melatonin is normally produced during the dark hours of each day. During the winter months when the nights are longer and there are fewer hours of bright sunlight, melatonin and melatonin-stimulating hormone (MSH) levels are increased. This can trigger seasonal affective disorder, a mood disorder characterized by depression, weight gain, and an increased desire for food and sleep. [*see also*: Beck Depression Inventory, melatonin, pineal gland] A

sebaceous gland
An exocrine gland of the skin that secretes sebum through a duct. Sebaceous glands are located in the dermis. The duct joins with a hair, and sebum coats the hair shaft as it moves toward the surface of the skin. [*see also*: blepharitis, seborrhea, stye] S

seborrhea [706.xx]
Overproduction of sebum, particularly on the face and scalp, that occurs at a time other than puberty. [*see also*: acne rosacea, acne vulgaris, comedo]

secondary hypertension [405.xx; 642.xx]
An elevated blood pressure which has a known cause, (for example, from a disease such as renal failure). [*see also*: hypertension]

secondary site
When a cancerous tumor spreads or metastasizes via the blood or lymphatic system to a distant part of the body, that area is known as the secondary site. There is always just one primary site, but there may be several secondary sites. [*see also*: in situ, primary site]

second-degree burn [948.xx]
Involves the epidermis and the upper layer of the dermis. Heat (fire, hot objects, steam, boiling water), electrical current (lightning, electrical outlets or cords), chemicals, or radiation or x-rays (sunshine or prescribed radiation therapy) can injure superficial or deep tissues. [*see also*: burns]

second-degree heart block [426.xx]
Arrhythmia in which only some of the electrical impulses traveling from the SA node reach the Purkinje fibers. [*see also*: conduction system, dysrhythmia, heart block]

secretory phase	Days 15–26 of the menstrual cycle when the ruptured follicle becomes the corpus luteum and secretes progesterone to increase the thickness of the endometrium. If the ovum is not fertilized, the corpus luteum begins to disintegrate. The menstrual cycle consists of the menstrual phase, proliferative phase, secretory phase, ovulation, and ischemic phase.
seizure [345.xx]	Recurring condition in which a group of neurons in the brain spontaneously sends out electrical impulses in an abnormal, uncontrolled way. Impulses spread from neuron to neuron, causing altered consciousness and abnormal muscle movements. The type and extent of the symptoms depend on the number and location of the affected neurons. Types of seizures include absence (petit mal), complex partial (psychomotor), simple partial (focal motor), and tonic-clonic (grand mal). [*see also*: aura, eclampsia, postictal state, status epilepticus]
semen	Fluid expelled from the penis during ejaculation. Semen contains spermatozoa, seminal fluid, prostatic fluid, and mucus from the bulbourethral glands. [*see also*: ejaculatory duct]
semen analysis	Microscopic examination of the spermatozoa. A semen analysis is done as part of a workup for infertility. After not ejaculating for 36 hours, the man gives a semen specimen. A normal sperm count is greater than 50 million/mL. The motility and morphology of the spermatozoa are evaluated. A semen analysis is also done after a vasectomy to verify aspermia and a successful sterilization. [*see also*: antisperm antibody test, infertility]
semicircular canals	Three separate but intertwined canals in the inner ear that are oriented in different planes (horizontally, vertically, obliquely). They help the body keep its balance. They relay information to the brain via the vestibular branch of the auditory nerve. [*see also*: Romberg's sign, vertigo]
seminal vesicles	Glands along the posterior wall of the bladder that secrete seminal fluid, a source of energy for the spermatozoa and the main component of semen.
seminiferous tubules	Tubules within each testis where spermatozoa develop. [*see also*: testes]
senile lentigo	Light-to-dark brown macules with irregular edges. They occur most often on the hands and face, areas that are chronically exposed to the sun.
sensorineural hearing loss [389.xx]	Progressive, permanent decline in the ability to hear sounds in one or both ears. Otosclerosis, damage to the inner ear from excessive noise, or aging prevents generation of nerve impulses to the auditory nerve. [*see also*: audiometry, conductive hearing loss, Ménière's disease, mixed hearing loss]
sentinel node biopsy	The sentinel lymph node, which is the first lymph node that receives drainage from the site of the primary cancerous tumor, is removed and sent to the laboratory. [*see also*: primary site, secondary site]
septal deviation	Lateral displacement of the nasal septum, significantly narrowing one of the nasal airways. This can be a congenital condition or it can be caused by trauma to the nose.
septicemia [038.xx]	Severe bacterial infection of the tissues that spreads to the blood. Both the bacteria and their toxins cause severe systemic symptoms. [*see also*: adult respiratory distress syndrome, disseminated intravascular coagulation, toxic shock syndrome]

Marginal section markers (right column): S (seizure), F (semicircular canals), F (seminal vesicles), S (senile lentigo), S (septicemia)

septum	A structure dividing or separating a cavity or space. [*see also*: heart, nasal septum]	
serotonin	Neurotransmitter between neurons in the limbic system, hypothalamus, cerebellum, and spinal cord. [*see also*: carcinoid syndrome, premenstrual syndrome]	S
serum	Fluid portion of the plasma that remains after the clotting factors are activated to form a blood clot. [*see also*: plasma]	
severe acute respiratory syndrome [079.xx]	Acute viral respiratory illness that can be fatal. [*see also*: adult respiratory distress syndrome]	A
sexually transmitted disease	Contagious disease that is contracted during sexual intercourse with an infected individual, or it can be passed to the newborn infant *in utero* or as it travels through the birth canal. It can cause serious illness, blindness, and even death. [*see also*: bacteriuria, blindness, chlamydia, dysuria, epididymitis, genital herpes, genital warts, gonorrhea, human immunodeficiency virus, pelvic inflammatory disease, prostatitis, syphilis, urethritis, vaginitis]	A S
shaken baby syndrome [995.xx]	Caused by vigorously shaking an infant, usually in anger or to discipline the child. Because the infant's head is large and the neck muscles are weak, severe shaking causes the head to whip back and forth. This can cause a cerebral contusion, concussion, hemorrhaging, mental retardation, coma, or even death.	
shave biopsy	Uses a scalpel or razor blade to remove a superficial lesion of the epidermis and/or dermis to send to the laboratory for examination.	
shin splints	Pain and inflammation of the tendons of the flexor muscles of the lower leg over the anterior tibia. An overuse injury common to athletes who run.	
shingles [053.xx]	Causes the skin rash of chickenpox during childhood. The virus remains dormant in the body until it is activated in later life by illness or emotional stress. Then it forms painful vesicles and crusts along some dermatomes. [*see also*: herpes, Tzanck test]	S
sialolithiasis [527.xx]	A stone that forms in the salivary gland and becomes lòdged in the duct, blocking the flow of saliva.	
sick sinus syndrome [427.xx]	Arrhythmia in which bradycardia alternates with tachycardia. Occurs when the sinoatrial node and ectopic sites elsewhere in the myocardium take turns being the heart's pacemaker. [*see also*: conduction system, dysrhythmia, radiofrequency catheter ablation]	
sickle cell anemia [282.xx]	Inherited genetic abnormality of an amino acid in hemoglobin. Low oxygen levels in the blood cause the erythrocyte to become distorted into a crescent or sickle shape. Sickle cells do not move easily through the capillaries, blocking the flow of blood, causing small clots and pain, particularly in the joints and abdomen. Sickle cells are fragile (because they frequently change shape), and they have a shortened life span, which results in anemia. [*see also*: anemia, anoxia, blood dyscrasia]	L S
	Dx H&P. Pregnant women at high risk often have an amniocentesis done.	
	Tx Treatment is directed at the symptoms the patient is having, as there is no cure or treatment to stop the cells from becoming distorted. Often oxygen is provided to saturate the blood and IV fluids are given to help flush out distorted cells.	

simple partial seizures — Involuntary contractions of one or several muscle groups (jerking of one hand, turning of the head). No impairment of consciousness. The patient is aware of the seizure but is unable to stop the motor activity. May also include sensory hallucinations. [*see also*: epilepsy, seizure]   S

single-photon emission computed tomography scan — During a myocardial perfusion scan or a MUGA scan, the gamma camera is normally kept in a stationary position above the patient's chest. However, if the gamma camera is moved in a circle around the patient, then this becomes a SPECT scan. The computer creates many individual images or "slices" (tomography) and compiles them into a three-dimensional image of the heart. [*see also*: radionuclide ventriculography]   A

sinoatrial node — Pacemaker of the heart. Small knot of tissue located in the posterior wall of the right atrium. The SA node dictates the heart rate at 70 to 80 beats per minute when the body is at rest. It originates the electrical impulse for the entire conduction system of the heart. [*see also*: conduction system, dysrhythmia]   S F

sinus — Hollow cavity within a bone of the cranium. The paranasal sinuses include all of the sinuses. [*see also*: ethmoid sinuses, frontal sinuses, maxillary sinuses, sphenoid sinuses, sinusitis]   F

sinus series — Plain x-rays are taken from various angles to show all of the sinuses and confirm or rule out a diagnosis of sinusitis. Sinusitis shows as cloudy, opacified sinuses with thickened mucous membranes. Sometimes an air-fluid level can be seen within the sinus.

sinus tachy-cardia [427.xx] — Arrhythmia in which there is a fast but regular rhythm (up to 200 beats/minute), due to an abnormality in the sinoatrial (SA) node. [*see also*: conduction system, dysrhythmia]

sinusitis [461.xx; 473.xx] — Acute or chronic bacterial infection in one or all of the sinus cavities [*see also*: pansinusitis].

    Sx Headache, pain in the face over the sinus, postnasal drainage, fatigue, and fever.

skeletal muscles — One of three types of muscles in the body, but the only muscles that are under voluntary, conscious control. Under the microscope, skeletal muscle has a striated appearance. [*see also*: striated]   F

skeletal system — Body system that includes the bones, cartilage, ligaments, and joints. It supports the body.

skeleton — The bony framework of the body that consists of all the bones.   F

skin — Tissue covering of the body that consists of two layers (epidermis and dermis). Skin is categorized as an epithelial tissue. The skin is one part of the integumentary system.

skin grafting — Surgical procedure that uses human, animal, or artificial skin to provide a temporary covering or permanent layer of skin over a burn or wound. A dermatome is used to remove (harvest) a thin layer of skin to be used as a graft. A split-thickness skin graft contains the epidermis and part of the dermis. A full-thickness skin graft contains the epidermis and all of the dermis. Tiny holes can be cut in the skin graft to stretch it like mesh and cover a larger area. These holes allow fluid from damaged tissue to flow out and provide spaces into which the new skin can grow. [*see also*: allograft, autograft, debridement, dermatoplasty, xenograft]

skin resurfacing — Removal of superficial and deep acne scars, fine or deep wrinkles, or tattoos, and correction of large pores and skin tone irregularities by means of topical chemicals, abrasion, or laser treatments. [*see also*: chemical peel, dermabrasion, exfoliation, laser skin resurfacing]

skin scraping
A skin scraping is done with the edge of a scalpel to obtain material from skin lesions to examine under a microscope and make a diagnosis of ringworm. [*see also*: ringworm]

sleep apnea
[327.xx; 780.xx]
Brief or prolonged absence of spontaneous respirations during sleep, usually at night, because of obstruction of the airway by the soft palate or neck tissues. Apnea is followed by a gasping breath that often awakens the patient. Patients experience sleep deprivation, fatigue, and difficulty concentrating during the day. Occurs most often in middle-aged, obese men who snore excessively. [*see also*: apnea, polysomnography]

slit-lamp examination
Diagnostic procedure to look for abnormalities of the cornea, anterior chamber, iris, or lens. The slit lamp combines a low-power microscope for magnification with a high-intensity light beam whose width can be adjusted down to a slit. [*see also*: gonioscopy]

small intestine
Organ of digestion between the stomach and the large intestine. The duodenum, jejunum, and ileum are the three parts of the small intestine. [*see also*: barium swallow, chyme, gluten enteropathy, villi]   S

sodium
Ion that plays a role in the contraction of the myocardium. The chemical symbol is Na^+. [*see also*: metabolic panel]   A
L

solar keratoses
[702.xx]
Raised, irregular, rough areas of skin that are dry and feel like sandpaper. These develop in middle-aged persons in areas chronically exposed to the sun and can become squamous cell carcinoma.   S

> **Dx** H&P. Possible biopsy to determine presence of squamous cell carcinoma.

> **Tx** Cryosurgery to freeze the areas or electrosurgery to burn the areas, making them easier to remove.

somatic nervous system
Division of the nervous system that uses the neurotransmitter acetylcholine and carries nerve impulses to the voluntary skeletal muscles.

somatostatin
Hormone secreted by the delta cells of the islets of Langerhans in the pancreas. It inhibits the release of growth hormone, glucagon, and insulin. [*see also*: inhibition]

spastic paralysis
After an injury to the spinal cord, without nerve impulses the muscles lose their tone and firmness and eventually atrophy. However, the reflex arc of the lower spinal cord often remains intact and, in response to pain or a full bladder, the spinal cord below the injury will send nerve impulses that cause the muscles to spasm. [*see also*: flaccid paralysis, paraplegia, quadriplegia]

spermatic cord
Muscular tube that contains arteries, veins, and nerves for each testis as well as the vas deferens. It passes through the inguinal canal. [*see also*: varicocele]

spermatocyte
Immature spermatozoon in the wall of the seminiferous tubule.

spermatogenesis
Process of producing a mature spermatozoon through the processes of mitosis and meiosis. [*see also*: oogenesis, spermatozoon]

spermatozoon
An individual mature sperm. It contains 23 chromosomes and is known as a gamete. [*see also*: gamete]   S
F

sphenoid sinuses	Sinuses in the sphenoid bone posterior to the nasal cavity and next to the pituitary gland of the brain. [*see also*: pansinusitis, transsphenoidal hypophysectomy]	
sphincter	Muscular ring around a tube. The sphincter in the bladder neck is not under conscious control. The external urethral sphincter at the end of the urethra is under voluntary, conscious control.	
spina bifida [741.xx]	Congenital abnormality of the neural tube where the vertebrae form incompletely. There is an abnormal opening in the vertebral column through which the spinal cord and nerves may protrude to the outside of the body. This defect is covered only by the meninges. [*see also*: neural tube defect]	
spinal cavity	Hollow cavity that is surrounded by the vertebral column and contains the spinal cord, spinal nerves, and spinal fluid.	S
spinal cord	Part of the central nervous system. It joins the medulla oblongata of the brain and extends down the back in the spinal cavity. It ends at L2 and separates into individual nerves (cauda equina). [*see also*: cauda equina, Lou Gehrig's disease, meninges, neural tube injury, reflex, spinal cord injury]	
spinal cord injury	Trauma to the spinal cord with a partial or complete transection of the cord, which interrupts nerve impulses, causing partial or complete anesthesia and paralysis. [*see also*: cystometry, flaccid paralysis, incontinence, paraplegia, priapism, quadriplegia, neurogenic bladder, spastic paralysis]	A
spinal nerves	Thirty-one pairs of nerves. Each pair comes out from the spinal cord between two vertebrae. An individual spinal nerve consists of dorsal nerve roots and ventral nerve roots. [*see also*: dermatome]	
spinal tap	Medical procedure to obtain cerebrospinal fluid (CSF) for testing. A needle is inserted in the space between the L3–4 or L4–5 vertebrae and into the subarachnoid space. Cerebrospinal fluid flows through the needle and is collected and sent to the laboratory. Before the spinal needle is removed, a calibrated manometer may be attached to the needle to measure the intracranial pressure as the CSF rises in the manometer. [*see also*: cerebrospinal fluid examination]	S
spinal traction	Medical procedure in which a fracture of the vertebra is immobilized while it heals. Two metal pins are surgically inserted into the cranium and attached to a set of tongs with a rope and pulley and 7–10 pounds of weight. A patient with a partially healed fracture of the vertebra can be fitted for a halo vest with pins in the cranium attached to a metal ring (halo).	
spine	Bony vertical column of vertebrae. It is divided into five regions: cervical, thoracic, lumbar, sacrum, and coccyx. [*see also*: bone density tests, dextroscoliosis, kyphosis, levoscoliosis, lordosis, myelography, scoliosis, spondylolisthesis, vertebra]	S F
spiral computerized axial tomography	Uses an x-ray beam that is controlled by a computer and moves around the body axis of a patient inside the CT scanner. Produces individual images as "slices," as well as a composite three-dimensional view. During a spiral or helical CT scan, the patient's bed moves through the scanner while the x-ray beam rotates, creating a spiral. [*see also*: computerized axial tomography, multidetector-row computerized tomography]	S
spiral fracture	Bone is broken in a spiral because of a twisting force. [*see also*: fracture]	

A = Abbreviations Section   **F** = Figures Section   **L** = Laboratory Section   **S** = Synonyms Section
Sx (Symptoms)   **Dx** (Diagnosis)   **Tx** (Treatment)

spleen	Lymphoid organ located in the abdominal cavity behind the stomach. The spleen destroys old erythrocytes, breaking their hemoglobin into heme and globins. It also acts as a storage area for whole blood. Its white pulp is lymphoid tissue that contains B and T lymphocytes. [see also: lymphatic system, splenomegaly]	F
splenomegaly [789.xx]	Enlargement of the spleen, felt on palpation of the abdomen. Can be caused by mononucleosis, Hodgkin's disease, hemolytic anemia, polycythemia vera, or leukemia. [see also: portal hypertension]	
spondylolisthesis [756.xx]	Degenerative condition of the spine in which one vertebra moves anteriorly over another vertebra and slips out of proper alignment due to degeneration of the intervertebral disk. [see also: ankylosing spondylitis]	S
sprain	Overstretching or tearing of a ligament. [see also: ligament]	
squamous cell carcinoma	Arises from the flat squamous cells of the outer part of the epidermis. It often begins as an actinic keratosis. It most often appears as a red bump or ulcer. It is the second most common type of cancer, but it grows slowly. [see also: solar keratoses]	A
staging	Medical (or surgical) procedure that classifies cancer by how far it has spread in the body. The TNM staging system is used to describe the size of the tumor and whether the tumor has spread to lymph nodes and other sites.	
status asthmaticus [493.xx]	A prolonged, extremely severe, life-threatening asthma attack. [see also: asthma]	
status epilepticus [345.xx]	A state of prolonged, continuous seizure activity or frequently repeated individual seizures that occur without the patient regaining consciousness. [see also: epilepsy, postictal state, seizure]	
steatorrhea	Greasy, frothy, and foul-smelling stools that contain undigested fats. [see also: defecation]	
stem cell	Extremely immature cell in the red marrow that is the precursor to all types of blood cells. [see also: bone marrow testing, pancytopenia, stem cell transplantation, thrombocytopenia]	F
stem cell transplantation	Stem cells (rather than bone marrow) from the patient or a matched donor are collected by apheresis of the peripheral blood. Matched stem cells from umbilical cord blood can also be given. [see also: apheresis, bone marrow transplantation]	
stereoscopic vision	Three-dimensional vision with depth perception.	
stereotactic biopsy and neurosurgery	Surgical procedure that uses three-dimensional excision of a tumor deep within the cerebrum. A CT or MRI scan is used to show the tumor in three dimensions and obtain its precise coordinates. The patient's head is fixed in a stereotactic apparatus that acts as a guidance system to guide the biopsy needle or to position an electrode within the brain.	
stimulation	Action of a hormone to cause an organ or gland to release its hormones. [see also: hormones]	
stomach	Organ of digestion between the esophagus and the small intestine. Areas of the stomach: cardia, fundus, body, antrum, and pylorus. The stomach secretes hydrochloric acid, pepsinogen, gastrin, and intrinsic factor needed to absorb vitamin B_{12}. [see also: barium swallow, cholecystokinin, chyme, emesis, gastrectomy, gastric analysis, gastric bypass, gastrin, gastritis, gastroenteritis,	F

gastroesophageal reflux disease, gastroplasty, gastrostomy, heartburn, hiatal hernia, hydrochloric acid, nausea, omentum, pepsin, pepsinogen, pernicious anemia, sudden infant death syndrome, varices]

stomatitis [528.xx]   Inflammation of the oral mucosa. [*see also*: aphthous stomatitis]

stone basketing   Surgical procedure in which a cystoscope is inserted into the bladder. A stone basket (a long-handled instrument with several interwoven wires at its end) is then passed through the cystoscope to a kidney stone to remove it.

strabismus [378.xx]   Deviation of one or both eyes medially or laterally. Medial deviation is known as esotropia or cross-eye. Lateral deviation is known as exotropia or wall-eye. [*see also*: amblyopia, convergence, esotropia, exotropia]   S

straight catheter   Medical procedure in which a catheter (flexible tube) is inserted through the urethra and into the bladder to drain urine each time the bladder becomes full, or it can also be used to obtain a single urine specimen for testing. [*see also*: condom catheter, Foley catheter, neurogenic bladder, suprapubic catheter]   S

strep throat [034.xx]   Bacterial infection of the throat caused by the bacterium group A beta-hemolytic streptococcus. It is important to diagnose strep throat and treat it with an antibiotic drug so that it does not cause the complication of rheumatic heart disease. [*see also*: rapid strep test, rheumatic heart disease]

stress test   Diagnostic procedure performed to evaluate the heart's response to exercise in patients with chest pain, palpitations, or arrhythmias. The patient walks on a motorized treadmill or rides a stationary bike. The speed, incline, or resistance is gradually increased while the patient's heart rate, blood pressure, and EKG are monitored. [*see also*: angina pectoris, Cardiolite stress test, myocardial perfusion scan, pharmacologic stress test]   S

striated   Having stripes. This is a characteristic of skeletal muscle cells at the cellular level. The stripes are alternating strands of actin and myosin. [*see also*: muscle]

stridor [786.xx]   A high-pitched, harsh, crowing sound due to obstruction in the trachea or larynx.

stye [373.xx]   Red, painful swelling or pimple containing pus near the edge of the eyelid. Caused by a bacterial infection (staphylococcus) in a sebaceous (meibomian) gland. Also known as a hordeolum. [*see also*: blepharitis, chalazion]   S

subarachnoid space   Space beneath the arachnoid layer of the meninges. It is filled with cerebrospinal fluid. [*see also*: arachnoid, cerebrospinal fluid, lumbar puncture, myelography]   F

subcutaneous tissue   Loose, connective tissue directly beneath the dermis. It is composed of adipose tissue. [*see also*: adipose tissue]

subdural hematoma [432.xx]   Localized collection of blood that forms between the dura mater and the arachnoid in the brain because of the rupture of an artery or vein.

Dx   H&P. The patient will have rapid neurological changes on exam. A CT scan and MRI will be performed to visualize the brain.

Tx   Directed toward relieving the pressure, which usually means trephination (drilling a hole through the skull) to drain the fluid and relieve the pressure. [*see also*: craniotomy]

substantia nigra	A darkly pigmented area in the midbrain of the brainstem that produces the neurotransmitter dopamine. [see also: dopamine]
sudden infant death syndrome [798.xx]	The exact cause is unknown, but it has been attributed to respiratory arrest from aspiration of stomach contents or asphyxiation from soft bedding blocking the flow of air. [see also: aspiration pneumonia]	A S
sudoriferous gland	An exocrine gland of the skin that secretes sweat through a duct. These glands are located in the dermis. The duct opens at a pore on the surface of the skin. [see also: anhidrosis]
sulcus	One of many large grooves between the gyri in the cerebrum and cerebellum. Plural: sulci. [see also: gyrus]
superficial	On or near the surface of the body or the surface of an organ or structure.
superior	Pertaining to the upper half of the body or a position above an organ or structure. Opposite of inferior. [see also: transverse plane]
supination	Turning the palm of the hand upward. Opposite of pronation.
supinator	Muscle that produces supination when it contracts.
supine	Position of lying on the posterior part of the body. Opposite of prone.	S
suppressor genes	Group of genes in the DNA of each cell that inhibits mitosis. The p53 gene is the most important suppressor gene.
suprapubic catheter	A catheter is inserted through the abdominal wall (just above the pubic bone) and into the bladder to drain the urine. It is sometimes inserted after bladder or prostate gland surgery. [see also: condom catheter, Foley catheter, straight catheter, urination]
supraventricular tachycardia [727.xx]	Arrhythmia in which there is a fast but regular rhythm (up to 200 beats/minute) when the ectopic group of cells is located superior to the ventricles. [see also: automatic implantable cardiac defibrillator, cardiac cycle, defibrillator, dysrhythmia]	A
surfactant	Protein-fat compound that creates surface tension and keeps the walls of the alveolus from collapsing inward with each exhalation. [see also: hyaline membrane disease, lecithin/sphingomyelin ratio]	S
suture	Immoveable joint between two bones of the cranium.
sympathetic nervous system	Division of the autonomic nervous system that uses the neurotransmitter epinephrine and carries nerve impulses to the heart, involuntary muscles, and glands during times of increased activity, danger, or stress. [see also: autonomic nervous system, epinephrine, hypothalamus]
synapse	Space between the axon of one neuron and the dendrites of the next neuron. [see also: neuron]
syncope [780.xx]	Temporary loss of consciousness. A syncopal episode is one in which the patient becomes lightheaded and then faints and briefly remains unconscious. Most often due to diseases that cause decreased blood flow to the brain.
syndactyly [755.xx]	Congenital abnormality in which the skin and soft tissues are joined between the fingers or toes. [see also: polydactyly]
syndrome of inappropriate antidiuretic hormone [253.xx]	Hypersecretion of antidiuretic hormone (ADH). ADH moves water from the renal tubules back into the blood. Too much ADH causes a fluid and electrolyte imbalance. [see also: antidiuretic hormone, diabetes insipidus]	A L

A = Abbreviations Section   F = Figures Section   L = Laboratory Section   S = Synonyms Section
Sx (Symptoms)   Dx (Diagnosis)   Tx (Treatment)

synergism

Process in which two hormones work together to accomplish the same, but enhanced, result. [*see also*: hormone]

synovial joint

Fully moveable joints. There are two types: hinge-type and ball-and-socket joints. Ligaments hold the bone ends together. The entire joint is enclosed in a joint capsule. The inner surface of the joint capsule is lined by a synovial membrane that produces synovial fluid to lubricate the joint. [*see also*: arthroscopy, bursa]

syphilis [092.xx; 096.xx–097.xx]

A sexually transmitted disease caused by *Treponema pallidum,* a spirochete (spiral) bacterium.

Sx   Single, painless chancre (lesion that ulcerates, forms a crust, and then heals) on the penis in men and on the female genitalia in women. Later symptoms include fever, rash, and various symptoms that mimic other diseases. Fluid from a lesion viewed with special illumination under darkfield microscopy shows the spiral bacterium.

Dx   Blood tests for antibodies (RPR, VDRL).

Tx   Oral antibiotic drugs.

systematic desensitization

Technique in which patients imagine about 10 different scenarios involving a specific phobia (for example, fear of spiders). Each scenario is associated with progressively greater anxiety. The patient practices relaxation techniques before and after visualizing the first scenario. When the first scenario no longer causes anxiety, patients move on to the second, and so forth until they are no longer sensitive to that phobia.

systemic circulation

The blood vessels (arteries, capillaries, and veins) everywhere in the body, except the lungs. [*see also*: pulmonary circulation]

systemic lupus erythematosus [710.xx]

Autoimmune disorder characterized by deterioration of collagen in the skin and connective tissues. There is a rash, joint pain, sensitivity to sunlight, and fatigue. Often there is a characteristic butterfly-shaped, erythematous rash that covers the nose and cheeks. [*see also*: autoimmune disease]

A
L
S

Dx   H&P. There is no diagnostic test for SLE. Clinicians use a variety of criteria to make a definitive diagnosis. [*see also*: C-reactive protein, enzyme-linked immunosorbent assay]

Tx   Treatment depends on the severity, the symptoms, and which organ is affected.

systemic reaction

Allergic reaction that takes place throughout the body in a hypersensitive person after contact with an allergen that was ingested, inhaled, or injected. [*see also*: anaphylactic shock]

systole

Combined contractions of the atria and the ventricles. [*see also*: asystole, diastole]

T

T cell

Type of lymphocyte that matures in the thymus. There are four subsets of T cells: helper T cells (CD4 cells), memory T cells, cytotoxic T cells, and suppressor T cells (CD8 cells).

tachycardia [427.xx]

Arrhythmia in which there is a fast but regular rhythm (up to 200 beats/minute). [*see also*: atrial tachycardia, conduction system, dysrhythmia, paroxysmal tachycardia, sinus tachycardia, and supraventricular tachycardia]

S

tachypnea [786.xx]	Abnormally rapid rate of breathing caused by lung disease. [*see also*: dyspnea]	**S**
talipes [754.xx]	Congenital deformity of one or both feet in which the foot is pulled downwards and laterally to the side. The plantar surface of the foot never rests on the ground.	
Tanner staging	System used to describe the development of the female breasts from childhood through puberty. There are five different stages, from Tanner stage 1 (nipple and areola are flat against the chest wall) to Tanner stage 5 (enlargement of the entire breast). The Tanner system is also used to describe the development of the female external genitalia.	
technetium-99m	Given intravenously for nuclear medicine imaging of many different areas of the body. It is the most common radiopharmaceutical used in nuclear imaging. Technetium, a rare silvery gray metal, is used commercially to prevent corrosion in steel. [*see also*: Cardiolite stress test, hydroxyiminodiacetic acid scan, radiopharmaceutical]	
telemetry	Diagnostic procedure to monitor a patient's heart rate and rhythm in the hospital. The patient wears electrodes that continuously transmit the ECG tracing to a central monitoring station. [*see also*: conduction system, electrocardiography]	
temporal lobe	Lobe of the cerebrum that receives and analyzes sensory information. Contains the auditory cortex for the sense of hearing and the olfactory cortex for the sense of smell. [*see also*: anosmia, auditory cortex]	**F**
temporo-mandibular joint syndrome [524.xx]	Dysfunction of the temporomandibular joint with clicking, pain, muscle spasm, and difficulty opening the jaw. Caused by chewing on only one side of the mouth, clenching or grinding the teeth (often during sleep), or misalignment of the teeth.	
tendon	Cordlike white band of nonelastic fibrous connective tissue that attaches a muscle to a bone. [*see also*: avulsion, bursa, deep tendon reflexes, fascia, ganglion, ligament, shin splints, tendonitis, tenorrhaphy]	
tendonitis	Inflammation of any tendon from injury or overuse. [*see also*: repetitive strain injury, tenosynovitis]	
tenorrhaphy	Surgical procedure to suture together the torn ends of a tendon following an injury. [*see also*: avulsion, tendon]	
tenosynovitis	Inflammation and pain due to overuse of the tendon and inability of the tendon sheath to produce enough lubricating fluid. [*see also*: pain management]	
Tensilon test	Diagnostic procedure in which the drug Tensilon is given to confirm a diagnosis of myasthenia gravis. The drug blocks the enzyme that breaks down acetylcholine, and patients with myasthenia gravis show increased muscle strength. [*see also*: myasthenia gravis]	
testes	Endocrine glands on either side of the scrotum. FSH from the anterior pituitary gland stimulates their seminiferous tubules to produce sperm. LH from the anterior pituitary gland stimulates their interstitial cells to produce and secrete testosterone. [*see also*: alpha fetoprotein, cryptorchism, follicle-stimulating hormone, FSH assay and LH assay, gonads, human chorionic gonadotropin, inguinal canal, oligospermia, orchiectomy, orchitis, scrotum, semen, testicular self-examination, testosterone, vasectomy]	**F** **S**

testicular self-examination	Systematic palpation of the testes and scrotum to detect lumps, masses, or enlarged lymph nodes. TSE should be done monthly to detect early signs of testicular cancer. [*see also*: testes]
testosterone	Male hormone that is the most abundant and most biologically active of the androgens. Testosterone is produced and secreted by the interstitial cells of the testes when stimulated by LH from the anterior pituitary gland. [*see also*: androgens, gynecomastia, hormone testing, impotence, infertility, luteinizing hormone, precocious puberty] L
tetralogy of Fallot [745.xx]	Syndrome of four congenital heart defects: ventricular septal defect, narrowing of the pulmonary artery valve and trunk, hypertrophy of the right ventricle, and malposition of the aorta.
thalamus	Relay station in the brain that receives sensory nerve impulses from the optic nerves and sends them to the visual centers in the occipital lobes of the brain. Cranial nerves II, III, and IV originate from the thalamus. [*see also*: cranial nerves, limbic system, hypothalamus]
thalassemia [282.xx]	Inherited genetic abnormality that affects the synthesis of globin chains in the hemoglobin molecule. The erythrocytes are small, pale, and of variable size. Target cells (erythrocytes with a central dark spot) are seen. [*see also*: anisocytosis]
Thematic Apperception Test	Assesses personality, emotions, attitudes, motivation, and conflicts. The patient is shown 31 different pictures of social or interpersonal situations. The patient describes what is happening in the picture or what the theme of the picture is. A
therapeutic milieu	Stable, structured, and safe emotional and physical environment that provides ongoing therapy of various types for a psychiatric patient.
third-degree burn [948.xx]	Involves the epidermis and entire dermis. The subcutaneous tissue and even the muscle layer may be involved. Heat (fire, hot objects, steam, boiling water), electrical current (lightning, electrical outlets or cords), chemicals, or radiation or x-rays (sunshine or prescribed radiation therapy) can injure superficial or deep tissues. [*see also*: burn, eschar]
third-degree heart block [426.xx]	Arrhythmia in which no electrical impulses travel from the SA node to the Purkinje fibers. [*see also*: conduction system, dysrhythmia, heart block] S
thoracentesis	Surgical procedure that uses a needle and syringe to remove pleural fluid from the pleural space. Used to treat pleural effusion or obtain fluid for the diagnosis of lung cancer. [*see also*: pleural effusion, pneumothorax, pyothorax]
thoracic cavity	Major body cavity in the chest that is surrounded by the sternum, ribs, and spinal column. It contains the lungs, mediastinum, heart, and great vessels. The diaphragm makes up the inferior side of the cavity.
thoracic vertebrae	Vertebrae T1 through T12 in the thoracic part of the spine in the chest. A F
thoracotomy	Incision into the thoracic cavity is the first step in some surgical procedures on the thoracic cavity and lungs. [*see also*: lung resection]
thrombocyte	Cell fragment that does not have a nucleus. It is active in the blood clotting process. [*see also*: aggregation, clotting factors, coagulation, leukemia, megakaryocyte, thrombocytopenia] F S

thrombocytopenia
[287.xx]

Deficiency in the number of thrombocytes due to damaged stem cells in the bone marrow, when leukemia cells take over the red bone marrow and crowd out the stem cells or a patient's antibodies destroy their own thrombocytes. [*see also*: blood dyscrasia]

L

thrombophlebitis
[451.xx]

Inflammation of a vein caused by a thrombus (blood clot). The area around the vein is painful and can partially occlude the vein and slow the flow of blood. [*see also*: phlebitis]

thromboplastin

Blood clotting factor III. Also known as tissue factor. [*see also*: clotting factors, partial thromboplastin time]

S

thrombus

A blood clot. [*see also*: cerebrovascular accident, deep vein thrombosis, myocardial infarction, phlebitis, prothrombin]

L
S

thrush [112.xx]

Oral infection caused by the yeast-like fungus *Candida albicans*. It coats the tongue and oral mucosa. Common in infants, but is also seen in the mouths of immunocompromised patients with AIDS because their immune response cannot control its growth. Also seen after a course of antibiotic drugs kills bacteria in the mouth, allowing overgrowth of *Candida albicans*.

S

thymectomy

Surgical removal of the thymus because of a benign or cancerous tumor. Thymectomy is also performed on patients with myasthenia gravis. After a thymectomy, the level of antibodies against acetylcholine receptors falls, and patients with myasthenia gravis can be treated with fewer immunosuppressant drugs. The reason for the improvement is not known. [*see also*: myasthenia gravis]

thymoma
[212.xx]

Usually benign tumor of the thymus. May cause cough and chest pain. Often seen in patients who already have an autoimmune disorder, such as myasthenia gravis. [*see also*: autoimmune disease]

thymus

Endocrine gland posterior to the sternum that produces and secretes the group of hormones known as thymosins. They cause immature T lymphocytes in the thymus to mature. [*see also*: lymphatic system, lymphocyte, T cell, thymectomy, thymoma]

F

thyroid function test

Blood test that measures the levels of T_3, T_4, and TSH. Used to evaluate the function of the thyroid gland and the anterior pituitary gland. The test uses radioimmunoassay in which antibodies labeled with radioactive isotopes combine with the hormone and the amount of radioactivity is measured. Another value, the free thyroxine index (FTI) or T_7, can be calculated from this.

A
L

thyroid gland

Endocrine gland in the neck that produces and secretes the hormones T_3, T_4, and calcitonin. Its two lobes and narrow connecting bridge (isthmus) give it a shieldlike shape. [*see also*: thyroid function tests]

thyroid storm
[242.xx]

Severe and sudden hypersecretion of T_3 and T_4 thyroid hormones. Caused by an adenoma or a nodule in the thyroid gland. (It can also be caused by hypersecretion of TSH from an adenoma in the anterior pituitary gland.)

S

thyroiditis
[245.xx]

Chronic inflammation and progressive destruction of the thyroid gland. The thyroid becomes inflamed and enlarged (goiter). Over time, the patient develops hypothyroidism as thyroid tissue is destroyed and replaced by fibrous tissue. [*see also*: Hashimoto's thyroiditis]

L

thyroid-stimulating hormone

Hormone secreted by the anterior pituitary gland that stimulates the thyroid to secrete T_3 and T_4.

A
L
S

thyroxine

Hormone (T_4) secreted by the thyroid gland, but mostly changed into T_3 by the liver. [*see also*: antithyroglobulin antibodies, hyperthyroidism, hypothyroidism, thyroid function tests, thyroid storm, thyroid-stimulating hormone, triiodothyronine]

A
L

tic douloureux [350.xx]

Characterized by stabbing pain for a few seconds on one side of the face or jaw along the distribution of the trigeminal nerve. [*see also*: neuralgia, pain management]

S

tinea [110.xx]

Skin infection caused by a microscopic fungus that feeds on epidermal cells. It multiplies quickly in the warm, moist environment of body creases and areas enclosed by clothing or shoes. Tinea is named according to where it occurs on the body: tinea capitis occurs on the scalp, tinea corporis (ringworm) occurs on any part of the body and produces a round lesion, tinea cruris (jock itch) occurs in the groin and perineum, and tinea pedis (athlete's foot) occurs on the feet and toes.

tinnitus [388.xx]

Sounds (buzzing, ringing, hissing, or roaring) that are heard constantly or intermittently in one or both ears, even in a quiet environment. It is caused by exposure to excess noise and associated with hearing loss. It can also be related to overuse of aspirin. [*see also*: conductive hearing loss, Ménière's disease, mixed hearing loss, sensorineural hearing loss]

S

TNM system

Used to characterize the size of a cancerous tumor and its spread throughout the body. T = size of the primary tumor (T1 through T4), N = number of regional lymph nodes affected (N1 through N4), M = presence or absence of metastases to other sites in the body (M0 or M1).

A

tongue

Large muscle that fills the oral cavity and assists with eating and talking. It contains taste buds and receptors for the sense of taste. [*see also*: glossitis, glottis, gustatory cortex, hypoglossal nerve, lingual tonsils, mastication, thrush]

F

tonic-clonic seizure [345.xx]

Unconsciousness with excessive motor activity. The body alternates between excessive muscle tone with rigidity (tonic) and jerking muscle contractions (clonic) in the extremities, with tongue biting and sometimes incontinence. [*see also*: epilepsy, seizures]

S

tonometry

Diagnostic procedure for increased intraocular pressure and glaucoma. The small, flat disk of the tonometer is pressed against the cornea to record the intraocular pressure. Alternatively, air-puff tonometry emits a short burst of air and measures the pressure of the air rebounding from the cornea without touching the patient's eye. [*see also*: glaucoma]

tonsillitis [463.xx; 474.xx]

Acute or chronic bacterial infection of the pharynx and palatine tonsils, with sore throat, difficulty swallowing, mouth breathing, and snoring. The tonsils hypertrophy and the tonsillar crypts contain pus and debris. The adenoids may also hypertrophy and block the eustachian tubes. [*see also*: lingual tonsils, palatine tonsils, pharyngeal tonsils]

torn meniscus [836.xx]

Tear of the cartilage pad of the knee because of an injury. [*see also*: arthrography, arthroscopy, articular cartilage]

torticollis [333.xx; 723.xx]

Painful contraction of the muscles on one side of the neck. [*see also*: pain management]

S

total iron binding capacity	Blood chemistry test that measures the level of transferrin, a protein that carries iron in the blood. Used to diagnose iron deficiency anemia. [*see also*: iron deficiency anemia]	A
total mastectomy	Surgical resection where the entire breast, the overlying skin, and nipple are removed, but not the chest muscle or axillary nodes. [*see also*: mastectomy]	S
Tourette's syndrome [703.xx]	Frequent, spontaneous, involuntary movement tics and vocal tics or comments that are socially inappropriate, vulgar, obscene, or racist. The patient can only temporarily suppress these tics. There may also be echolalia, obsessive-compulsive disorder, and hyperactivity. [*see also*: autism, dyskinesia, obsessive-compulsive disorder]	
toxic shock syndrome [040.xx]	Patients use super-absorbent tampons that allow the normally harmless vaginal bacterium *Staphylococcus aureus* to multiply in the old menstrual blood and release toxins. The tampon itself creates small tears in the vaginal wall that allow the toxins to enter the blood. [*see also*: sepsis]	
trabecular meshwork	Area of interlacing fibers through which the aqueous humor is filtered. It is located in the anterior chamber in the angle where the edges of the iris and the cornea meet. [*see also*: gonioscopy, trabeculoplasty]	
trabeculoplasty	Surgical procedure to treat open-angle glaucoma. An argon laser is used to create small holes in half of the trabecular meshwork to increase the flow of aqueous humor. The procedure is usually effective for five years, at which time another trabeculoplasty can be performed on the untreated half of the trabecular meshwork. [*see also*: open-angle glaucoma, trabecular meshwork]	
tracer	Nuclear medicine radiopharmaceutical whose presence in the body can be traced by the gamma rays it produces. [*see also*: Cardiolite stress test, myocardial perfusion scan, radioactive iodine uptake and thyroid scan, radionuclide ventriculography, Schilling test, scintigraphy]	S
trachea	Rigid, tubular air passageway between the larynx and the bronchi. It carries inhaled and exhaled air to and from the bronchi. [*see also*: bronchoscopy, endotracheal intubation, stridor, tracheostomy]	F S
tracheobronchial tree	Branching structures of the respiratory system that resemble an upside-down tree and its branches. It includes the trachea, bronchi, and bronchioles. [*see also*: bronchoscopy, endotracheal intubation]	S
tracheostomy	Incision into the trachea and creation of a permanent opening. A plastic or metal tube is then inserted to keep the opening patent. Tracheostomies are performed to provide permanent access to the lungs in patients who need long-term respiratory support, usually with a ventilator.	A
tragus	Triangular cartilage anterior to the external auditory meatus.	
transarterial chemoem-bolization	Surgical procedure in which an intra-arterial catheter is threaded through the femoral artery, aorta, and into the hepatic artery to deliver a one-time dose of chemotherapy. After the drug is administered, an inert substance is injected to block the flow of blood and to keep the drug concentrated at the site of the cancerous tumor. [*see also*: internal radiotherapy, interstitial radiotherapy, intracavitary radiotherapy]	A

A = Abbreviations Section   **F** = Figures Section   **L** = Laboratory Section   **S** = Synonyms Section
Sx (Symptoms)   **Dx** (Diagnosis)   **Tx** (Treatment)

transcutaneous electrical nerve stimulation unit	Medical procedure that uses an electrical device to control chronic pain. A battery produces regular, preset electrical impulses that travel through wires to electrodes on the skin. These impulses block the transmission of pain sensations to the brain. The impulses also stimulate the body to produce its own natural pain-relieving endorphins. [*see also*: pain management]	A
transesophageal echocardiography	A patient swallows an endoscopic tube that contains a tiny sound-emitting transducer. This is positioned in the esophagus directly behind the heart. Used when a standard echocardiogram produces a poor quality image. [*see also*: echocardiography, color flow duplex ultrasonography, Doppler ultrasonography]	A
transfusion reaction [999.xx]	Reaction that occurs when a patient receives a blood transfusion with an incompatible blood type. Antibodies in the patient's serum attack antigens on the erythrocytes of the donor blood, causing hemolysis of the donor erythrocytes. Transfusion reactions can be fatal. [*see also*: blood transfusion]	L S
transient ischemic attack [435.xx]	A temporary lack of oxygenated blood to an area of the brain. It is like a RIND, but its effects only last 24 hours. [*see also*: cerebral angiography, cerebrovascular accident, reversible ischemic neurologic deficit]	A
translocation	Damage to the DNA that breaks off a gene segment from one chromosome and puts it into another chromosome. [*see also*: genetic mutation]	
transsexualism [302.xx]	Person's belief that he or she has been assigned (by anatomy, parents, or society) the wrong gender identity. The patient desires to change his or her outward appearance to the opposite sex in order to match what is already felt in the mind as being the true personal identity.	
transsphenoidal hypophysectomy	Surgical procedure to remove an adenoma from the pituitary gland. The pituitary gland is difficult to visualize through an incision in the cranium, so the incision is made through the sphenoid sinus.	
transurethral resection of the prostate	Surgical procedure to reduce the size of the prostate gland. A special cystoscope known as a resectoscope is inserted through the urethra. It has built-in cutting instruments and cautery to resect pieces of the prostate and cauterize bleeding vessels. Chips of prostatic tissue are then irrigated out. [*see also*: benign prostatic hypertrophy]	A
transverse fracture [829.xx]	Bone is broken in a transverse plane perpendicular to its long axis. [*see also*: fracture]	
transverse plane	Plane that divides the body into top and bottom sections, superior and inferior. [*see also*: coronal plane, midsagittal plane, oblique, projection]	
transverse rectus abdominis muscle flap	The transverse rectus abdominis muscle flap is used in conjunction with reconstructive mammaplasty. Skin, fat and muscle are excised, except for one end that is left attached to blood vessels (pedicle graft). Alternatively, the latissimus dorsi muscle of the back can be used. Then the flap is tunneled under the skin of the upper abdomen to the site of the previous mastectomy. Later, a tattoo can be done on the skin to create an areola and nipple. [*see also*: mastectomy, reconstructive mammaplasty]	A
transvestism [302.xx]	Obtaining sexual arousal by wearing clothes belonging to the opposite sex or posing as someone of the opposite sex. [*see also*: transsexualism]	S

A = Abbreviations Section **F** = Figures Section **L** = Laboratory Section **S** = Synonyms Section
Sx (Symptoms) **Dx** (Diagnosis) **Tx** (Treatment)

tremor	Small, involuntary, sometimes jerky, back-and-forth movements of the hands, neck, jaw, or extremities. These are continuous movements that cannot be suppressed by the patient. [*see also*: delirium tremens]
trichotillomania [312.xx]	Repetitive pulling out of hair from the head.
tricuspid valve	Heart valve located between the right atrium and right ventricle. It has three (tri-) pointed leaflets or cusps. [*see also*: chordae tendineae, endocarditis, valve] F
trigeminal nerve	Cranial nerve V. Sensation in the eyeball, lower eyelid, scalp, face, lips, and tongue. Controls movement of the muscles in these areas. Composed of three nerve branches: ophthalmic nerve, maxillary nerve, mandibular nerve. [*see also*: blepharoptosis] S
trigger point injections	Medical procedure to treat fibromyalgia and myofascial pain syndrome. A local anesthetic and a corticosteroid drug are injected into each trigger point to relieve pain and decrease inflammation. [*see also*: pain management]
trigone	Triangular-shaped area in the bladder that is formed by the two ureteral orifices and the opening to the urethra.
triiodothyronine	Hormone (T_3) secreted by the thyroid gland. Increases the rate of cellular metabolism. It is dependent on adequate iodine in the diet. A L
trimester	A period of three months. The time of gestation is divided into three equal trimesters. [*see also*: gestation]
trochlear nerve	Cranial nerve IV. Controls movement of the eyeball. [*see also*: convergence] S
troponin	Blood test to measure the level of two proteins that are released into the blood when myocardial cells die. Troponin I and troponin T are only found in the myocardium. The troponin levels begin to rise 4–6 hours after a myocardial infarction. More importantly, they remain elevated for up to 10 days, so they can be used to diagnose a myocardial infarction many days after it occurred. Troponin levels are done in conjunction with CK-MB and LDH levels. [*see also*: cardiac enzymes] A L
tubal ligation	Surgical procedure to prevent pregnancy. A short segment of each fallopian tube is removed. The cut ends are sutured and then crushed or cauterized. The woman continues to ovulate, but the ovum cannot travel through the blocked fallopian tube. A tubal anastomosis is the procedure to rejoin the fallopian tube segments so that the woman can get pregnant again. [*see also*: vasectomy] S
tuberculosis [010.xx–018.xx]	Lung infection caused by the bacterium *Mycobacterium tuberculosis* and spread by airborne droplets expelled by coughing. Initially, the infection may cause few symptoms. If the patient's immune system is strong, the bacteria can remain dormant for years without causing symptoms. If the patient's immune system is depressed, the bacteria multiply, producing tubercles (soft nodules of necrosis) in the lungs. [*see also*: adult respiratory distress syndrome, Mantoux test] A L
tubules	Small tubes within the nephron. [*see also*: distal convoluted tubules, loop of Henle, proximal convoluted tubules]
tumor markers	Blood test that detects antigens on the surface of cancer cells. Tumor markers are used to evaluate the extent of the cancer

A = Abbreviations Section   F = Figures Section   L = Laboratory Section   S = Synonyms Section
Sx (Symptoms)   Dx (Diagnosis)   Tx (Treatment)

	and the effectiveness of the treatment being given. They include CA 15-3 (breast cancer), CA 19-9 (cancer of the pancreas and bile ducts), CA 27.29 (cancer of the breast), and CA 125 (cancer of the ovary). AFP, CEA, and HCG are also classified as tumor markers.	
tumor necrosis factor	Substance released by macrophages. It destroys endotoxins produced by certain bacteria. It also destroys cancerous cells.	A
turbinates	Three long projections (superior, middle, inferior) of the ethmoid bone that jut into the nasal cavity and are covered with mucous membranes. They disperse the flow of air and moisturize as it enters the nose. [see also: allergic rhinitis, hay fever]	S F
tympanic membrane	Membrane that divides the external ear from the middle ear. [see also: conductive hearing loss, hemotympanum, mixed hearing loss, myringotomy, ossicles, otitis media, otoscopy, ruptured tympanic membrane, sensorineural hearing loss, tympanometry]	A F S
tympanometry	Hearing test that measures the ability of the tympanic membrane and the bones of the middle ear to move back and forth. Air pressure (rather than sound vibration) is applied to the external auditory canal. If infection or disease has fixed the middle ear bones, then the tympanic membrane will move very little. [see also: audiometry, tympanic membrane]	
type and crossmatch	Performed when a patient needs to receive a blood transfusion. The donor's blood was typed when it was stored in the blood bank. The patient's (recipient's) blood is then typed. The patient's plasma is mixed with the donor's red blood cells (crossmatching). If the donor's red blood cells clump together, the blood types are not compatible. [see also: blood transfusion]	A
Tzanck test	A skin scraping is done to obtain fluid from a vesicle. A smear of the fluid is placed on a slide, stained, and examined under a microscope. Herpes virus infections and shingles show characteristic giant cells with viruses in them. [see also: herpes]	

U

ulcerative colitis [556.xx]	A type of inflammatory bowel disease that affects the colon and rectum and causes inflammation and ulcers. [see also: barium enema, colon, inflammatory bowel disease]	
ultrasonography	Radiologic procedure that uses ultra high-frequency sound waves emitted by a transducer or probe that bounce off organs, creating echoes that are changed into an image by a computer. Three-dimensional ultrasonography couples the ultrasound with a position sensor to generate a high-resolution image in three dimensions.	S
umbilical cord	Rubbery cord that connects the placenta to the umbilicus (navel) of the fetus. It contains two arteries and one vein. [see also: nuchal cord, prolapsed cord]	
umbilical hernia [551.xx–553.xx]	A weakness in the muscles of the abdominal wall that allows loops of intestine to balloon outward, occurring next to the umbilicus. [see also: omphalocele]	
umbilical region	One of nine regions on the surface of the anterior abdominal area. The centered umbilical region is located around the umbilicus. [see also: epigastric region, hypochondriac region, hypogastric region, inguinal region, lumbar region, quadrant]	
undifferentiated	Cells that are immature and embryonal in appearance and behavior. [see also: differentiated]	

A = Abbreviations Section   **F** = Figures Section   **L** = Laboratory Section   **S** = Synonyms Section
Sx (Symptoms)   **Dx** (Diagnosis)   **Tx** (Treatment)

upper respiratory infection
[465.xx; 487.xx]

Bacterial or viral infection of the nose that can spread to the throat and ears. The nose is a part of the respiratory system as well as the ENT system.

A
S

urea

Waste product from protein metabolism. It is removed from the blood by the kidneys. [*see also*: blood urea nitrogen, metabolism, uremia]

uremia
[585.xx–586.xx]

Excessive amounts of urea in the blood because of renal failure. The kidneys are unable to remove the waste product urea, which reaches toxic levels in the blood. It is then excreted through the sweat glands, making white deposits on the skin that look like ice. [*see also*: blood urea nitrogen, renal failure, urea]

L

ureter

Tube that carries urine from the pelvis of the kidney to the bladder. [*see also*: hydronephrosis, KUB x-ray, nephrolithiasis, pyelography, pyelonephritis, renal colic]

F

ureteral orifice

Opening at the end of the ureter as it enters the bladder. [*see also*: ureter]

urethra

Tube that carries urine from the bladder to the outside of the body. [*see also*: benign prostatic hypertrophy, bladder neck suspension, bulbourethral glands, cystitis, ejaculatory duct, prostate gland, pyelography, transurethral resection of the prostate, urethritis, urinary meatus, urinary tract infection, voiding cystourethrography]

F

urethral meatus

The opening to the outside of the body that is at the end of the urethra. [*see also*: epispadias, hypospadias, urethroplasty]

F

urethritis

Inflammation or infection of the urethra, most often caused by a sexually transmitted disease. [*see also*: bacteriuria, nonspecific urethritis, sexually transmitted disease]

S

urethroplasty

Surgical procedure that involves plastic surgery to reposition the urethra. [*see also*: epispadias, hypospadias]

urgency [788.xx]

Strong urge to urinate and a sense of pressure in the bladder. It is caused by obstruction from an enlarged prostate gland, a kidney stone, or inflammation from a urinary tract infection. [*see also*: urination]

uric acid

Waste product from purine metabolism. It is removed from the blood by the kidneys. Elevated uric acid levels in the blood are found in patients with gout and gouty arthritis. [*see also*: gout, metabolic panel]

L

urinalysis

Urine test to describe the characteristics of the urine and detect substances in it. A quick urinalysis can be done with a dipstick test or the urine specimen can be sent to the laboratory for a full analysis. [*see also*: 24-hour creatinine test, ADH stimulation test, Bence Jones protein, drug screening, glucose tolerance test, leukocyte esterase, pregnancy test, Schilling test, vanillylmandelic acid]

A

urinary retention
[788.xx]

Inability to empty the bladder because of an obstruction, nerve damage, or as a side effect of certain types of drugs. Even when the bladder contracts, a large amount of postvoid residual urine remains in the bladder. [*see also*: neurogenic bladder, urination]

urinary system

Body system that includes the kidneys, ureters, bladder, and urethra. Its function is to produce urine. It also helps regulate the internal environment of the body by secreting the enzyme renin and the hormone erythropoietin. [*see also*: edema, urination]

S

A = Abbreviations Section   F = Figures Section   L = Laboratory Section   S = Synonyms Section
Sx (Symptoms)   **Dx** (Diagnosis)   **Tx** (Treatment)

urinary tract infection [599.xx]	General category of an infection anywhere in the urinary tract. Urinary infections are caused by bacteria, most often by *Escherichia coli* (*E. coli*), which is commonly found in the intestines and rectum. Because of the short length of the urethra in women and its location close to the anus, women are more prone than men to develop urinary tract infections. Catheterization can also introduce bacteria into the urinary tract. [*see also*: bacteriuria, cystitis, epididymitis, leukocyte esterase, prostatitis, pyelonephritis, pyuria, urethritis]	A
urination	The process of producing urine and expelling it from the body. [*see also*: anuria, bladder neck suspension, dysuria, enuresis, frequency, hematuria, hesitancy, incontinence, nocturia, nocturnal enuresis, oliguria, overactive bladder, polyuria, urgency, urinary retention, voiding cystourethrography]	S
urine	Water, waste products, and other substances excreted by the kidneys. [*see also*: albuminuria, bacteriuria, glycosuria, hematuria, ketonuria, pyuria, urination]	
urticaria [708.xx]	Caused by an allergic reaction. Edema and wheals appear suddenly and may also disappear rapidly. Scratching tends to cause the areas to enlarge. [*see also*: histamine, pruritus]	S
uterine artery embolization	Surgical and radiologic procedure used to treat uterine fibroids. A catheter is inserted into the femoral artery in the groin and threaded to the uterine artery. Radiopaque contrast dye is injected to identify the smaller artery that supplies blood to a fibroid. Tiny particles are injected to block that artery. Without a blood supply, the fibroid shrinks in size. [*see also*: uterine fibroid]	
uterine fibroid [218.xx]	Benign tumor of the myometrium. It can be small or as large as a soccer ball. There is pelvic pain, excessive uterine bleeding, and painful sexual intercourse. [*see also*: endometrial ablation, dysmenorrhea, dyspareunia, endometrium, leiomyoma, myomectomy, uterine artery embolization]	S
uterine inertia [661.xx; 763.xx]	Weak or uncoordinated contractions during labor. Caused by decreased levels of oxytocin from the posterior pituitary gland. Can also occur if the uterus is very distended and unable to contract normally because of multiple fetuses. [*see also*: dystocia]	
uterine prolapse [618.xx]	Descent of the uterus from its normal position. Caused by stretching of ligaments and weakness in the muscles of the floor of the pelvic cavity. The cervix may be visible at the vaginal introitus. [*see also*: broad ligament, uterine suspension]	S
uterine suspension	Surgical procedure to suspend and fix the uterus into an anatomically correct position. Used to correct a retroverted uterus or uterine prolapse. The uplift procedure uses sutures inserted through the abdomen and into the round ligament. Then the suture ends are pulled to shorten the round ligaments, which pulls the uterus up into a normal position. [*see also*: broad ligament, uterine prolapse]	S
uterus	Internal female organ of menstruation and pregnancy. [*see also*: anteflexion, broad ligament, culdoscopy, dilation and curettage, hysterectomy, involution, menstruation, oxytocin, pelvic inflammatory disease, retroversion of the uterus, uterine prolapse, uterine suspension, vernix caseosa]	F S
uveal tract	Collective word for the iris, choroid, and ciliary body. [*see also*: choroid, uveitis]	S F

uveitis	Inflammation or infection of the uveal tract. Can be caused by infection in the eye or another part of the body, allergy, trauma, or autoimmune disorders. [*see also*: autoimmune disease]
uvula	Fleshy, hanging part of the soft palate that activates the gag reflex when food touches it. [*see also*: oral cavity] F

V

vaccination	Medical procedure that injects a vaccine into the body. The vaccine consists of killed or attenuated (weakened) bacterial cells, viruses, or cell fragments. The body produces antibodies and memory B lymphocytes specific to that pathogen. If the vaccinated patient encounters that pathogen again, the patient will have mild or no symptoms of the disease. Vaccinations are routinely used to prevent diseases that could be fatal or cause serious disability if contracted. Immunoglobins against some diseases can be given to provide passive immunity if the person has just been exposed. S
vacuum-assisted biopsy	A probe with a cutting device is inserted through the skin and rotated around to take multiple specimens. The specimens are then suctioned out and sent to the lab for analysis. [*see also*: biopsy]
vagina	Short, tubular structure connected at its superior end to the cervix and at its inferior end to the outside of the body. It contains the vaginal canal. The external entrance is known as the vaginal introitus. The vagina is where semen is deposited during sexual intercourse. [*see also*: bacterial vaginosis, colporrhaphy, colposcopy, episiotomy, introitus, rectocele, vaginal candidiasis, vaginitis, vesicocele, vesicovaginal fistula] F
vaginal candidiasis [112.xx]	Yeast infection of the vagina due to *Candida albicans*. There is vaginal itching and leukorrhea. Usually occurs after taking an antibiotic drug for a bacterial infection. The drug kills the pathogen and the normal bacteria, and this allows the yeast to flourish.
vaginitis	Vaginal inflammation or infection. It can be caused by irritation from the chemicals in spermicidal jelly or douches or caused by candidiasis, trichomonas, bacterial infection, or an STD. [*see also*: bacterial vaginosis, sexually transmitted disease]
vagus nerve	Cranial nerve X. Sensation in the throat, ears, and the internal organs of the chest and abdomen. Controls the beating of the heart. Controls the movement of the muscles of respiration and digestion. [*see also*: accessory nerve] S
valve	Structure that opens and closes to control the flow of blood. The heart valves include the tricuspid valve, pulmonary valve, mitral valve, and aortic valve. There are also valves in some of the large veins that prevent backflow of blood. [*see also*: chordae tendineae, endocarditis, valve replacement]
valve replacement	Surgical procedure to replace a severely damaged or prolapsed heart valve. There are several types of replacement heart valves that can be used. [*see also*: allograft, endocarditis, valve, xenograft]
valvuloplasty	Surgical procedure to reconstruct a heart valve to correct stenosis or prolapse. A valvulotome is used to cut the valve. [*see also*: valve replacement] S
vanillylmandelic acid	A 24-hour urine test that measures the levels of vanillylmandelic acid, a byproduct of epinephrine and norepinephrine. Used to A

evaluate the function of the adrenal medulla. [*see also*: adrenal medulla]

varices [456.xx]
: Swollen, protruding veins in the mucosa of the lower esophagus or stomach. [*see also*: portal hypertension]

varicocele [456.xx]
: Varicose vein in the spermatic cord to the testis. The valves in the vein leak, allowing blood to back up in them. This causes pooling of the blood. The vein becomes distended and painful. Can cause a low sperm count and infertility. [*see also*: infertility, spermatic cord]

varicose vein [454.xx–456.xx; 671.xx]
: Damaged or incompetent valves in a vein that let blood flow backward and collect in the preceding section of vein. Eventually the vein becomes engorged with blood, twisting and bulging under the surface of the skin. [*see also*: color flow duplex ultrasonography, radiofrequency catheter ablation, sclerotherapy, varicocele]   **S**

vas deferens
: Long tube that receives spermatozoa from the epididymis and carries them to the seminal vesicles. [*see also*: vasectomy]   **F**   **S**

vasculature
: Network of blood vessels in a particular organ.

vasectomy
: Surgical procedure in the male to prevent pregnancy in the female. Through a small incision at the base of the scrotum, both vas deferens are divided, a length of each tube is removed, and the cut ends are sutured and crushed or electrocoagulated. Spermatozoa continue to be produced by the testes, but they are absorbed back into the body. [*see also*: antisperm antibody test, vasovasostomy]

vasoconstriction
: Constriction of the smooth muscle in the artery wall causes the artery to become smaller in diameter.

vasodilation
: Relaxation of the smooth muscle in the artery wall causes the artery to become larger in diameter.

vasovasostomy
: A reversal of a vasectomy. The cut ends of the vas deferens are rejoined so that spermatozoa are again present in the ejaculate so that the man can again impregnate a woman. [*see also*: antisperm antibody test, vasectomy]

veins
: Blood vessels that carry blood back to the heart. They carry carbon dioxide and waste products of cellular metabolism away from the cells and back to the heart. All but one contain oxygen-poor blood. The exception is the pulmonary vein, which carries oxygenated blood from the lungs to the heart.

vena cava
: Largest vein in the body. The superior vena cava receives blood from the head, neck, arms, and chest and takes it to the heart. The inferior vena cava receives blood from the abdomen, pelvis, and legs and takes it to the heart.   **F**

venography
: Radiologic procedure in which radiopaque contrast dye is injected into a vein to fill and outline it. It shows weakened valves and dilated walls. [*see also*: angiography, aortography, arteriography, coronary angiography, rotational angiography]

ventilation-perfusion scan
: Nuclear medicine procedure that uses inhaled radioactive gas to show air flow (ventilation) in the lungs. Areas of decreased uptake ("cold spots") indicate pneumonia, atelectasis, or pleural effusion. A radioactive solution is given intravenously for the perfusion part of the scan. Areas of decreased uptake indicate poor blood flow to that part of the lung. If the same area shows decreased uptake on both scans, this indicates a pulmonary   **A**

A = Abbreviations Section   **F** = Figures Section   **L** = Laboratory Section   **S** = Synonyms Section
Sx (Symptoms)   **Dx** (Diagnosis)   **Tx** (Treatment)

embolus. [*see also*: atelectasis, pulmonary embolism, pleural effusion, pneumonia]

ventral	Pertaining to the anterior of the body, particularly the abdomen.	S
ventral hernia [552.xx–553.xx]	A weakness in the muscles of the abdominal wall that allows loops of intestine to balloon outward, occurring anywhere on the anterior abdominal wall except at the umbilicus. [*see also*: hernia, umbilical hernia]	
ventral nerve roots	Group of spinal nerve roots that exit from the anterior (ventral) part of the spinal cord and carry motor nerve impulses to the body. [*see also*: amyotrophic lateral sclerosis, dorsal nerve roots]	
ventricle	Hollow chamber that is filled with fluid. Found in the heart and brain.	F
ventricular septal defect [754.xx]	Congenital defect in which there is a permanent hole in the heart's interventricular septum. [*see also*: tetralogy of Fallot]	A
ventriculoperi-toneal shunt	Surgical procedure to insert a plastic tube to connect the ventricles of the brain to the peritoneal cavity. The shunt continuously removes excess cerebrospinal fluid associated with hydrocephalus. [*see also*: hydrocephalus]	
vermillion border	Pink-red edge around the lips.	
vernix caseosa	Thick, white, cheesy substance that covers the skin of the fetus to protect it from the amniotic fluid.	
verruca	Irregular, rough skin lesion caused by the human papillomavirus. Commonly found on the hand and fingers or the sole of the foot. [*see also*: cryosurgery, electrodesiccation]	S
vertebra	Bony structure of the spine. Most vertebrae have a vertebral body (flat, central area), spinous process (bony projection along the midback), two transverse processes (bony projections to the side), and a foramen (hole where the spinal cord passes through). [*see also*: ankylosing spondylitis, bone density test]	F
vertigo	Sensation of being off balance when the body is not moving. Caused by upper respiratory infection, middle or inner ear infection, head trauma, degenerative changes of the semicircular canals, or Ménière's disease. [*see also*: labyrinthitis, Ménière's disease, motion sickness, Romberg's sign, semicircular canals]	S
vesicocele [618.xx]	Hernia in which the bladder bulges through a weakness in the muscular wall of the vagina or rectum. This causes urinary retention in the part of the bladder that pouches into the vagina or rectum. Also known as a cystocele.	S
	Dx H&P.	
	Tx Depending on severity, monitoring or surgery. [*see also*: colporrhaphy]	
vesicovaginal fistula	Formation of an abnormal passageway connecting the bladder to the vagina. Urine flows from the bladder into the vagina and is excreted through the vagina. [*see also*: vagina]	
vestibule	First structure of the inner ear. Tubular structure filled with fluid that contacts the oval window and round window. The ends of the vestibule become the semicircular canals and the cochlea.	F
villi	Microscopic projections of the mucosa within the lumen of the small intestine. The site where nutrients are absorbed into the blood.	
viral load test	Measures tiny amounts of HIV RNA that are present in the serum during the six weeks before antibodies against HIV can be	

A = Abbreviations Section   **F** = Figures Section   **L** = Laboratory Section   **S** = Synonyms Section
Sx (Symptoms)   **Dx** (Diagnosis)   **Tx** (Treatment)

detected. Uses the RT-PCR or bDNA test. Also used to monitor the progression of the disease and response to antiretroviral drugs. [*see also*: enzyme-linked immunosorbent assay, OraSure, p24 antigen test, Western blot]

viscera	All of the internal organs in a body cavity.
visceral pleura	One of the two membranes of the pleura. It covers the surface of the lung. [*see also*: parietal pleura]
visual acuity testing	Diagnostic procedure for near and distance vision. Each eye is tested separately. Normal visual acuity is 20/20. The numerator stands for 20 feet, the standard distance between the chart and the patient. The denominator stands for the distance at which a person with normal vision could see that line on the chart. Children or patients who are illiterate are tested with charts that use pictures. [*see also*: fovea]
visual cortex	Areas in the right and left occipital lobes of the brain that receive and analyze sensory nerve impulses from the eye. They merge images from both eyes to create a single image that is right side up and in its original direction, matching the original object that was seen.
vital signs	Medical procedure during a physical examination in which the temperature, pulse, and respirations are measured. Sometimes an evaluation of pain is also included and is known as the fourth vital sign.
vitiligo [709.xx]	White, depigmented patches interspersed with normally pigmented skin. An autoimmune response slowly destroys melanocytes in ever-enlarging patches of skin, the rate of which varies. [*see also*: autoimmune disease]
vitreous humor	Clear, gel-like substance that fills the posterior cavity of the eye. [*see also*: flashers and floaters, retinal detachment]
vocal cords	Connective tissue bands in the larynx that vibrate and produce sounds for speaking and singing.
voiding cystourethrography	Radiologic procedure that uses x-rays and radiopaque contrast dye. The dye is inserted into the bladder through a cystoscope. It outlines the bladder and urethra. An x-ray image is taken while the patient is urinating.
voluntary muscle	Skeletal muscle. It contracts and relaxes in response to conscious thought.
volvulus [560.xx]	Twisting of a loop of intestine around itself or around another segment of intestine because of a structural abnormality of the mesentery. [*see also*: bowel resection and anastomosis]
voyeurism	Obtaining power, control, and sexual arousal by secretively viewing other people who are naked or having sexual relations. The elements of risk and danger as well as knowingly violating another's privacy are part of the experience.
vulva	Area between the inner thighs that includes the female external genitalia as well as the mons pubis and urethral meatus.

The vital signs entry is marked **A**, visual acuity testing marked nothing, vitreous humor marked **F**, voiding cystourethrography marked **A**, volvulus marked **S**.

W

walking pneumonia [486.xx]	Mild form of pneumonia caused by the bacterium *Mycoplasma pneumoniae*. The patient does not feel well but can continue daily activities. [*see also*: pneumonia]
Western blot	Serum test for antibodies against HIV. Used to confirm the findings of a positive ELISA and make a diagnosis of HIV

A = Abbreviations Section   **F** = Figures Section   **L** = Laboratory Section   **S** = Synonyms Section
Sx (Symptoms)   **Dx** (Diagnosis)   **Tx** (Treatment)

infection. [*see also*: enzyme-linked immunosorbent assay, OraSure, p24 antigen test, viral load test]

wet mount
Cytology test for yeasts, parasites, or bacteria. A swab is taken of the area and sent to the laboratory, where its contents are placed on a slide, mixed with saline solution, and examined under the microscope. [*see also*: ova and parasites]
  S

wheezes
High-pitched whistling or squeaking sounds during inspiration or expiration.

whiplash [847.xx]
Injury that occurs, most commonly in a car accident, as a person's head snaps backward and then forward. This can cause muscle strain or a muscle tear, as well as damage to the nerves.
  S

Dx H&P. X-ray, CT, MRI.

Tx Medication for pain and swelling. Physical therapy to strengthen the neck muscles, Soft cervical collar. Some patients may seek chiropractic treatments and adjustments.

white matter
Areas of white tissue in the brain and spinal cord that are composed of axons covered with myelin. [*see also*: myelin]

Wood's lamp or light
Ultraviolet light used to highlight areas of skin abnormality. In a darkened room, ultraviolet light makes vitiligo appear bright white and tinea capitis (ringworm) appear blue-green because the fungus fluoresces.

wound
Any area of visible damage to the skin that is caused by physical means (such as rubbing or trauma). [*see also*: debridement]

X–Z

xanthelasma [374.xx]
Benign growth that occurs as a yellow nodule or plaque on the eyelid. It is most often seen in patients who have high levels of lipids in the blood or diabetes mellitus. [*see also*: xanthoma]

xanthoma [272.xx]
Benign growth that occurs as a yellow nodule or plaque on the hands, elbows, knees, or feet. It is most often seen in patients who have high levels of lipids in the blood or diabetes mellitus. [*see also*: xanthelasma]

xenograft
A graft taken from an animal and used in a human patient. Example: Temporary skin graft to protect a burned area from infection and fluid loss, a permanent heart valve. [*see also*: allograft, autograft, graft-versus-host disease]

xenon-133
A gas that is inhaled for nuclear medicine imaging of the lungs. Xenon is a colorless, odorless gas that is present in trace amounts in the atmosphere.

xeroderma [757.xx]
Excessive dryness of the skin that can result in a fissure.

xeromammo-graphy
Uses an x-ray beam to expose a special x-ray plate and dry chemical to create an image of the breast on paper. [*see also*: mammography]

xerophthalmia [264.xx]
Insufficient production of tears with eye irritation. Associated with the aging process or an ectropion. Can also be caused by certain medications. [*see also*: ectropion, lacrimal gland]
  S

x-ray
Radiologic procedure that uses x-rays to diagnose bony abnormalities of any part of the body. X-rays are the primary means for diagnosing fractures, dislocations, and bone tumors. [*see also*: radiology, radiolucent, scout film]
  S

A = Abbreviations Section   **F** = Figures Section   **L** = Laboratory Section   **S** = Synonyms Section
Sx (Symptoms)   **Dx** (Diagnosis)   **Tx** (Treatment)

zygote   Cell that is the product of the union of a spermatozoon and an ovum. It is the fertilized ovum that is produced at the time of conception. This cell has 46 chromosomes.

Medical Word Synonyms

Identify Medical Word Synonyms

People often are familiar with medical words, but sometimes know them by different medical names or a common name. Also, some healthcare professionals call a disease by one name while others call it by a different name, even though both are correct.

This section provides an alphabetical listing of medical words with their matching names or medical word synonyms.

Note: This table has been fully cross-referenced so that each word's matching reference also has an entry in the table to assist students in quick referencing and cross-referencing.

MEDICAL WORD SYNONYMS

Medical Word	Synonym, the Same As, or Commonly Known As
0–9	
3-hydroxytyramine	**dopamine**
5-hydroxytryptamine	**serotonin**
A	
abducens nerve	cranial nerve VI, sixth cranial nerve
abnormal presentation	**malpresentation of the fetus**
abrasion	brush burn, carpet burn, rug burn
absence seizure	**petit mal seizure**

Bolded and blue medical words have a matching entry in the Glossary Section.

Medical Word	Synonym, the Same As, or Commonly Known As
acceleration-deceleration injury	hyperextension-hyperflexion injury, **whiplash**
accelerator globulin (AcG)	clotting factor V, labile factor, proaccelerin, prothrombin accelerator
accelerin	clotting factor VI
accessory nerve	cranial nerve XI, eleventh cranial nerve, spinal accessory nerve
acetonuria	**ketonuria**
achromasia	ashen, paleness, **pallor**, wanness
acoustic neuroma	vestibular schwannoma
acquired immune deficiency syndrome	**acquired immunodeficiency syndrome**
acquired immunodeficiency syndrome	acquired immune deficiency syndrome
actinic keratoses	**solar keratoses**
acute brain syndrome	acute confusional state, **delirium**
acute confusional state	acute brain syndrome, **delirium**
acute idiopathic polyneuritis	**Guillain-Barré syndrome**, Landry's syndrome, polyradiculoneuritis
acute ischemic stroke	brain attack, **cerebrovascular accident**, stroke
Adam's apple	**larynx**, voice box
Addison's anemia	malignant anemia, **pernicious anemia**
Addison's disease	chronic adrenocortical insufficiency, hypocorticalism, hypocorticoidism
adenohypophysis	anterior hypophysis, **anterior pituitary gland**
adenoids	nasopharyngeal tonsils, **pharyngeal tonsils**
adenomatous goiter	nodular goiter
ADH stimulation test	water deprivation test
adhesions	synechiae
adiaphoresis	**anhidrosis**
adipocere	grave wax
adipose tissue	subcutaneous fat
adipose tumor	**lipoma**
adolescence	**puberty**, pubescence
adrenal glands	suprarenal glands
adrenaline	**epinephrine**
adrenocorticotropic hormone	adrenotropin, corticotropin
adrenotropin	**adrenocorticotropic hormone**, corticotropin
adult-onset diabetes mellitus	**diabetes mellitus type 2**, non–insulin-dependent diabetes mellitus
afterbirth	**placenta**
age spots	liver spots, **senile lentigo**
air contrast barium enema	**double contrast barium enema**
albinism	depigmentation, hypomelanosis, hypopigmentation, leukoderma

Bolded and blue medical words have a matching entry in the Glossary Section.

Medical Word	Synonym, the Same As, or Commonly Known As
albuminuria	proteinuria
aldosteronism	**hyperaldosteronism**
alimentary canal	digestive tract, **gastrointestinal system**, gastrointestinal tract
allergic reaction	allergy
allergy	**allergic reaction**
allergy skin test	**scratch test**
allogeneic graft	**allograft**, homologous graft, homoplastic graft
allograft	allogeneic graft, homologous graft, homoplastic graft
alopecia	baldness
Alzheimer's disease	amentia, **dementia**
amblyopia	lazy eye
amentia	**dementia**, mental retardation
amnesia	memory loss
amnion	amniotic sac, bag of waters
amniotic sac	**amnion**, bag of waters
amniotomy	artificial rupture of membranes
amyotrophic lateral sclerosis	**Lou Gehrig's disease**
anacusis	deafness
anaphylactic shock	systemic anaphylaxis
anaplasia	dedifferentiation
anencephaly	neuroanencephaly
anesthesia	numbness
angina	**angina pectoris**, chest pain
angina pectoris	angina, chest pain
anhidrosis	adiaphoresis
ankylosing spondylitis	rheumatoid spondylitis
anosmia	anosphresia, olfactory anesthesia
anosphresia	**anosmia**, olfactory anesthesia
anterior	**ventral**
anterior hypophysis	adenohypophysis, **anterior pituitary gland**
anterior pituitary gland	adenohypophysis, anterior hypophysis
anterolisthesis	**spondylolisthesis**
anthracosis	black lung disease, coal miner's lung, collier's lung, melanedema, miner's lung
antibody	immunoglobulin
antigen	immunogen
antihemophilic factor A	antihemophilic globulin A, clotting factor VIII
antihemophilic factor B	Christmas factor, clotting factor IX, plasma thromboplastin component, plasma thromboplastin factor
antihemophilic globulin A	antihemophilic factor A, clotting factor VIII

Bolded and blue medical words have a matching entry in the Glossary Section.

Medical Word	Synonym, the Same As, or Commonly Known As
antisocial personality	**psychopath**, sociopath
anvil	incus
aphasia	speechlessness
aphtha	**aphthous stomatitis**, canker sore
aphthous stomatitis	aphtha, canker sore
aplastic anemia	Ehrlich's anemia
appendicitis	typhlitis
arch	**fornix**, trigonum cerebrale, vault
arm or leg	**extremity**, limb
armpit	axilla
arrest of labor	**failure to progress**
arrhythmia	**dysrhythmia**
arthrometer	fleximeter, **goniometer**
arthroplasty	**joint replacement surgery**
articulation	joint
artificial rupture of membranes	**amniotomy**
ascites	hydroperitonia, hydroperitoneum, peritoneal dropsy
ashen	achromasia, paleness, **pallor**, wanness
asthma	reactive airway disease
astrocyte	astroglia, macroglia
astroglia	**astrocyte**, macroglia
asystole	cardiac arrest, cardiac standstill
ataxia	incoordination
ataxic aphasia	Broca's aphasia, **expressive aphasia**, motor aphasia, nonfluent aphasia
atelectasis	collapsed lung, **pneumothorax**, punctured lung
athlete's foot	tinea pedis
atlas	C1 (first cervical vertebra)
atrioventricular bundle	**bundle of His**
atrium of the heart	auricle
atrophic arthritis	rheumatism, **rheumatoid arthritis**
atrophy	muscle wasting
attention deficit disorder	attention-deficit hyperactivity disorder, minimal brain dysfunction
attention-deficit hyperactivity disorder	**attention deficit disorder**, minimal brain dysfunction
auditory brainstem response	**brainstem auditory evoked response**
auditory nerve	cranial nerve VIII, eighth cranial nerve, vestibulocochlear nerve
augmentation mammaplasty	breast augmentation
auricle	atrium of the heart, pinna
autoallergy	**autoimmune disease**
autogeneic graft	**autograft**, autologous graft, autoplastic graft, autotransplant

Bolded and blue medical words have a matching entry in the Glossary Section.

Medical Word	Synonym, the Same As, or Commonly Known As
autograft	autogeneic graft, autologous graft, autoplastic graft, autotransplant
autoimmune disease	autoallergy
autologous graft	autogeneic graft, **autograft**, autologous graft, autotransplant
autoplastic graft	autogeneic graft, **autograft**, autologous graft, autotransplant
autotransplant	autogeneic graft, **autograft**, autologous graft, autoplastic graft
avulsion	evulsion
axilla	armpit
axis	C2 (second cervical vertebra)

B

Babinski's sign	great-toe reflex, paradoxical extensor reflex
baby	neonate, newborn
back of the knee	**popliteal space**
backbone	**spine**, spinal column, vertebral column
bag of waters	**amnion**, amniotic sac
baldness	**alopecia**
band	stab
barfing	puking, **regurgitation**, vomiting
barium enema	lower gastrointestinal series
barium swallow	upper gastrointestinal series
Basedow's disease	**Graves' disease**, Parry's disease
bedsore	decubitus ulcer, pressure sore
bedwetting	**nocturnal enuresis**
Bell's palsy	facial nerve palsy, peripheral facial paralysis
belly button	umbilicus
benign prostatic hyperplasia	**benign prostatic hypertrophy**
benign prostatic hypertrophy	benign prostatic hyperplasia
beta-D-galactosidase	**lactase**
biceps	biceps brachii muscle
biceps brachii muscle	biceps
bicuspid valve	**mitral valve**
big toe	great toe, hallux
bile ducts	biliary ducts, biliary tree
biliary ducts	**bile ducts**, biliary tree
biliary tree	**bile ducts**, biliary ducts
binge-eating syndrome	**bulimia**
bipolar disorder	**manic-depressive disorder**
birthmark	port-wine stain
black lung disease	**anthracosis**, coal miner's lung, collier's lung, melanedema, miner's lung

Bolded and blue medical words have a matching entry in the Glossary Section.

Medical Word	Synonym, the Same As, or Commonly Known As
blackhead	comedo
bleeder's disease	hemophilia
bleeding	hemorrhage
blister	bulla, vesicle
blood blister	hematoma
blood cancer	cancer of the blood, leukemia
blood clot	embolus, embolism, thrombus
blood poisoning	sepsis, septicemia
blood sugar	glucose
blood vessels	vascular structures
boil	furuncle
bone densitometry	bone density test
bone density test	bone densitometry
bone spur	osteophyte
bovine spongiform encephalopathy	Creutzfeldt-Jakob disease, mad cow disease, transmissible spongiform encephalopathy
bowel movement	defecation, elimination
bowel movement	feces, stool
bowleg	genu varum
Bowman's capsule	glomerular capsule
brain attack	acute ischemic stroke, cerebrovascular accident, stroke
brainstem auditory evoked response	auditory brainstem response
Braxton Hicks contractions	false labor
breaking wind	flatulence, flatus, gas, passing gas
breast augmentation	augmentation mammaplasty
breast bone	sternum
breasts	mammary glands
Broca's aphasia	ataxic aphasia, expressive aphasia, motor aphasia, nonfluent aphasia
bronchial tree	tracheobronchial tree
bruise	contusion
brush burn	abrasion, carpet burn, rug burn
bulbourethral glands	Cowper's glands
bulimia	binge-eating syndrome
bulla	blister
bundle of His	atrioventricular bundle
bursitis	housemaid's knee
buttocks	gluteus maximus muscle

C	
C1	atlas, first cervical vertebra
C2	axis, second cervical vertebra
calcaneus	heel bone
calcitonin	thyrocalcitonin

Bolded and blue medical words have a matching entry in the Glossary Section.

Medical Word	Synonym, the Same As, or Commonly Known As
calcium factor	clotting factor IV
calculogenesis	**lithogenesis**
calculus	kidney stone, **nephrolithiasis**
calf muscle	gastrocnemius muscle
callosity	**callus**
callus	callosity
cancer	malignancy, **metastases**
cancer of the blood	blood cancer, **leukemia**
canker sore	aphtha, **aphthous stomatitis**
capillary hemangioma	cavernous hemangioma, **hemangioma**, strawberry birthmark, strawberry nevus
carcinomatosis	carcinosis
carcinosis	**carcinomatosis**
cardiac arrest	**asystole**, cardiac standstill
cardiac exercise stress test	**stress test**, treadmill exercise stress test
cardiac hypertrophy	**cardiomegaly**, enlarged heart, macrocardia, megalocardia
cardiac sphincter	lower esophageal sphincter
cardiac standstill	**asystole**, cardiac arrest
Cardiolite stress test	thallium stress test
cardiomegaly	cardiac hypertrophy, enlarged heart, macrocardia, megalocardia
cardiomyopathy	myocardiopathy
carpet burn	**abrasion**, brush burn, rug burn
catamenia	emmenia, flow, **menses, menstruation**, period
caudad	inferior
cavernous hemangioma	capillary hemangioma, **hemangioma**, strawberry birthmark, strawberry nevus
celiac disease	celiac sprue, **gluten enteropathy**
celiac sprue	celiac disease, **gluten enteropathy**
central osteitis	**osteomyelitis**
cephalad	superior
cephalgia	headache
cerebrovascular accident	acute ischemic stroke, brain attack, stroke
cerumen	earwax
cervical smear	**Pap smear**
chalazion	meibomian cyst
change of life	climacteric, **menopause**
cheek bone	zygoma, zygomatic process
Chem 20	**metabolic panel**, SMA 20, SMAC 20
chest	rib cage, thorax
chest pain	angina, **angina pectoris**
chewing	**mastication**
chickenpox	herpes varicella-zoster, **shingles**

Bolded and blue medical words have a matching entry in the Glossary Section.

Medical Word	Synonym, the Same As, or Commonly Known As
childbirth	parturition
chin	mentum
chlamydia	nongonococcal urethritis
chloasma	circumscribed facial hyperpigmentation, mask of pregnancy, melasma
choked disk	**papilledema**
cholelithiasis	gallstones
cholescintigraphy	**hydroxyiminodiacetic acid scan**
chondromalacia patellae	patellofemoral syndrome
chordee	gryposis penis, penis lunatus
chorionic gonadotropin	**human chorionic gonadotropin**
Christmas factor	antihemophilic factor B, clotting factor IX, plasma thromboplastin component, plasma thromboplastin factor
chromosomal mutation	**genetic mutation**, mutation, translocation
chronic adrenocortical insufficiency	**Addison's disease**, hypocorticalism, hypocorticoidism
cicatrix	scar
cingulate gyrus	**limbic lobe**
circumscribed facial hyperpigmentation	**chloasma**, mask of pregnancy, melasma
cistron	**gene**
clap	**gonorrhea**
clavicle	collar bone
climacteric	change of life, **menopause**
clotting	**coagulation**
clotting factor I	**fibrinogen**
clotting factor II	**prothrombin**
clotting factor III	**thromboplastin**, tissue factor
clotting factor IV	calcium factor
clotting factor V	accelerator globulin (AcG), labile factor, proaccelerin, prothrombin accelerator
clotting factor VI	accelerin
clotting factor VII	cothromboplastin, proconvertin, prothrombin conversion accelerator, serum prothrombin conversion accelerator
clotting factor VIII	antihemophilic factor A, antihemophilic globulin A
clotting factor IX	antihemophilic factor B, Christmas factor, plasma thromboplastin component, plasma thromboplastin factor
clotting factor X	Stuart-Prower factor
clotting factor XI	plasma thromboplastin antecedent
clotting factor XII	Hageman factor
clotting factor XIII	fibrin-stabilizing factor, protransglutaminase

Bolded and blue medical words have a matching entry in the Glossary Section.

Medical Word	Synonym, the Same As, or Commonly Known As
clubfoot	talipes equinovarus
coagulation	clotting
coal miner's lung	**anthracosis**, black lung disease, collier's lung, melanedema, miner's lung
coccyx	tail bone
coitus	sexual intercourse
cold sores	fever blisters, herpes labialis, herpes simplex virus type 1, oral herpes
colic	intestinal colic, renal colic
collapsed lung	**atelectasis, pneumothorax**, punctured lung
collar bone	clavicle
collier's lung	**anthracosis**, black lung disease, coal miner's lung, melanedema, miner's lung
combat fatigue	**posttraumatic stress disorder**, shell shock
comedo	blackhead
common cold	head cold, **upper respiratory infection**
complete heart block	**third-degree heart block**
complex partial seizure	psychomotor seizure
compound fracture	open fracture
conception	**fertilization**
condylomata acuminata	**genital warts**, venereal warts, verruca acuminata
conjunctivitis	**pink eye**
conjunctivitis arida	dry eye syndrome, keratoconjunctivitis sicca, xeroma, **xerophthalmia**
contact dermatitis	irritant dermatitis
contusion	bruise
convergent strabismus	cross-eye, **esotropia**
convulsion	**epilepsy, seizure**
cord (umbilical) around the neck	**nuchal cord**
corneal ulcer	ulcerative keratitis
coronal plane	frontal plane
corticotropin	**adrenocorticotropic hormone**, adrenotropin
cortisol	hydrocortisone
cothromboplastin	clotting factor VII, proconvertin, prothrombin conversion accelerator, serum prothrombin conversion accelerator
Cowper's glands	**bulbourethral glands**
cradle cap	**eczema**, seborrheic dermatitis
cramp	**muscle spasm**, spasm
cranial nerve I	first cranial nerve, **olfactory nerve**
cranial nerve II	**optic nerve**, second cranial nerve
cranial nerve III	**oculomotor nerve**, third cranial nerve
cranial nerve IV	fourth cranial nerve, **trochlear nerve**
cranial nerve V	fifth cranial nerve, **trigeminal nerve**

Bolded and blue medical words have a matching entry in the Glossary Section.

Medical Word	Synonym, the Same As, or Commonly Known As
cranial nerve VI	**abducens nerve**, sixth cranial nerve
cranial nerve VII	**facial nerve**, seventh cranial nerve
cranial nerve VIII	**auditory nerve**, eighth cranial nerve, vestibulocochlear nerve
cranial nerve IX	**glossopharyngeal nerve**, ninth cranial nerve
cranial nerve X	tenth cranial nerve, **vagus nerve**
cranial nerve XI	**accessory nerve**, eleventh cranial nerve, spinal accessory nerve
cranial nerve XII	**hypoglossal nerve**, twelfth cranial nerve
crazy bone	funny bone, ulnar nerve
crescent cell anemia	drepanocytic anemia, **sickle cell anemia**
Creutzfeldt-Jakob disease	bovine spongiform encephalopathy, mad cow disease, transmissible spongiform encephalopathy
crib death	**sudden infant death syndrome**
Crohn's disease	granulomatous colitis, granulomatous enteritis, regional enteritis, segmental enteritis, terminal ileitis
cross-dressing	**transvestism**
cross-eye	convergent strabismus, **esotropia**
crotch	**genitalia**, genital organs, genitals, privates
cryptorchidism	**cryptorchism**
cryptorchism	cryptorchidism
cumulative trauma disorder	repetitive strain injury
cusp of a valve	leaflet of a valve
cystocele	**vesicocele**
cytokeratin	keratin

D

deafness	**anacusis**
decubitus ulcer	bedsore, pressure sore
dedifferentiation	**anaplasia**
defecation	bowel movement, elimination
degenerative joint disease	osteoarthritis
deglutition	swallowing
delirium	acute brain syndrome, acute confusional state
delirium tremens	rum fits, shakes, shaking delirium
delta hepatitis	hepatitis D
dementia	**Alzheimer's disease**, amentia
dementia praecox	**schizophrenia**
depigmentation	**albinism**, hypomelanosis, hypopigmentation, leukoderma
detached retina	**retinal detachment**
diabetes mellitus type 1	insulin-dependent diabetes mellitus, juvenile-onset diabetes mellitus

Bolded and blue medical words have a matching entry in the Glossary Section.

Medical Word	Synonym, the Same As, or Commonly Known As
diabetes mellitus type 2	adult-onset diabetes mellitus, non–insulin-dependent diabetes mellitus
diaphoresis	hidrosis, **perspiration**, sudation, sudoresis, sweating
diarrhea	loose stools
dictyosome	**Golgi apparatus**, Golgi body, Golgi complex
digestive tract	alimentary canal, **gastrointestinal system**, gastrointestinal tract
digit	finger or toe, **phalanx**, ray
digital herpes simplex	finger herpes, hand herpes, herpes whitlow
diplopia	double vision
disseminated lupus erythematosus	**systemic lupus erythematosus**
disseminated sclerosis	**multiple sclerosis**
dissociative identity disorder	identity disorder, **multiple personality disorder**, split personality
diverticular disease	diverticulosis
diverticulosis	diverticular disease
dizygotic twins	**fraternal twins**
dizziness	lightheadedness, **vertigo**
doctor of medicine	physician
doctor of podiatric medicine	foot doctor, podiatrist
dopamine	3-hydroxytyramine
dorsal	**posterior**
dorsal supine position	**supine**
double contrast barium enema	air contrast barium enema
double vision	**diplopia**
Down syndrome	amentia, mental retardation, mongolism, trisomy 21
drepanocytic anemia	crescent cell anemia, **sickle cell anemia**
dry eye syndrome	conjunctivitis arida, keratoconjunctivitis sicca, xeroma, **xerophthalmia**
ductus deferens	**vas deferens**
dwarfism	nanism, short stature
dyslipidemia	**hyperlipidemia**, hyperlipoproteinemia
dyspepsia	indigestion
dysphagia	odynophagia
dyspnea	shortness of breath
dysrhythmia	**arrhythmia**

E

ear canal	**external auditory canal**
eardrum	**tympanic membrane**
earwax	**cerumen**

Bolded and blue medical words have a matching entry in the Glossary Section.

Medical Word	**Synonym, the Same As, or Commonly Known As**
echocardiography	two-dimensional echocardiography
ectopic pregnancy	tubal pregnancy
eczema	cradle cap, seborrheic dermatitis
eczema marginatum	**jock itch**, tinea cruris
efflorescence	**rash**
egg	**ovum**
egotism	**narcissistic personality**, self-loving personality
Ehrlich's anemia	**aplastic anemia**
eighth cranial nerve	**auditory nerve**, cranial nerve VIII, vestibulocochlear nerve
elasticin	**elastin**
elastin	elasticin
elbow	olecranon
elective abortion	therapeutic abortion
electroconvulsive therapy	**electroshock therapy**
electroshock therapy	electroconvulsive therapy
eleventh cranial nerve	**accessory nerve**, cranial nerve XI, spinal accessory nerve
elimination	bowel movement, **defecation**
embolism	blood clot, embolus, **thrombus**
embolus	blood clot, embolism, **thrombus**
emesis	vomit, vomitus
emmenia	catamenia, flow, **menses**, **menstruation**, period
empyema	**pyothorax**
endothelium	intima
engagement	lightening
enlarged heart	cardiac hypertrophy, **cardiomegaly**, macrocardia, megalocardia
enterogastritis	**gastroenteritis**, intestinal flu, stomach flu
eosinophil	eosinophilic leukocyte, oxyphil, oxyphilic leukocyte
eosinophilic leukocyte	**eosinophil**, oxyphil, oxyphilic leukocyte
ephelis	**freckle**, lentigo
epicardium	visceral pericardium
epilepsy	convulsion, **seizure**
epinephrine	adrenaline
epiphysial plate	growth plate
epiphysis cerebri	pineal body, **pineal gland**
epistaxis	nosebleed
epithelial tissue	epithelium
epithelium	epithelial tissue
erectile dysfunction	**impotence**
erythema	redness
erythremia	Osler-Vaquez disease, polycythemia rubra, **polycythemia vera**

Bolded and blue medical words have a matching entry in the Glossary Section.

Medical Word	Synonym, the Same As, or Commonly Known As
erythrocyte	red blood cell, red corpuscle
esophageal reflux	**gastroesophageal reflux disease**
esotropia	convergent strabismus, cross-eye
evulsion	**avulsion**
excretory system	genitourinary system, **urinary system**, urogenital system
excretory urography	intravenous pyelography, **pyelography**
exhalation	expiration
exomphalos	**omphalocele**, umbilical hernia
exotropia	**strabismus**, wall-eye
expiration	exhalation
expressive aphasia	ataxic aphasia, Broca's aphasia, motor aphasia, nonfluent aphasia
external auditory canal	ear canal
extracorporeal shock wave lithotripsy	lithotripsy
extrasystole	**premature contraction**
extremity	arm or leg, limb
eye doctor	ophthalmologist, optometrist

F

face lift	**rhytidectomy**
facial nerve	cranial nerve VII, seventh cranial nerve
facial nerve palsy	**Bell's palsy**, peripheral facial paralysis
factor	clotting factor
failure to progress	arrest of labor
faint	swoon, **syncope**
fallopian tube	oviduct
false labor	**Braxton Hicks contractions**
farsightedness	**hyperopia**
fat-storing cell	**lipocyte**
feces	bowel movement, stool
femur	thigh bone
ferritin	iron
fertilization	conception
fever blisters	**cold sores**, herpes labialis, herpes simplex virus type 1, oral herpes
fibrinogen	clotting factor I
fibrin-stabilizing factor	clotting factor XIII, protransglutaminase
fibromyalgia	fibromyositis, fibrositis
fibromyositis	**fibromyalgia**, fibrositis
fibrositis	**fibromyalgia**, fibromyositis
fifth cranial nerve	cranial nerve V, **trigeminal nerve**
finger herpes	digital herpes simplex, hand herpes, herpes whitlow

Bolded and blue medical words have a matching entry in the Glossary Section.

Medical Word	Synonym, the Same As, or Commonly Known As
finger or toe	digit, **phalanx**, ray
first cervical vertebra	atlas, C1
first cranial nerve	cranial nerve I, **olfactory nerve**
flatulence	breaking wind, **flatus**, gas, passing gas
flatus	breaking wind, gas, passing gas
fleximeter	arthrometer, **goniometer**
flow	catamenia, emmenia, **menses**, **menstruation**, period
flu	**influenza**
focal motor seizure	**simple partial seizure**
follicle-stimulating hormone	follitropin
follitropin	**follicle-stimulating hormone**
fontanel	soft spot
foot doctor	doctor of podiatric medicine, podiatrist
fornix	arch, trigonum cerebrale, vault
fourth cranial nerve	cranial nerve IV, **trochlear nerve**
fraternal twins	dizygotic twins
freckle	ephelis, lentigo
frontal plane	**coronal plane**
funny bone	crazy bone, ulnar nerve
furuncle	**boil**

G

galactorrhea	lactorrhea
gallbladder	vesica biliaris
gallstones	**cholelithiasis**
gamma ray	photon
ganglion	myxoid cyst, synovial cyst
gangrene	mortification, slough, sloughing, sphacelus
gas	breaking wind, **flatulence**, **flatus**, passing gas
gastric bypass	gastric stapling, **gastroplasty**
gastric stapling	**gastric bypass**, **gastroplasty**
gastrocnemius muscle	calf muscle
gastroenteritis	enterogastritis, intestinal flu, stomach flu
gastroesophageal reflux disease	esophageal reflux
gastrointestinal system	alimentary canal, digestive tract, gastrointestinal tract
gastrointestinal tract	alimentary canal, digestive tract, **gastrointestinal system**
gastroplasty	**gastric bypass**, gastric stapling
gated blood pool scan	multiple-gated acquisition scan, **radionuclide ventriculography**
Gélineau syndrome	**narcolepsy**

Bolded and blue medical words have a matching entry in the Glossary Section.

Medical Word	Synonym, the Same As, or Commonly Known As
gene	cistron
genetic mutation	chromosomal mutation, mutation, translocation
genital herpes	herpes, herpes genitalis, herpes simplex virus type 2
genital organs	crotch, genitalia, genitals, privates
genital warts	condylomata acuminata, venereal warts, verruca acuminata
genitalia	crotch, genital organs, genitals, privates
genitals	crotch, genital organs, genitalia, privates
genitourinary system	excretory system, urinary system, urogenital system
genu valgum	knock-knee
genu varum	bowleg
getting your tubes tied	tubal ligation, tubes tied
giantism	gigantism
gigantism	giantism
glandular fever	infectious mononucleosis, kissing disease, mononucleosis
global amnesia	total amnesia
global aphasia	mixed aphasia, total aphasia
glomerular capsule	Bowman's capsule
glossopharyngeal nerve	cranial nerve IX, ninth cranial nerve
glucocorticoid	glycocorticoid
glucose	blood sugar
glucose tolerance test	oral glucose tolerance test
glucosuria	glycosuria, glycuresis
gluten enteropathy	celiac disease, celiac sprue
gluteus maximus muscle	buttocks
glycocorticoid	glucocorticoid
glycohemoglobin	glycosylated hemoglobin, hemoglobin A$_{1C}$
glycosuria	glycuresis, glucosuria
glycosylated hemoglobin	glycohemoglobin, hemoglobin A$_{1C}$
glycuresis	glucosuria, glycosuria
goiter	struma, thyromegaly
Goldflam's disease	myasthenia gravis
golfer's elbow	little leaguer's elbow, medial epicondylitis, pitcher's elbow
Golgi apparatus	dictyosome, Golgi body, Golgi complex
Golgi body	dictyosome, Golgi apparatus, Golgi complex
Golgi complex	dictyosome, Golgi apparatus, Golgi body
gonads	ovaries and testes, sex glands
goniometer	arthrometer, fleximeter
gonorrhea	clap
gout	gouty arthritis, urarthritis

Bolded and blue medical words have a matching entry in the Glossary Section.

Medical Word	Synonym, the Same As, or Commonly Known As
gouty arthritis	**gout**, urarthritis
grand mal seizure	**tonic-clonic seizure**
granulomatous colitis	**Crohn's disease**, granulomatous enteritis, regional enteritis, segmental enteritis, terminal ileitis
granulomatous enteritis	**Crohn's disease**, granulomatous colitis, regional enteritis, segmental enteritis, terminal ileitis
grave wax	adipocere
Graves' disease	Basedow's disease, Parry's disease
great toe	big toe, hallux
great-toe reflex	**Babinski's sign**, paradoxical extensor reflex
growth hormone	somatotropin
growth plate	epiphysial plate
gryposis penis	**chordee**, penis lunatus
guaiac-positive stool	**hematochezia**, **melena**, tarry stool
Guillain-Barré syndrome	acute idiopathic polyneuritis, Landry's syndrome, polyradiculoneuritis
gynecomastia	pseudogynecomastia

H

Hageman factor	clotting factor XII
half moon	**lunula**
hallux	big toe, great toe
hammer	malleus
hamstrings	biceps femoris, semimembranosus, semitendinosus
hand herpes	digital herpes simplex, finger herpes, herpes whitlow
handicapped	physically challenged
hay fever	seasonal allergies
head cold	common cold, **upper respiratory infection**
headache	**cephalgia**
heart attack	**myocardial infarction**
heart murmur	valvular regurgitation
heartburn	**pyrosis**
heel bone	calcaneus
helical computerized axial tomography	**spiral computerized axial tomography**
hemangioma	capillary hemangioma, cavernous hemangioma, strawberry birthmark, strawberry nevus
hematochezia	guaiac-positive stool, **melena**, tarry stool
hematopoiesis	hemopoiesis
hematuria	hemoglobinuria
heme	reduced hematin
hemianopia	hemianopsia
hemianopsia	**hemianopia**

Bolded and blue medical words have a matching entry in the Glossary Section.

Medical Word	Synonym, the Same As, or Commonly Known As
hemicephalalgia	hemicrania, megrim, migraine, **migraine headache**, sick headache
hemicrania	hemicephalalgia, megrim, migraine, **migraine headache**, sick headache
hemoglobin A$_{1C}$	glycohemoglobin, **glycosylated hemoglobin**
hemoglobinuria	**hematuria**
hemolytic reaction	**transfusion reaction**
hemophilia	bleeder's disease
hemopoiesis	**hematopoiesis**
hemorrhage	bleeding
hemorrhoids	piles
hepatitis	viral hepatitis
hepatitis A	infectious hepatitis
hepatitis B	serum hepatitis
hepatitis D	delta hepatitis
hepatocellular carcinoma	hepatoma, liver cancer
hepatoma	hepatocellular carcinoma, liver cancer
hepatomegaly	megalohepatia
hereditary chorea	**Huntington's chorea**
herniated nucleus pulposis	radiculopathy, **sciatica**, slipped disk
herpes	**genital herpes**, herpes genitalis, herpes simplex virus type 2
herpes genitalis	**genital herpes**, **herpes**, herpes simplex virus type 2
herpes labialis	**cold sores**, fever blisters, herpes simplex virus type 1, oral herpes
herpes simplex virus type 1	**cold sores**, fever blisters, herpes labialis, oral herpes
herpes simplex virus type 2	**genital herpes**, **herpes**, herpes genitalis
herpes varicella-zoster	chickenpox, **shingles**
herpes whitlow	digital herpes simplex, finger herpes, hand herpes
heterophil antibody test	MonoSpot test
hiatal hernia	hiatus hernia
hiatus hernia	**hiatal hernia**
hidrosis	**diaphoresis**, **perspiration**, sudation, sudoresis, sweating
hilum	porta
hirsutism	hypertrichosis
hives	**urticaria**
Hodgkin's disease	**Hodgkin's lymphoma**
Hodgkin's lymphoma	Hodgkin's disease
homologous graft	allogeneic graft, **allograft**, homoplastic graft
homoplastic graft	allogeneic graft, **allograft**, homologous graft
hordeolum	**stye**
Hortega cells	**microglia**

Bolded and blue medical words have a matching entry in the Glossary Section.

Medical Word	Synonym, the Same As, or Commonly Known As
housemaid's knee	**bursitis**
human chorionic gonadotropin	chorionic gonadotropin
humpback	hunchback, **kyphosis**
hunchback	humpback, **kyphosis**
Huntington's chorea	hereditary chorea
hyaline membrane disease	respiratory distress syndrome
hydatid mole	**hydatidiform mole**, molar pregnancy
hydatidiform mole	hydatid mole, molar pregnancy
hydrocephalus	water on the brain
hydrocortisone	**cortisol**
hydronephrosis	uronephrosis
hydroperitonia, hydroperitoneum	**ascites**, peritoneal dropsy
hydroxyiminodiacetic acid scan	cholescintigraphy
hymen	maidenhead, virginal membrane
hyperactivity	hyperkinesia, **hyperkinesis**
hyperaldosteronism	aldosteronism
hypercapnea	hypercarbia
hypercarbia	hypercapnea
hypercholesteremia	**hypercholesterolemia**
hypercholesterolemia	hypercholesteremia
hyperdactyly	**polydactyly**
hyperemesis gravidarum	**morning sickness**, nausea gravidarum
hyperesthesia	oxyesthesia
hyperextension-hyperflexion injury	acceleration-deceleration injury, **whiplash**
hyperinsulinemia	**hyperinsulinism**
hyperinsulinism	hyperinsulinemia
hyperkinesia	hyperactivity, **hyperkinesis**
hyperkinesis	hyperactivity, hyperkinesia
hyperlipidemia	dyslipidemia, hyperlipoproteinemia
hyperlipoproteinemia	dyslipidemia, **hyperlipidemia**
hypermenorrhea	**menorrhagia**
hyperopia	farsightedness
hyperpnea	hyperventilation, polypnea, **tachypnea**
hyperthyroidism	thyrotoxicosis
hypertrichosis	**hirsutism**
hypertrophic rosacea	**rhinophyma**, rum nose, toper's nose
hyperventilation	hyperpnea, polypnea, **tachypnea**
hypnosis	hypnotherapy
hypnotherapy	**hypnosis**
hypocorticalism	**Addison's disease**, chronic adrenocortical insufficiency, hypocorticoidism
hypocorticoidism	**Addison's disease**, chronic adrenocortical insufficiency, hypocorticalism
hypoglossal nerve	cranial nerve XII, twelfth cranial nerve

Bolded and blue medical words have a matching entry in the Glossary Section.

Medical Word	Synonym, the Same As, or Commonly Known As
hypokalemia	hypopotassemia
hypomelanosis	albinism, depigmentation, hypopigmentation, leukoderma
hypomenorrhea	oligomenorrhea
hypophysial cachexia	panhypopituitarism
hypophysis	master gland, pituitary gland
hypopigmentation	albinism, depigmentation, hypomelanosis, leukoderma
hypopotassemia	hypokalemia
hypospadias	urogenital sinus anomaly
hypoxemia	hypoxia
hypoxia	hypoxemia
hysteropexy	uterine suspension

I

icterus	jaundice
identical twins	monozygotic twins
identity disorder	dissociative identity disorder, multiple personality disorder, split personality
iliac region	inguinal region
ilium	pelvic bone
immunization	vaccination
immunogen	antigen
immunoglobulin	antibody
impotence	erectile dysfunction
in place	*in situ*
in situ	in place
incisional biopsy	open biopsy
incoordination	ataxia
incus	anvil
indigestion	dyspepsia
infectious hepatitis	hepatitis A
infectious mononucleosis	glandular fever, kissing disease, mononucleosis
inferior	caudad
infertility	sterility
influenza	flu
inguinal region	iliac region
inhalation	inspiration
initis	myositis
inkblot test	Rorschach test
inspiration	inhalation
insulin-dependent diabetes mellitus	diabetes mellitus type 1, juvenile-onset diabetes mellitus

Bolded and blue medical words have a matching entry in the Glossary Section.

Medical Word	Synonym, the Same As, or Commonly Known As
integument	skin
interstitial cell-stimulating hormone	**luteinizing hormone**, lutropin
intestinal colic	**colic**
intestinal flu	enterogastritis, **gastroenteritis**, stomach flu
intima	**endothelium**
intravenous pyelography	excretory urography, **pyelography**
involutional melancholia	**postpartum depression**
iron	**ferritin**
irritable bowel syndrome	mucous colitis, spastic colon
irritant dermatitis	**contact dermatitis**
ischium	pelvic bone
itching	**pruritus**

J

Medical Word	Synonym, the Same As, or Commonly Known As
jaundice	icterus
jaw bone (lower)	mandible
jaw bone (upper)	maxilla
jock itch	eczema marginatum, tinea cruris
joint	**articulation**
joint replacement surgery	arthroplasty
juvenile-onset diabetes mellitus	diabetes mellitus type 1, insulin-dependent diabetes mellitus

K

Medical Word	Synonym, the Same As, or Commonly Known As
keratin	cytokeratin
keratoconjunctivitis sicca	conjunctivitis arida, dry eye syndrome, xeroma, **xerophthalmia**
ketonuria	acetonuria
kidney stone	calculus, **nephrolithiasis**
kinesia	kinetosis, **motion sickness**
kinetosis	kinesia, **motion sickness**
kissing disease	glandular fever, infectious mononucleosis, **mononucleosis**
knee jerk	patellar reflex
kneecap	patella
knock-knee	**genu valgum**
kyphosis	hunchback, humpback

L

Medical Word	Synonym, the Same As, or Commonly Known As
labyrinthitis	otitis interna
labile factor	accelerator globulin (AcG), clotting factor V, proaccelerin, prothrombin accelerator
lacrimal gland	tear gland

Bolded and blue medical words have a matching entry in the Glossary Section.

Medical Word	Synonym, the Same As, or Commonly Known As
lactase	beta-D-galactosidase
lactation	suckling
lactogenic hormone	prolactin
lactorrhea	galactorrhea
Landry's syndrome	acute idiopathic polyneuritis, Guillain-Barré syndrome, polyradiculoneuritis
large bowel	large intestine
large intestine	large bowel
larynx	Adam's apple, voice box
laser peel	laser skin resurfacing
laser skin resurfacing	laser peel
lateral epicondylitis	tennis elbow
lazy eye	amblyopia
leaflet of a valve	cusp of a valve
leaky valve	prolapsed valve
leg or arm	extremity, limb
leiomyoma	uterine fibroid
lentigo	ephelis, freckle
lesion	wound
leukemia	blood cancer, cancer of the blood
leukocyte	white blood cell, white corpuscle
leukoderma	albinism, depigmentation, hypomelanosis, hypopigmentation
lice	pediculosis
lightening	engagement
lightheadedness	dizziness, vertigo
limb	arm or leg, extremity
limbic lobe	cingulate gyrus
lipocyte	fat-storing cell
lipoma	adipose tumor
liposuction	suction-assisted lipectomy
lithogenesis	calculogenesis
lithotripsy	extracorporeal shock wave lithotripsy
little leaguer's elbow	golfer's elbow, medial epicondylitis, pitcher's elbow
liver cancer	hepatocellular carcinoma, hepatoma
liver spots	age spots, senile lentigo
loose stools	diarrhea
lordosis	swayback
Lou Gehrig's disease	amyotrophic lateral sclerosis
lower esophageal sphincter	cardiac sphincter
lower gastrointestinal series	barium enema
lower jaw bone	mandible

Bolded and blue medical words have a matching entry in the Glossary Section.

Medical Word	Synonym, the Same As, or Commonly Known As
lumbar puncture	spinal tap
lung scan	ventilation-perfusion scan
lunula	half moon
luteinizing hormone	interstitial cell-stimulating hormone, lutropin
lutropin	interstitial cell-stimulating hormone, luteinizing hormone
Lyme arthritis	Lyme disease
Lyme disease	Lyme arthritis

M	
macrocardia	cardiac hypertrophy, cardiomegaly, enlarged heart, megalocardia
macroglia	astrocyte, astroglia
macrophage	monocyte
mad cow disease	bovine spongiform encephalopathy, Creutzfeldt-Jakob disease, transmissible spongiform encephalopathy
maidenhead	hymen, virginal membrane
malignancy	cancer, metastases
malignant anemia	Addison's anemia, pernicious anemia
malleus	hammer
malpresentation of the fetus	abnormal presentation
malrotation of the intestines	volvulus
mammaplasty	mammoplasty
mammary glands	breasts
mammoplasty	mammaplasty
mandible	jaw bone (lower)
manic-depressive disorder	bipolar disorder
mask of pregnancy	chloasma, circumscribed facial hyperpigmentation, melasma
master gland	hypophysis, pituitary gland
mastication	chewing
maxilla	jaw bone (upper)
medial epicondylitis	golfer's elbow, little leaguer's elbow, pitcher's elbow
megalocardia	cardiac hypertrophy, cardiomegaly, enlarged heart, macrocardia
megalohepatia	hepatomegaly
megrim	hemicephalalgia, hemicrania, migraine, migraine headache, sick headache
meibomian cyst	chalazion
meibomian glands	oil glands, sebaceous glands
melanedema	anthracosis, black lung disease, coal miner's lung, collier's lung, miner's lung
melasma	chloasma, circumscribed facial hyperpigmentation, mask of pregnancy

Bolded and blue medical words have a matching entry in the Glossary Section.

Medical Word	Synonym, the Same As, or Commonly Known As
melena	guaiac-positive stool, hematochezia, tarry stool
memory loss	amnesia
meningomyelocele	myelomeningocele
menopause	change of life, climacteric
menorrhagia	hypermenorrhea
menses	catamenia, emmenia, flow, menstruation, period
menstruation	catamenia, emmenia, flow, menses, period
mental retardation	amentia, Down syndrome, mongolism, trisomy 21
mentum	chin
metabolic panel	Chem 20, SMA 20, SMAC 20
metastases	cancer, malignancy
microglia	Hortega cells
micturition	passing water, peeing, urination, voiding
migraine, migraine headache	hemicephalalgia, hemicrania, megrim, sick headache
miner's lung	anthracosis, black lung disease, coal miner's lung, collier's lung, melanedema
minimal brain dysfunction	attention deficit disorder, attention-deficit hyperactivity disorder
miscarriage	spontaneous abortion
mites	scabies
mitral valve	bicuspid valve
mixed aphasia	global aphasia, total aphasia
molar pregnancy	hydatid mole, hydatidiform mole
mole	nevus, nevus pigmentosus
mongolism	amentia, Down syndrome, mental retardation, trisomy 21
monocyte	macrophage
mononucleosis	glandular fever, infectious mononucleosis, kissing disease
MonoSpot test	heterophil antibody test
monozygotic twins	identical twins
morning sickness	hyperemesis gravidarum, nausea gravidarum
mortification	gangrene, slough, sloughing, sphacelus
motion sickness	kinesia, kinetosis
motor aphasia	ataxic aphasia, Broca's aphasia, expressive aphasia, motor aphasia
motor strength	muscle strength
mouth	oral cavity, stoma
mucosa	mucous membrane
mucous colitis	irritable bowel syndrome, spastic colon
mucous membrane	mucosa
multiple myeloma	plasma cell myeloma
multiple personality disorder	dissociative personality disorder, identity disorder, split personality

Bolded and blue medical words have a matching entry in the Glossary Section.

Medical Word	Synonym, the Same As, or Commonly Known As
multiple sclerosis	disseminated sclerosis
multiple-gated acquisition scan	gated blood pool scan, radionuclide ventriculography
muscle spasm	cramp, spasm
muscle strain	pulled muscle
muscle strength	motor strength
muscle wasting	atrophy
muscles	musculature
muscular dystrophy	myodystrophy
musculature	muscles
musculoskeletal system	skeletomuscular system
mutation	chromosomal mutation, genetic mutation, translocation
myalgia	myodynia
myasthenia gravis	Goldflam's disease
myelomeningocele	meningomyelocele
myocardial infarction	heart attack
myocardiopathy	cardiomyopathy
myodynia	myalgia
myodystrophy	muscular dystrophy
myopia	nearsightedness
myositis	initis
myxoid cyst	ganglion, synovial cyst

N

nail (fingernail; toenail)	nail plate
nail bed	quick
nail plate	nail (fingernail; toenail)
nanism	dwarfism, short stature
narcissistic personality	egotism, self-loving personality
narcolepsy	Gélineau syndrome
nares	nostrils
nasal conchae	turbinates
nasopharyngeal tonsils	adenoids, pharyngeal tonsils
nausea gravidarum	hyperemesis gravidarum, morning sickness
nearsightedness	myopia
neonate	baby, newborn
neoplasm	tumor
nephroblastoma	Wilm's tumor
nephrolithiasis	calculus, kidney stone
neurilemma	Schwann cell
neuroanencephaly	anencephaly
neurofibromatosis	von Recklinghausen's disease

Bolded and blue medical words have a matching entry in the Glossary Section.

Medical Word	Synonym, the Same As, or Commonly Known As
neurohypophysis	**posterior pituitary gland**
neutrophil	polymorphonucleated leukocyte, seg, segmented neutrophil, segmenter
nevus	mole, nevus pigmentosus
nevus pigmentosus	**nevus**, mole
newborn	baby, neonate
ninth cranial nerve	cranial nerve IX, **glossopharyngeal nerve**
nocturnal enuresis	bedwetting
nodular goiter	adenomatous goiter
nonfluent aphasia	ataxic aphasia, Broca's aphasia, **expressive aphasia**, motor aphasia
nongonococcal urethritis	**chlamydia**
non–insulin-dependent diabetes mellitus	adult-onset diabetes mellitus, **diabetes mellitus type 2**
nonspecific urethritis	**urethritis**
noradrenaline	**norepinephrine**
norepinephrine	noradrenaline
nosebleed	**epistaxis**
nostrils	nares
nuchal cord	umbilical cord around the neck
nuchal rigidity	stiff neck
numbness	**anesthesia**
nursing home	skilled nursing facility

O

occupational lung disease	**pneumoconiosis**
oculomotor nerve	cranial nerve III, third cranial nerve
odynophagia	**dysphagia**
oil glands	**sebaceous glands**, meibomian glands
olecranon	elbow
olfactory anesthesia	**anosmia**, anosphresia
olfactory nerve	cranial nerve I, first cranial nerve
oligoamnios	**oligohydramnios**
oligohydramnios	oligoamnios
oligomenorrhea	hypomenorrhea
omphalocele	exomphalos, umbilical hernia
open biopsy	**incisional biopsy**
open fracture	**compound fracture**
ophthalmologist	eye doctor, optometrist
optic nerve	cranial nerve II, second cranial nerve
optometrist	eye doctor, ophthalmologist
oral candidiasis	**thrush**
oral cavity	mouth, stoma

Bolded and blue medical words have a matching entry in the Glossary Section.

Medical Word	Synonym, the Same As, or Commonly Known As
oral glucose tolerance test	**glucose tolerance test**
oral herpes	**cold sores**, fever blisters, herpes labialis, herpes simplex virus type 1
orange peel breast	peau d' orange
orchitis	testitis
Osler-Vaquez disease	erythremia, polycythemia rubra, **polycythemia vera**
os coxae	pelvic bones, pelvic girdle, pelvis
ossicles	ossicular chain
ossicular chain	**ossicles**
osteoarthritis	**degenerative joint disease**
osteogenic sarcoma	osteosarcoma
osteomalacia	rickets
osteomyelitis	central osteitis
osteophyte	bone spur
osteosarcoma	osteogenic sarcoma
otitis externa	swimmer's ear
otitis interna	**labyrinthitis**
ovaries and testes	**gonads**, sex glands
oviduct	**fallopian tube**
ovum	egg
oxyesthesia	**hyperesthesia**
oxyphil	**eosinophil**, eosinophilic leukocyte, oxyphilic leukocyte
oxyphilic leukocyte	**eosinophil**, eosinophilic leukocyte, oxyphil

P

pacemaker of the heart	**sinoatrial node**
palate	roof of the mouth
paleness	achromasia, ashen, **pallor**, wanness
pallor	achromasia, ashen, paleness, wanness
panhypopituitarism	hypophysial cachexia
Pap smear	cervical smear
papilledema	choked disk
papilloma	villoma
paradoxical extensor reflex	**Babinski's sign**, great-toe reflex
paralysis agitans	parkinsonism, **Parkinson's disease**, shaking palsy
parathormone	**parathyroid hormone**
parathyroid hormone	parathormone
parkinsonism	paralysis agitans, **Parkinson's disease**, shaking palsy
Parkinson's disease	paralysis agitans, parkinsonism, shaking palsy
Parry's disease	Basedow's disease, **Graves' disease**
parturition	childbirth

Bolded and blue medical words have a matching entry in the Glossary Section.

Medical Word	Synonym, the Same As, or Commonly Known As
passing gas	breaking wind, **flatulence, flatus,** gas
passing water	micturition, peeing, **urination,** voiding
patella	kneecap
patellar reflex	knee jerk
patellofemoral syndrome	**chondromalucia** patellae
peau d' orange	orange peel breast
pediculosis	lice
peeing	micturition, passing water, **urination,** voiding
pelvic bones	os coxae, pelvic girdle, pelvis
pelvic girdle	os coxae, pelvic bones, pelvis
pelvis	os coxae, pelvic bones, pelvic girdle
penis	phallus
penis lunatus	**chordee,** gryposis penis
pepsinogen	propepsin
peptidase	proteolytic enzyme
period	catamenia, emmenia, flow, **menses, menstruation**
peripheral facial paralysis	**Bell's palsy,** facial nerve palsy
peristalsis	vermiculation
peritoneal dropsy	**ascites,** hydroperitonia, hydroperitoneum
pernicious anemia	Addison's anemia, malignant anemia
perspiration	**diaphoresis,** hidrosis, sudation, sudoresis, sweating
petit mal seizure	absence seizure
phagocyte	scavenger cell
phalanx	digit, finger or toe, ray
phallus	**penis**
pharyngeal tonsils	adenoids, nasopharyngeal tonsils
pharyngitis	sore throat
pharynx	throat
phlebotomy	venipuncture
photalgia	**photophobia**
photon	**gamma ray**
photophobia	photalgia
physically challenged	handicapped
physician	doctor of medicine
piles	**hemorrhoids**
pineal body	epiphysis cerebri, **pineal gland**
pineal gland	epiphysis cerebri, pineal body
pink eye	**conjunctivitis**
pinna	auricle
pitcher's elbow	golfer's elbow, little leaguer's elbow, **medial epicondylitis**
pituitary gland	hypophysis, master gland
placenta	afterbirth

Bolded and blue medical words have a matching entry in the Glossary Section.

Medical Word	Synonym, the Same As, or Commonly Known As
plantar wart	**verruca**, verruca plantaris
plasma cell myeloma	**multiple myeloma**
plasma thromboplastin antecedent	clotting factor XI
plasma thromboplastin component	antihemophilic factor B, Christmas factor, clotting factor IX, plasma thromboplastin factor
plasma thromboplastin factor	antihemophilic factor B, Christmas factor, clotting factor IX, plasma thromboplastin component
platelet	**thrombocyte**
pleurisy	pleuritis
pleuritis	**pleurisy**
pneumoconiosis	occupational lung disease
pneumothorax	**atelectasis**, collapsed lung, punctured lung
podiatrist	doctor of podiatric medicine, foot doctor
polycythemia rubra	erythremia, Osler-Vaquez disease, **polycythemia vera**
polycythemia vera	erythremia, Osler-Vaquez disease, polycythemia rubra
polydactyly	hyperdactyly
polymorphonucleated leukocyte	**neutrophil**, seg, segmented neutrophil, segmenter
polypnea	hyperpnea, hyperventilation, **tachypnea**
polyradiculoneuritis	**acute idiopathic polyneuritis, Guillain-Barré syndrome**, Landry's syndrome
polysomnography	sleep study
popliteal space	back of the knee
porta	**hilum**
port-wine stain	birthmark
posterior	**dorsal**
posterior pituitary gland	neurohypophysis
postmortem rigidity	**rigor mortis**
postpartum depression	involutional melancholia
posttraumatic stress disorder	combat fatigue, shell shock
premature contraction	extrasystole
pressure sore	bedsore, decubitus ulcer
primary site	site of tumor
privates	crotch, **genitalia**, genital organs, genitals
proaccelerin	accelerator globulin (AcG), clotting factor V, labile factor
proconvertin	clotting factor VII, cothromboplastin, prothrombin conversion accelerator, serum prothrombin conversion accelerator
proctocele	**rectocele**
prolactin	lactogenic hormone
prolapsed uterus	uterine descensus, **uterine prolapse**
prolapsed value	leaky valve

Bolded and blue medical words have a matching entry in the Glossary Section.

Medical Word	Synonym, the Same As, or Commonly Known As
prone	prostrate
propepsin	pepsinogen
prosthesis	prosthetic device
prosthetic device	prosthesis
prostrate	prone
proteinuria	albuminuria
proteolytic enzyme	peptidase
prothrombin	clotting factor II
prothrombin accelerator	accelerator globulin (AcG), clotting factor V, labile factor, proaccelerin, prothrombin accelerator
prothrombin conversion accelerator	clotting factor VII, cothromboplastin, proconvertin, serum prothrombin conversion accelerator
protransglutaminase	clotting factor XIII, fibrin-stabilizing factor
pruritus	itching
pseudogynecomastia	gynecomastia
psychomotor seizure	complex partial seizure
psychopath	antisocial personality, sociopath
puberty	adolescence, pubescence
pubescence	adolescence, puberty
pubis	pelvic bone
puking	barfing, regurgitation, vomiting
pulled muscle	muscle strain
punctured lung	atelectasis, collapsed lung, pneumothorax
pustule	whitehead
pyelography	excretory urography, intravenous pyelography
pyothorax	empyema
pyrosis	heartburn

Q

quick	nail bed

R

radiculopathy	herniated nucleus pulposis, sciatica, slipped disk
radiograph	roentgenogram, x-ray
radionuclide ventriculography	gated blood pool scan, multiple-gated acquisition scan
radiopharmaceutical	tracer
rash	efflorescence
ray	digit, finger or toe, phalanx
reactive airway disease	asthma
rectocele	proctocele
red blood cell	erythrocyte, red corpuscle
red corpuscle	erythrocyte, red blood cell
reduced hematin	heme

Bolded and blue medical words have a matching entry in the Glossary Section.

Medical Word	Synonym, the Same As, or Commonly Known As
regional enteritis	**Crohn's disease**, granulomatous colitis, granulomatous enteritis, segmental enteritis, terminal ileitis
regurgitation	barfing, puking, vomiting
regurgitation (valvular)	heart murmur
renal colic	**colic**
repetitive strain injury	**cumulative trauma disorder**
respirator	ventilator
respiratory distress syndrome	**hyaline membrane disease**
retinal detachment	detached retina
retinopathy of prematurity	**retrolental fibroplasia**
retroflexion of the uterus	**retroversion of the uterus**
retrolental fibroplasia	retinopathy of prematurity
retroversion of the uterus	retroflexion of the uterus
rheumatic fever	**rheumatic heart disease**
rheumatic heart disease	rheumatic fever
rheumatism	atrophic arthritis, **rheumatoid arthritis**
rheumatoid arthritis	atrophic arthritis, rheumatism
rheumatoid spondylitis	**ankylosing spondylitis**
rhinophyma	hypertrophic rosacea, rum nose, toper's nose
rhytidectomy	face lift
rib cage	chest, thorax
rickets	**osteomalacia**
rigor mortis	postmortem rigidity
ringing in the ears	**tinnitus**
ringworm	tinea capitis, tinea corporis
roentgenogram	radiograph, **x-ray**
roof of the mouth	**palate**
Rorschach test	inkblot test
rug burn	**abrasion**, brush burn, carpet burn
rum fits	**delirium tremens**, shakes, shaking delirium
rum nose	hypertrophic rosacea, **rhinophyma**, toper's nose

S

saliva	spit, spittle
scabies	mites
scapula	shoulder blade
scar	**cicatrix**
scavenger cell	**phagocyte**
schizophrenia	dementia praecox
schizotrichia	split ends
Schwann cell	neurilemma

Bolded and blue medical words have a matching entry in the Glossary Section.

Medical Word	Synonym, the Same As, or Commonly Known As
sciatica	herniated nucleus pulposis, radiculopathy, slipped disk
sclera	white of the eye
scratch test	allergy skin test
seasonal allergies	hay fever
sebaceous glands	meibomian glands, oil glands
seborrheic dermatitis	cradle cap, eczema
second cervical vertebra	axis, C2
second cranial nerve	cranial nerve II, optic nerve
seg	neutrophil, polymorphonucleated leukocyte, segmented neutrophil, segmenter
segmental enteritis	Crohn's disease, granulomatous enteritis, regional enteritis, segmental enteritis, terminal ileitis
segmented neutrophil	neutrophil, polymorphonucleated leukocyte, seg, segmenter
segmenter	neutrophil, polymorphonucleated leukocyte, seg, segmented neutrophil
seizure	epilepsy, convulsion
self-loving personality	egotism, narcissistic personality
senile lentigo	age spots, liver spots
sepsis	blood poisoning, septicemia
septicemia	blood poisoning, sepsis
serotonin	5-hydroxytryptamine
serum hepatitis	hepatitis B
serum prothrombin conversion accelerator	clotting factor VII, cothromboplastin, proconvertin, prothrombin conversion accelerator
seventh cranial nerve	cranial nerve VII, facial nerve
sex glands	gonads, ovaries and testes
sexual intercourse	coitus
sexually transmitted disease	venereal disease
shakes	delirium tremens, rum fits, shaking delirium
shaking delirium	delirium tremens, rum fits, shakes
shaking palsy	paralysis agitans, parkinsonism, Parkinson's disease
shell shock	combat fatigue, posttraumatic stress disorder
shin bone	tibia
shingles	chickenpox, herpes varicella-zoster
short stature	dwarfism, nanism
shortness of breath	dyspnea
shoulder blade	scapula
sick headache	hemicephalalgia, hemicrania, megrim, migraine migraine headache
sickle cell anemia	crescent cell anemia, drepanocytic anemia
simple mastectomy	total mastectomy

Bolded and blue medical words have a matching entry in the Glossary Section.

Medical Word	Synonym, the Same As, or Commonly Known As
simple partial seizure	focal motor seizure
sinoatrial node	pacemaker of the heart
site of tumor	primary site
sixth cranial nerve	abducens nerve, cranial nerve VI
skeletomuscular system	musculoskeletal system
skilled nursing facility	nursing home
skin	integument
sleep study	polysomnography
slipped disk	herniated nucleus pulposis, radiculopathy, sciatica
slough, sloughing	gangrene, mortification, sphacelus
SMA 20	Chem 20, metabolic panel, SMAC 20
SMAC 20	Chem 20, metabolic panel, SMA 20
small bowel	small intestine
small intestine	small bowel
sociopath	antisocial personality, psychopath
soft spot	fontanel
solar keratoses	actinic keratoses
somatotropin	growth hormone
sonography	ultrasonography
sore throat	pharyngitis
spasm	cramp, muscle spasm
spastic colon	irritable bowel syndrome, mucous colitis
speechlessness	aphasia
sperm	spermatozoon
spermatozoon	sperm
sphacelus	gangrene, mortification, slough, sloughing
spinal accessory nerve	accessory nerve, cranial nerve XI, eleventh cranial nerve
spinal canal	spinal cavity
spinal cavity	spinal canal
spinal column	backbone, spine, vertebral column
spinal tap	lumbar puncture
spine	backbone, spinal column, vertebral column
spiral computerized axial tomography	helical computerized axial tomography
spit	saliva, spittle
spittle	saliva, spit
split ends	schizotrichia
split personality	dissociative identity disorder, identity disorder, multiple personality disorder
spondylolisthesis	anterolisthesis
spontaneous abortion	miscarriage
stab	band
stapes	stirrup

Bolded and blue medical words have a matching entry in the Glossary Section.

Medical Word	Synonym, the Same As, or Commonly Known As
sterility	**infertility**
sternum	breast bone
stiff neck	nuchal rigidity
stirrup	stapes
stoma	mouth, **oral cavity**
stomach flu	enterogastritis, **gastroenteritis**, intestinal flu
stool	bowel movement, **feces**
strabismus	exotropia, wall-eye
straight cath	**straight catheterization**
straight catheterization	straight cath
strawberry birthmark, strawberry nevus	capillary hemangioma, cavernous hemangioma, **hemangioma**
stress test	cardiac exercise stress test, treadmill exercise stress test
stretch marks	striae
striae	stretch marks
stroke	acute ischemic stroke, brain attack, **cerebrovascular accident**
struma	**goiter**, thyromegaly
Stuart-Prower factor	clotting factor X
stye	hordeolum
subcutaneous fat	**adipose tissue**
subtotal thyroidectomy	thyroid lobectomy
suckling	**lactation**
suction-assisted lipectomy	**liposuction**
sudation	**diaphoresis**, hidrosis, **perspiration**, sudoresis, sweating
sudden infant death syndrome	crib death
sudoresis	**diaphoresis**, hidrosis, **perspiration**, sudation, sweating
sudoriferous glands	sweat glands
superior	**cephalad**
supine	dorsal supine position
suprarenal glands	**adrenal glands**
surface-active agent	**surfactant**
surfactant	surface-active agent
swallowing	**deglutition**
swayback	**lordosis**
sweat glands	sudoriferous glands
sweating	**diaphoresis**, hidrosis, **perspiration**, sudation, sudoresis
swimmer's ear	**otitis externa**
swoon	faint, **syncope**

Bolded and blue medical words have a matching entry in the Glossary Section.

Medical Word	Synonym, the Same As, or Commonly Known As
syncope	faint, swoon
synechiae	**adhesions**
synovial cyst	**ganglion**, myxoid cyst
systemic anaphylaxis	**anaphylactic shock**
systemic lupus erythematosus	disseminated lupus erythematosus

T

tachycardia	tachyrhythmia, tachysystole
tachypnea	hyperpnea, hyperventilation, polypnea
tachyrhythmia	**tachycardia**, tachysystole
tachysystole	**tachycardia**, tachyrhythmia
tail bone	coccyx
talipes equinovarus	clubfoot
tarry stool	guaiac-positive stool, **hematochezia**, **melena**
tear gland	**lacrimal gland**
tennis elbow	**lateral epicondylitis**
tenth cranial nerve	cranial nerve X, **vagus nerve**
terminal ileitis	**Crohn's disease**, granulomatous colitis, granulomatous enteritis, regional enteritis, segmental enteritis
testes	testicles
testes and ovaries	**gonads**, sex glands
testicles	testes
testitis	**orchitis**
thallium stress test	**Cardiolite stress test**
therapeutic abortion	**elective abortion**
thigh bone	femur
third cranial nerve	cranial nerve III, **oculomotor nerve**
third-degree heart block	complete heart block
thorax	chest, rib cage
throat	**pharynx**
thrombocyte	platelet
thromboplastin	clotting factor III, tissue factor
thrombus	blood clot, embolus, embolism
thrush	oral candidiasis
thyrocalcitonin	**calcitonin**
thyroid lobectomy	subtotal thyroidectomy
thyroid-stimulating hormone	thyrotropin
thyroid storm	thyrotoxic crisis
thyromegaly	**goiter**, struma
thyrotoxic crisis	**thyroid storm**
thyrotoxicosis	**hyperthyroidism**

Bolded and blue medical words have a matching entry in the Glossary Section.

Medical Word	Synonym, the Same As, or Commonly Known As
thyrotropin	**thyroid-stimulating hormone**
tibia	shin bone
tic douloureux	trigeminal neuralgia
tinea capitis	**ringworm**
tinea corporis	**ringworm**
tinea cruris	eczema marginatum, **jock itch**
tinea pedis	athlete's foot
tinnitus	ringing in the ears
tissue factor	clotting factor, **thromboplastin**
toe or finger	digit, **phalanx**, ray
tonic-clonic seizure	grand mal seizure
toper's nose	hypertrophic rosacea, **rhinophyma**, rum nose
torticollis	wryneck
total amnesia	global amnesia
total aphasia	**global aphasia**, mixed aphasia
total mastectomy	simple mastectomy
tracer	**radiopharmaceutical**
trachea	windpipe
tracheobronchial tree	bronchial tree
transfusion reaction	hemolytic reaction
translocation	chromosomal mutation, **genetic mutation**, mutation
transmissible spongiform encephalopathy	bovine spongiform encephalopathy, **Creutzfeldt-Jakob disease**, mad cow disease
transvestism	cross-dressing
treadmill exercise stress test	cardiac exercise stress test, **stress test**
triceps	triceps brachii muscle
triceps brachii muscle	triceps
trigeminal nerve	cranial nerve V, fifth cranial nerve
trigeminal neuralgia	**tic douloureux**
trigonum cerebrale	arch, **fornix**, vault
trisomy 21	amentia, **Down syndrome**, mental retardation, mongolism
trochlear nerve	cranial nerve IV, fourth cranial nerve
tubal ligation	getting your tubes tied, tubes tied
tubal pregnancy	**ectopic pregnancy**
tubes tied	getting your tubes tied, **tubal ligation**
tumor	**neoplasm**
turbinates	nasal conchae
twelfth cranial nerve	cranial nerve XII, **hypoglossal nerve**
two-dimensional echocardiography	**echocardiography**
tympanic membrane	eardrum
typhlitis	**appendicitis**

Bolded and blue medical words have a matching entry in the Glossary Section.

Medical Word	Synonym, the Same As, or Commonly Known As
U	
ulcerative keratitis	corneal ulcer
ulnar nerve	crazy bone, funny bone
ultrasonography	sonography
umbilical cord around the neck	**nuchal cord**
umbilical hernia	exomphalos, **omphalocele**
umbilicus	belly button
upper gastrointestinal series	**barium swallow**
upper respiratory infection	common cold, head cold
urarthritis	**gout**, gouty arthritis
urethritis	nonspecific urethritis
urinary system	excretory system, genitourinary system, urogenital system
urination	micturition, passing water, peeing, voiding
urogenital sinus anomaly	**hypospadias**
urogenital system	excretory system, genitourinary system, **urinary system**
uronephrosis	**hydronephrosis**
urticaria	hives
uterine descensus	prolapsed uterus, **uterine prolapse**
uterine fibroid	**leiomyoma**
uterine prolapse	prolapsed uterus, uterine descensus
uterine suspension	hysteropexy
uterus	womb
uvea	**uveal tract**
uveal tract	uvea
V	
vaccination	immunization
vagus nerve	cranial nerve X, tenth cranial nerve
valvoplasty	**valvuloplasty**
valvular regurgitation	heart murmur
valvuloplasty	valvoplasty
vas deferens	ductus deferens
vascular structures	**blood vessels**
vault	arch, **fornix**, trigonum cerebrale
venereal disease	**sexually transmitted disease**
venereal warts	condylomata acuminata, **genital warts**, verruca acuminata
venipuncture	**phlebotomy**
ventilation-perfusion scan	lung scan
ventilator	respirator
ventral	**anterior**

Bolded and blue medical words have a matching entry in the Glossary Section.

Medical Word	Synonym, the Same As, or Commonly Known As
vermiculation	peristalsis
verruca	plantar wart, verruca plantaris
vertebral column	backbone, **spine**, spinal column
vertigo	dizziness, lightheadedness
verruca acuminata	condylomata acuminata, **genital warts**, venereal warts
vesica biliaris	**gallbladder**
vesicle	**blister**
vesicocele	cystocele
vestibular schwannoma	**acoustic neuroma**
vestibulocochlear nerve	**auditory nerve**, cranial nerve VIII, eighth cranial nerve
villoma	**papilloma**, skin tag
viral hepatitis	**hepatitis**
virginal membrane	**hymen**, maidenhead
visceral pericardium	**epicardium**
voice box	Adam's apple, **larynx**
voiding	micturition, passing water, peeing, **urination**
volvulus	malrotation of the intestines
vomit	**emesis**, vomitus
vomiting	barfing, puking, **regurgitation**
vomitus	**emesis**, vomit
von Recklinghausen's disease	**neurofibromatosis**

W

wall-eye	**strabismus**, exotropia
wanness	achromasia, ashen, paleness, **pallor**
water deprivation test	**ADH stimulation test**
water on the brain	**hydrocephalus**
wet mount	wet prep
wet prep	**wet mount**
whiplash	acceleration-deceleration injury, hyperextension-hyperflexion injury
white blood cell	**leukocyte**, white blood corpuscle
white blood corpuscle	**leukocyte**, white blood cell
white of the eye	**sclera**
whitehead	pustule
Wilm's tumor	**nephroblastoma**
windpipe	**trachea**
womb	**uterus**
wound	**lesion**
wryneck	**torticollis**

Bolded and blue medical words have a matching entry in the Glossary Section.

X–Z

xeroma	conjunctivitis arida, dry eye syndrome, keratoconjunctivitis sicca, xerophthalmia
xerophthalmia	conjunctivitis arida, dry eye syndrome, keratoconjunctivitis sicca, xeroma
x-ray	radiograph, roentgenogram
zygoma	cheek bone, zygomatic process
zygomatic process	cheek bone, zygoma

Medical Abbreviations, Acronyms, and Symbols

Define Medical Abbreviations, Acronyms, and Symbols

Abbreviations are commonly used in all types of medical documents; however, they can mean different things to different people and their meanings can be misinterpreted.

This section consists of two parts.

PART A: ABBREVIATIONS/ACRONYMS AND DEFINITIONS

An alphabetical listing of abbreviations/acronyms with their definitions is provided so that you can quickly find an abbreviation and what that definition means.

PART B: MEDICAL SYMBOLS AND DEFINITIONS

A list of symbols commonly used in written medical language is provided so that you can quickly find a symbol and its definition.

Note: The far-right column in these tables is the cross-reference section that provides a cross-reference to other sections in this reference guide: ʟ = Laboratory Section and ꜱ = Synonyms Section.

---

* Commonly used medical jargon or slang
ʟ = Laboratory Section ꜱ = Synonyms Section
Bolded and blue medical words have a matching entry in the Glossary Section.

PART A: ABBREVIATIONS/ACRONYNMS AND DEFINITIONS

Abbreviation	Definition	
0-9		
5-HIAA	5-hydroxyindoleacetic acid	S
A	Blood type A in the ABO blood group assessment (heading in a SOAP note)	
A		
A fib	atrial fibrillation	
A&O	alert and orientated, alert and oriented	
A&P	anatomy and physiology auscultation and percussion	
AAA	abdominal aortic aneurysm	
AB	Blood type AB in the ABO blood group	
AB Ab	abortion	
ABD	abdomen	
ABG	**arterial blood gases**	
ABR	auditory brainstem response	S
ACE	angiotensin-converting enzyme (inhibitor)	
Ach	acetylcholine	
ACS	acute coronary syndrome	
ACT	**activated clotting time**	
ACTH	**adrenocorticotropic hormone**	
AD A.D.	auris dextra (right ear)	
ADA	American Dental Association American Diabetes Association American Dietetic Association Americans with Disabilities Act	
ADD	attention deficit disorder	S
ADH	**antidiuretic hormone**	
ADHD	**attention-deficit hyperactivity disorder**	S
ADLs	activities of daily living	
AED	**automatic external defibrillator**	
AFB	acid-fast bacillus	
AFP	**alpha fetoprotein**	
AGA	appropriate for gestational age	
AI	aortic insufficiency apical impulse artificial insemination artificial intelligence	

* Commonly used medical jargon or slang
L = Laboratory Section   S = Synonyms Section
Bolded and blue medical words have a matching entry in the Glossary Section.

Abbreviation	Definition	
AICD	**automatic implantable cardiac defibrillator**	
	automatic implantable cardioverter-defibrillator	
AIDS	**acquired immunodeficiency syndrome**	
AKA	**above-the-knee amputation**	
alk phos*	alkaline phosphatase	L
ALP	alkaline phosphatase	
ALL	acute lymphocytic leukemia	
ALS	amyotrophic lateral sclerosis	S
ALT	alanine aminotransferase	L
AMI	acute myocardial infarction	
AML	acute myelogenous leukemia	
ANS	**autonomic nervous system**	
AP	anteroposterior	
ARDS	acute respiratory distress syndrome	
	adult respiratory distress syndrome	
ARF	**acute renal failure**	
	acute respiratory failure	
	acute rheumatic fever	
ARM	artificial rupture of membrane	
ARMD	age-related macular degeneration	
AS	aortic stenosis	
AS	auris sinister (left ear)	
A.S.		
ASC	ambulatory surgery center	
ASC-H	atypical squamous cells, cannot exclude HSIL	
ASC-US	atypical squamous cells of undetermined significance	
ASCVD	arteriosclerotic cardiovascular disease	
ASD	**atrial septal defect**	
ASHD	arteriosclerotic heart disease	
ASIS	anterior–superior iliac spine	
AST	aspartate aminotransferase	L
ATN	**acute tubular necrosis**	
AU	auris unitas (both ears)	
A.U.	auris uterque (each ear)	
AV	**atrioventricular**	
AVM	**arteriovenous malformation**	

B		
B	Blood type B in the ABO blood group	
Ba	**barium**	
BAEP	brainstem auditory evoked potential	
BAER	**brainstem auditory evoked response**	
bagged*	manually ventilated with an Ambu bag	

* Commonly used medical jargon or slang
L = Laboratory Section   S = Synonyms Section
Bolded and blue medical words have a matching entry in the Glossary Section.

Abbreviation	Definition	
baso*	**basophil**	
BBT	basal body temperature	
BDI	**Beck Depression Inventory**	
BE	**barium enema**	
	base excess	L
BKA	**below-the-knee amputation**	
BM	bowel movement	S
BMD	bone mineral density	
BMT	**bone marrow transplantation**	
BOM	bilateral otitis media	
BP	blood pressure	
BPD	biparietal diameter (of fetal head)	
BPH	**benign prostatic hypertrophy**	
BPM bpm	beats per minute	
BPP	biophysical profile	
BRBPR	bright red blood per rectum	
BRCA	breast cancer (gene)	
BS	bowel sounds; breath sounds	
BSE	**breast self-examination**	
BSO	bilateral salpingo-oophorectomy	
BUN	**blood urea nitrogen**	L
Bx	**biopsy**	

C		
C&S	**culture and sensitivity**	
C1–C7	cervical vertebrae and the vertebral numbers	
Ca	cancer; **carcinoma**	
CA	cancer; **carcinoma**	
Ca Ca++	**calcium**	L
CABG	**coronary artery bypass graft** ("cabbage"*)	
CAD	**coronary artery disease**	
CAPD	**continuous ambulatory peritoneal dialysis**	
CAT	**computerized axial tomography** [see also: CT]	
cath*	catheterize catheterization	
CBC	**complete blood count**	
CBD	common bile duct	
CBT	**cognitive-behavioral therapy**	
CC	chief complaint	
cc	cubic centimeter (measure of volume)	
CCPD	**continuous cycling peritoneal dialysis**	

* Commonly used medical jargon or slang
L = Laboratory Section   S = Synonyms Section
Bolded and blue medical words have a matching entry in the Glossary Section.

Abbreviation	Definition
CCU	coronary care unit
CDC	Centers for Disease Control (and Prevention)
CDCP	Centers for Disease Control and Prevention
CDE	certified diabetes educator
CDH	**congenital dislocation of the hip**
CEA	carcinoembryonic antigen
CF	**cystic fibrosis**
chemo*	chemotherapy
CHF	**congestive heart failure**
CIN	cervical intraepithelial neoplasia (grading system on Pap smear)
CIS	carcinoma *in situ*
CK	conductive keratoplasty
	creatine kinase
CKD	chronic kidney disease
CK-MB	creatine kinase-MB bands [*see also*: CPK-MB]
Cl	chloride
Cl⁻	
CLL	chronic lymphocytic leukemia
CLO	*Campylobacter*-like organism
CML	chronic myelogenous leukemia
cmm	cubic millimeter
CN1–CN12	**cranial nerves and the cranial nerve numbers**
CNM	certified nurse midwife
CNS	**central nervous system**
CO	carbon monoxide
CO_2	**carbon dioxide**
COMT	catechol-*O*-methyltransferase
COPD	**chronic obstructive pulmonary disease**
COTA	certified occupational therapy assistant
CP	**cerebral palsy**
	cardiopulmonary
CPAP	continuous positive airway pressure
CPD	**cephalopelvic disproportion**
CPK	creatine phosphokinase
CPK-MB	**creatine phosphokinase MB bands**
CPK-MM	**creatine phosphokinase MM bands**
CPR	**cardiopulmonary resuscitation**
	computerized patient record
CRF	**chronic renal failure**
	cardiac risk factors
CRNA	certified registered nurse anesthetist
CRP	**C-reactive protein**
CRPS	chronic regional pain syndrome
	complex regional pain syndrome

The "Cl" / "chloride" row is marked **L** in the right margin; the "cmm" / "cubic millimeter" row is marked **S** in the right margin.

* Commonly used medical jargon or slang
L = Laboratory Section   S = Synonyms Section
Bolded and blue medical words have a matching entry in the Glossary Section.

Abbreviation	Definition	
CRT	certified radiation therapist	
CS	**cesarean section**	
C-section*	**cesarean section**	
CSF	**cerebrospinal fluid**	
CT	computerized tomography	
CTD	**cumulative trauma disorder**	
CTR	certified tumor registrar	
CTS	**carpal tunnel syndrome**	
CV	cardiovascular	
CVA	**cerebrovascular accident**	L
		S
CVS	**chorionic villus sampling**	
CXR	chest x-ray	
cysto*	**cystoscopy**	

D		
D&C	**dilation and curettage**	
D.C.	Doctor of Chiropractic	
D.D.S.	Doctor of Dental Surgery	
D.O.	Doctor of Osteopathy	
D.P.M.	Doctor of Podiatric Medicine	
dB db	decibel	
Derm*	**dermatology**	
DEXA	**dual energy x-ray absorptiometry**	
DI	**diabetes insipidus**	
DIC	**disseminated intravascular coagulation**	
diff*	differential count of WBCs	
DIP	distal interphalangeal (joint)	
DJD	**degenerative joint disease**	
DKA	**diabetic ketoacidosis**	
DM	**diabetes mellitus**	
DNA	deoxyribonucleic acid	
DOE	dyspnea on exertion	
Dr.	doctor	
DRE	**digital rectal examination**	
DS	discharge summary	
DSA	**digital subtraction angiography**	
DSM-IV	*Diagnostic and Statistical Manual of Mental Disorders,* 4th edition	
DT	**delirium tremens**	
DTR	**deep tendon reflex**	
DUB	**dysfunctional uterine bleeding**	

* Commonly used medical jargon or slang
L = Laboratory Section S = Synonyms Section
Bolded and blue medical words have a matching entry in the Glossary Section.

Abbreviation	Definition	
DVT	**deep vein thrombosis**	
Dx	diagnosis	
DXA	**dual energy x-ray absorptiometry**	

E		
EAC	**external auditory canal**	
EBT	electron beam tomography	
EBV	Epstein-Barr virus	
ECCE	extracapsular cataract extraction	
ECG	**electrocardiogram, electrocardiography**	
echo*	echocardiogram, echocardiography	
ECT	electroconvulsive therapy	S
ECV	**external cephalic version**	
ED	emergency department	
	erectile dysfunction	S
EDB	estimated date of birth	
EDC	estimated date of confinement	
	extensor digitorum communis	
EEG	**electroencephalogram, electroencephalography**	
EGA	estimated gestational age	
EGD	esophagogastroduodenoscopy	
EHR	electronic health record	
EKG	**electrocardiogram, electrocardiography**	
ELISA	**enzyme-linked immunosorbent assay**	
EMB	endometrial biopsy	
EMG	**electromyography**	
END	electroneurodiagnostic (technician)	
ENT	ears, nose, and throat	
EOM	extraocular movements	
EOMI	extraocular muscles intact	
eo*	**eosinophil**	
epi*	epithelial cell (in the urine specimen)	
	epinephrine	
EPO	**erythropoietin**	
EPR	electronic patient record	
EPS	**electrophysiologic study**	
ER	emergency room	
	estrogen receptor	
ERCP	**endoscopic retrograde cholangiopancreatography**	
ESRD	**end-stage renal disease**	
ESWL	**extracorporeal shock wave lithotripsy**	
ESWT	extracorporeal shock wave therapy	
ET	endotracheal tube [*see also*: ETT]	

* Commonly used medical jargon or slang
L = Laboratory Section   **S** = Synonyms Section
Bolded and blue medical words have a matching entry in the Glossary Section.

Abbreviation	Definition
ETOH	alcohol (liquor)
ETT	endotracheal tube [see also: ET]

F

Abbreviation	Definition
FBS	fasting blood sugar
Fe	ferritin (iron)
FEV_1	forced expiratory volume (in one second)
FHR	fetal heart rate
fib*	fibula
FIGO	Federation Internationale de Gynécologie et Obstétrique
FiO_2	fraction (percentage) of inspired oxygen
FOBT	fecal occult blood test
FSH	follicle-stimulating hormone
FTI	free thyroxine index (T_7)
FVC	forced vital capacity
Fx	fracture

G

Abbreviation	Definition	
G	gravid	
	gauge (of a needle)	
G/TPAL	gravida/ term, premature, abortion, living	
	G = number of pregnancies	
	T = number of term births	
	P = number of premature births	
	A = number of abortions (spontaneous or induced)	
	L = number of living children.	
GC	gonococcus (Neisseria gonorrhoeae)	
GCS	Glasgow Coma Scale	
G-CSF	granulocyte colony-stimulating factor	
GDM	gestational diabetes mellitus	
GERD	gastroesophageal reflux disease	
GGT	gamma-glutamyl transpeptidase	L
GH	growth hormone	
GI	gastrointestinal	
GIFT	gamete intrafallopian transfer	
GM-CSF	granulocyte-macrophage colony-stimulating factor	
gtt.	drops	
GTT	glucose tolerance test	
GU	genitourinary	
	gonococcal urethritis	
GVHD	graft-versus-host disease	
GYN	gynecology	

* Commonly used medical jargon or slang
L = Laboratory Section   S = Synonyms Section
Bolded and blue medical words have a matching entry in the Glossary Section.

Abbreviation	Definition	
H		
H&H	hemoglobin and hematocrit	
H&P	history and physical history and physical examination	
HAV	hepatitis A virus	
Hb	**hemoglobin** [see also: Hgb]	
HbA$_{1C}$	hemoglobin A$_{1C}$	S
HbCO	**carboxyhemoglobin**	L
HBV	hepatitis B virus	
HCG hCG	**human chorionic gonadotropin**	
HCO$_3^-$	bicarbonate	
HCT	hematocrit	
HCV	hepatitis C virus	
HDL	high-density lipoprotein	
HEENT	head, eyes, ears, nose, and throat	
Hg	mercury	
Hgb	**hemoglobin** [see also: Hb]	
HIDA	**hydroxyiminodiacetic acid**	
HIPAA	Health Insurance Portability and Accountability Act	
HIV	**human immunodeficiency virus**	
HLA	human leukocyte antigen	
HMD	**hyaline membrane disease**	
HNP	herniated nucleus pulposus	
hpf	high-power field	
HPI	history of present illness	
HPV	human papillomavirus	
HRT	hormone replacement therapy	
HSG	**hysterosalpingogram, hysterosalpingography**	
HSIL	high-grade squamous intraepithelial lesion	
HSV	herpes simplex virus	S
HTN	**hypertension**	
Hx	history	
Hz	hertz	
I		
I&D	**incision and drainage**	
I&O	**intake and output**	
IBD	**inflammatory bowel disease**	
IBS	**irritable bowel syndrome**	
ICCE	intracapsular cataract extraction	
ICD-9	*International Classification of Diseases,* 9th edition	
ICP	intracranial pressure	

* Commonly used medical jargon or slang
L = Laboratory Section S = Synonyms Section
Bolded and blue medical words have a matching entry in the Glossary Section.

Abbreviation	Definition	
ICSI	intracytoplasmic sperm injection	
IDDM	insulin-dependent diabetes mellitus	S
IgA	**immunoglobulin A**	
IgD	**immunoglobulin D**	
IgE	**immunoglobulin E**	
IgG	**immunoglobulin G**	
IgM	**immunoglobulin M**	
IM	intramuscular	
INR	international normalized ratio	
IOL	intraocular lens	
IOP	intraocular pressure	
IRS	insulin resistance syndrome	
IUGR	**intrauterine growth retardation**	
IVC	**intravenous cholangiography**	
IVF	*in vitro* fertilization	
IVP	intravenous pyelogram intravenous pyelography	S

J		
JOD	juvenile onset diabetes (mellitus)	S
JVD	jugular venous distention	

K		
K, K+	**potassium**	L
KS	**Kaposi's sarcoma**	
KUB	**kidneys, ureters, bladder**	

L		
L&D	labor and delivery	
L/S	**lecithin/sphingomyelin (ratio)**	L
L1–L5	lumbar vertebrae and the vertebral numbers	
LA	left atrium	
LASIK	laser-assisted *in situ* keratomileusis	
Lat	**lateral**	
LBBB	**left bundle branch block**	
LDH	lactic dehydrogenase	L
LDL	low-density lipoprotein	
LEEP	loop electrocautery excision procedure	
LES	lower esophageal sphincter	S
LFTs	liver function tests	
LGA	large for gestational age	
LH	**luteinizing hormone**	

* Commonly used medical jargon or slang
L = Laboratory Section   **S** = Synonyms Section
Bolded and blue medical words have a matching entry in the Glossary Section.

Abbreviation	Definition	
LLE	left lower extremity	
LLL	left lower lobe (of the lung)	
LLQ	left lower quadrant (of the abdomen)	
LMP	last menstrual period	
LP	lumbar puncture	S
LPN	licensed practical nurse	
LSD	lysergic acid diethylamide (a street drug)	
LSIL	low-grade squamous intraepithelial lesion	
LTK	laser thermal keratoplasty	
LUE	left upper extremity	
LUL	left upper lobe (of the lung)	
LUQ	left upper quadrant (of the abdomen)	
LV	left ventricle	
LVAD	left ventricular assist device	
LVH	left ventricular hypertrophy	
lymph *	**lymphocyte**	

M

Abbreviation	Definition
M.D.	Doctor of Medicine
MAO	monoamine oxidase (inhibitor drug)
MCH	mean cell hemoglobin
MCHC	mean cell hemoglobin concentration
MCP	metacarpophalangeal (joint)
MCV	mean cell volume
MD	**muscular dystrophy**
MDCT	**multidetector-row computerized tomography**
MDI	metered-dose inhaler
mets	unit of measure during cardiac treadmill stress test
mets*	**metastases** or metastasis
MI	**myocardial infarction**
mL	milliliter (measure of volume)
mm Hg	millimeters of mercury
mm^3	cubic millimeter
MMSE	**mini mental status examination**
mono*	**mononucleosis**
mono*	**monocyte**
MR	mitral regurgitation
MRA	magnetic resonance angiography
MRI	**magnetic resonance imaging**
MS	**multiple sclerosis** magnesium sulfate morphine sulfate
MSH	**melanocyte-stimulating hormone**

* Commonly used medical jargon or slang
L = Laboratory Section **S** = Synonyms Section
Bolded and blue medical words have a matching entry in the Glossary Section.

Abbreviation	Definition	
MUGA	multiple-gated acquisition (scan)	S
MVP	**mitral valve prolapse**	

N

N&V	nausea and vomiting	
Na, Na⁺	**sodium**	L
NB	newborn	
NCS	**nerve conduction study**	
NG	nasogastric	
NICU	neonatal intensive care unit ("NIK-yoo"*)	
	neurologic intensive care unit ("NIK-yoo"*)	
NIDDM	**non–insulin-dependent diabetes mellitus**	
NK	**natural killer (cell)**	
NP	nurse practitioner	
NPH	neutral protamine Hagedorn (type of insulin)	
	normal pressure hydrocephalus	
NPO	nothing by mouth (nil per os)	
n.p.o.		
NSAID	nonsteroidal anti-inflammatory drug	
NSR	**normal sinus rhythm**	
NST	**nonstress test**	
NSVD	normal spontaneous vaginal delivery	

O

O	Blood type O in the ABO blood group	
	objective (heading in a SOAP note)	
O&P	**ova and parasites**	
O.D.	Doctor of Optometry; overdose; right eye	
O₂	**oxygen**	
OA	osteoarthritis	S
OB	**obstetrics**	
OCD	**obsessive-compulsive disorder**	
OCG	**oral cholecystography**	
OCP	oral contraceptive pill	
OD	overdose	
OD, O.D.	right eye (oculus dexter)	
OGTT	oral glucose tolerance test	S
OOB	out of bed	
ORIF	**open reduction and internal fixation**	
ortho*	**orthopedics**	
OS, O.S.	left eye (oculus sinister)	
OSHA	Occupational Safety and Health Administration	

* Commonly used medical jargon or slang
L = Laboratory Section   S = Synonyms Section
Bolded and blue medical words have a matching entry in the Glossary Section.

Abbreviation	Definition	
OT	occupational therapy occupational therapist	
OU, O.U.	both eyes (oculus unitas) each eye (oculus uterque)	

P

P	para phosphorus plan (heading in a SOAP note) **pulse**	L
P.O. p.o.	by mouth (per os)	
PA	physician's assistant **posteroanterior**	
PAC	**premature atrial contraction**	
PACU	postanesthesia care unit ("PAK-yoo" *)	
PAD	**peripheral artery disease**	
Pap*	**Papanicolaou** (smear or test)	
PAP	prostatic acid phosphatase	
PCO$_2$ pCO$_2$	partial pressure of carbon dioxide	
PCP	phencyclidine (angel dust, a street drug) *Pneumocystis carinii* pneumonia primary care physician	
PD	prism diopter	
PDA	**patent ductus arteriosus**	
PDT	photodynamic therapy	
PE	physical examination pressure-equalizing (tube) **pulmonary embolism**	
PEG	**percutaneous endoscopic gastrostomy**	
PEJ	percutaneous endoscopic jejunostomy	
PERRL	pupils equal, round, and reactive to light	
PERRLA	pupils equal, round, reactive to light and accommodation	
PET	**positron emission tomography**	
PFTs	**pulmonary function tests**	
pH	potential of hydrogen (acidity or alkalinity)	L
Pharm.D.	Doctor of Pharmacy	
PICC	peripherally inserted central catheter	
PICU	pediatric intensive care unit ("PIK-yoo" *)	
PID	**pelvic inflammatory disease**	
PIP	proximal interphalangeal (joint)	
PM&R	physical medicine and rehabilitation	
PMDD	**premenstrual dysphoric disorder**	
PMH	past medical history	

* Commonly used medical jargon or slang
L = Laboratory Section   S = Synonyms Section
Bolded and blue medical words have a matching entry in the Glossary Section.

Abbreviation	Definition	
PMI	point of maximum impulse	
PMN	polymorphonucleated leukocyte	
PMS	**premenstrual syndrome**	
PND	**paroxysmal nocturnal dyspnea** postnasal drip postnasal drainage	
PO$_2$ pO$_2$	partial pressure of oxygen	
PO$_4$	phosphorus	
poly*	polymorphonucleated leukocyte	S
PPD	protein purified derivative (TB test) packs per day (of cigarettes)	
PR	progesterone receptor	
PRBCs	packed red blood cells	
PRK	photorefractive keratectomy	
PRN, p.r.n.	as needed (pro re nata)	
pro time*	**prothrombin time** [see also: PT]	
PROM	passive range of motion **premature rupture of membranes**	
PSA	**prostate-specific antigen**	
Psy* Psych*	**psychiatry** psychology	
PT	**physical therapy** physical therapist **prothrombin time** [see also: pro time]	
PTC	**percutaneous transhepatic cholangiography**	
PTCA	**percutaneous transluminal coronary angioplasty**	
PTSD	**posttraumatic stress disorder**	
PTT	**partial thromboplastin time**	
PUD	**peptic ulcer disease**	
PUVA	psoralen drug and ultraviolet A light (therapy)	
PVC	**premature ventricular contraction**	
PVD	**peripheral vascular disease**	

Q		
QCT	**quantitative computerized tomography**	

R		
R, r	roentgen (unit of exposure to x-rays or gamma rays)	S
RA	**rheumatoid arthritis** right atrium room air (no supplemental oxygen)	
rad	radiation absorbed dose	
RAIU	**radioactive iodine uptake**	

* Commonly used medical jargon or slang
L = Laboratory Section   S = Synonyms Section
Bolded and blue medical words have a matching entry in the Glossary Section.

Abbreviation	Definition	
RAST	**radioallergosorbent test**	
RBBB	**right bundle branch block**	
RBC	red blood cell	
RDS	respiratory distress syndrome	
rehab*	rehabilitation	
rem	roentgen-equivalent man	
RFA	**radiofrequency catheter ablation**	
RIA	radioimmunoassay	
RICE	rest, ice, compression, elevation	
RIND	**reversible ischemic neurological deficit**	
RLE	right lower extremity	
RLL	right lower lobe (of the lung)	
RLQ	right lower quadrant (of the abdomen)	
RML	right middle lobe (of the lung)	
RN	registered nurse	
RNA	ribonucleic acid	
RNV	**radionuclide ventriculography**	
ROM	range of motion rupture of membranes	
ROP	retinopathy of prematurity	
ROS	review of systems	
RP	**retinitis pigmentosa**	
RPR	rapid plasma reagin (test for syphilis)	
RRT	registered radiologic technologist registered respiratory therapist	
RSI	repetitive strain injury	S
RUE	right upper extremity	
RUL	right upper lobe (of the lung)	
RUQ	right upper quadrant (of the abdomen)	
RV	right ventricle	

S		
S	subjective (heading in a SOAP note)	
S1	first sacral vertebra	
S_1	first heart sound	
S_2	second heart sound	
S_3	third heart sound	
S_4	fourth heart sound	
SA	sinoatrial	
SAB	spontaneous abortion	S
SAD	**seasonal affective disorder**	
SARS	**severe acute respiratory syndrome**	
SBE	subacute bacterial endocarditis	

* Commonly used medical jargon or slang
L = Laboratory Section   S = Synonyms Section
Bolded and blue medical words have a matching entry in the Glossary Section.

Abbreviation	Definition	
SCC	**squamous cell carcinoma**	
SCI	**spinal cord injury**	
seg*	segmented neutrophil	S
SG	specific gravity	
SGA	small for gestational age	
SGOT	serum glutamic-oxaloacetic transaminase	
SGPT	serum glutamic-pyruvic transaminase	
SIADH	**syndrome of inappropriate ADH**	
SICU	surgical intensive care unit ("SIK-yoo")	
SIDS	**sudden infant death syndrome**	
SLE	**systemic lupus erythematosus**	
SMA	sequential multichannel analysis	S
SMAC	sequential multichannel analysis with computer	S
SNF	skilled nursing facility	
SOAP	subjective, objective, assessment, plan	
SOB	shortness of breath	S
SOM	serous otitis media	
sp gr	specific gravity [*see also:* SG]	
SPECT	**single-photon emission computerized tomography**	
SQ	subcutaneous [*see also:* subcu, subQ]	
SSEP	somatosensory evoked potential	
SSER	somatosensory evoked response	
SSRI	selective serotonin reuptake inhibitor	
STD	**sexually transmitted disease**	
subcu subQ	subcutaneous [*see also:* SQ, subQ]	
SVT	**supraventricular tachycardia**	
Sx	symptoms	

T		
T&A	tonsillectomy and adenoidectomy	
T1–T12	**thoracic vertebrae** and the vertebral numbers	
T_3	**triiodothyronine**	
T_4	**thyroxine**	
T_7	free thyroxine index (FTI)	
TAB	therapeutic abortion	S
TACE	**transarterial chemoembolization**	
TAH-BSO	total abdominal hysterectomy and bilateral salpingo-oophorectomy	
TAT	**Thematic Apperception Test**	
TB	**tuberculosis**	
TEE	**transesophageal echocardiogram transesophageal echocardiography**	

* Commonly used medical jargon or slang
L = Laboratory Section   S = Synonyms Section
Bolded and blue medical words have a matching entry in the Glossary Section.

Abbreviation	Definition	
TENS	transcutaneous electrical nerve stimulation (unit)	
TFTs	thyroid function tests	
THR	total hip replacement	
TIA	transient ischemic attack	
tib*	tibia	S
tib-fib*	tibia-fibula	
TIBC	total iron-binding capacity	
TM	tympanic membrane	
TMJ	temporomandibular joint	
TNF	tumor necrosis factor	
TNM	tumor, nodes, metastases (TNM system)	
TnT	troponin T	L
TNTC	too numerous to count	
TPA	tissue plasminogen activator (drug)	
TPAL	term, premature, abortions, living. [see also: G, G/TPAL] T = number of term births P = number of premature births A = number of abortions (spontaneous or induced) L = number of living children.	
TPR	temperature, pulse, and respiration	
trach*	tracheostomy	
TRAM	transverse rectus abdominis muscle (flap)	
TRUS	transrectal ultrasound	
TSE	testicular self-examination	
TSH	thyroid-stimulating hormone	
TURBT	transurethral resection of bladder tumor	
TURP	transurethral resection of the prostate	
TVH	total vaginal hysterectomy	
Tx	treatment	
TXM	type and crossmatch	

U		
UA	urinalysis	
UGI	upper gastrointestinal (GI) series	S
URI	upper respiratory infection	
US	ultrasound	S
UTI	urinary tract infection	

V		
V fib*	ventricular fibrillation	
V tach*	ventricular tachycardia	
V/Q	ventilation-perfusion (scan)	
VBAC	vaginal birth after cesarean section ("V-back"*)	

* Commonly used medical jargon or slang
L = Laboratory Section   S = Synonyms Section
Bolded and blue medical words have a matching entry in the Glossary Section.

Abbreviation	Definition	
VCUG	**voiding cystourethrography**	
VD	venereal disease	S
VDRL	Venereal Disease Research Laboratory (test for syphilis)	
VEP	visual evoked potential	
VER	visual evoked response	
VF	visual field	
VLDL	very low-density lipoprotein	
VMA	**vanillylmandelic acid**	
VS	vital signs	
VSD	**ventricular septal defect**	

W		
WBC	white blood cell	S

X–Z		
ZIFT	zygote intrafallopian transfer	

* Commonly used medical jargon or slang
L = Laboratory Section   **S** = Synonyms Section
Bolded and blue medical words have a matching entry in the Glossary Section.

PART B: MEDICAL SYMBOLS AND DEFINITIONS

Symbol	Meaning	Examples of Usage
®	right	® arm
Ⓛ	left	Ⓛ leg
♂	male	10-year-old Caucasian ♂
♀	female	45-year-old Hispanic ♀
1°	primary	1° diagnosis
2°	secondary	2° diagnosis
3°	tertiary	3° diagnosis
I	one (Roman numeral)	cranial nerve I EKG lead I Clark level I melanoma
II	two (Roman numeral)	cranial nerve II EKG lead II Clark level II melanoma
III	three (Roman numeral)	cranial nerve III EKG lead III Clark level III melanoma
IV	four (Roman numeral)	cranial nerve IV Clark level IV melanoma
V	five (Roman numeral)	cranial nerve V Clark level V melanoma
VI	six (Roman numeral)	cranial nerve VI
VII	seven (Roman numeral)	cranial nerve VII
VIII	eight (Roman numeral)	cranial nerve VIII
IX	nine (Roman numeral)	cranial nerve IX
X	ten (Roman numeral)	cranial nerve X
XI	eleven (Roman numeral)	cranial nerve XI
XII	twelve (Roman numeral)	cranial nerves II through XII
+	positive, plus	+ drawer sign on the right; reflexes +1 and symmetric
−	negative, minus	− drawer sign on the left knee with normal flexion but −10 degrees of extension
±	plus or minus, slightly more or slightly less	The average age was 68 ± 1.6 years.
=	equal	Right and left arms show = muscle strength.
≠	does not equal	Survival rate with chemotherapy ≠ survival rate with surgery and radiation.
Ø	no, none	Ø bowel sounds are heard
<	less than	left leg circumference < right leg circumference
>	greater than	right leg circumference > left leg circumference
≤	less than or equal to	a ≤ b

* Commonly used medical jargon or slang
L = Laboratory Section   **S** = Synonyms Section
Bolded and blue medical words have a matching entry in the Glossary Section.

Symbol	Meaning	Examples of Usage
≥	greater than or equal to	b ≥ a
×	by; times (times sign)	2 × 3 cm lesion; oriented × 3
x	magnification	microscope with an x30 lens
%	percent	limited to 50% weightbearing on the right leg
c/o	complains of; in care of	Patient c/o shortness of breath. Send this letter c/o Dr. Vaughn.
#	number pounds suture size	Proventil 2 mg #6 refills weight 125# #3-0 braided silk suture
Δ	change (Greek letter delta)	Δ Procardia 20 mg p.o. from b.i.d. to t.i.d.
&	and (ampersand)	T&A (tonsillectomy and adenoidectomy)
@	at	intravenous fluids of D5W @ 90 cc/hour
®	registered trademark	Calan SR®
c̄	with	Lungs c̄ decreased breath sounds throughout
s̄	without	Heart s̄ evidence of murmur, gallop, or rub
↑	up, above, increase	There is ↑ drainage from the wound.
↓	down, below, decrease	There is ↓ range of motion in the left arm.
→	to the right, caused or produced	Rotation of the head → causes pain. Her stroke has → weakness of her entire left side.
←	to the left, in the direction of	← Look here for the most recent laboratory test results.
/	or, over, out of (diagonal, slant, slash, virgule)	right/left; blood pressure 120/90; 2/3 (fraction); grade 2/6 murmur
′	foot	female who is 5′6″
″	inch	The wound is 2″ deep.
:	to, is to (ratio sign)	ANA positive at 1:160.
°	degree	98.6°F 30° flexion

Laboratory Tests and Values

Analyze Laboratory Tests, Values, and Their Meaning

Laboratory testing is commonplace in health care. Knowing what the different types of laboratory tests are will help you understand how and why they are used. Certain tests are grouped together because of a common element (such as blood tests or urine tests).

This section includes some common laboratory tests and their values, as used in medicine. If a test value is either high or low, it may indicate the presence of certain conditions or diseases. The normal range of laboratory test values is provided to assist you in determining what the values indicate.

Key to Formatting of Entries

test name			
Definition of the test and other related information.			
test item	♂ **(male)**[**]	♀ **(female)**[**]	Diseases or conditions associated with an abnormal level.
	normal ranges (measurement)[*]		

[*] Values and normal ranges differ from laboratory to laboratory, depending on the equipment used. These are provided as a guide only.

[**] Some test items have different normal ranges for males and females. If so, they are separated into different columns.

Bolded and blue medical words have a matching entry in the Glossary section.

LABORATORY TESTS AND VALUES

arterial blood gases (ABG)

Blood test on arterial blood to measure the pH and the partial pressure (p) of the gases oxygen (pO_2) and carbon dioxide (pCO_2). The lungs help regulate the amount of carbon dioxide in the blood. The more carbon dioxide, the more acidic the blood and the lower the pH. The kidneys help regulate the amount of bicarbonate in the blood. The more bicarbonate, the more alkalotic the blood and the higher the pH. Interpreting an ABG will assist the physician in determining whether the patient has an abnormal pH with acidosis or alkalosis, and whether the cause is the respiratory system or the renal system (metabolic).

				metabolic	respiratory
pH	**7.35–7.45**	High	alkalosis	**emesis** (excessive), metabolic alkalosis: **Cushing's syndrome**, diuretic use, steroid use	hyperventilation, respiratory alkalosis
		Low	acidosis	metabolic acidosis: **diabetic ketoacidosis, diarrhea** (severe), poisoning (alcohol), poisoning (aspirin), **renal failure**	**asthma, chronic obstructive pulmonary disease,** respiratory acidosis
pCO₂	**35–45**	High		asthma, chronic obstructive pulmonary disease, smoking	
		Low		respiratory compensation (possible overcompensation)	
pO₂	**70–100**	High		normal	
		Low		heart disease, pneumonia, **pulmonary edema, pulmonary embolism**	
HCO₃⁻	**19–25**	High		compensation for chronic acidosis	
		Low		**diabetes** (uncontrolled), **diarrhea** (excessive), exercise (strenuous), kidney disease, liver disease, poisoning (alcohol), poisoning (aspirin), shock	
BE	**± 2**			Base excess (BE) indicates the blood's total negative ions; only half of the negative ions in the blood are due to HCO_3^-. The base excess is correlated with the HCO_3^- level to assist in interpreting the ABG; therefore high or low levels don't indicate specific diseases or conditions.	
O₂ sat	**90–100**			The percentage of heme units that are carrying oxygen. This gives an indication of how well saturated the blood is with oxygen.	

Bolded and blue medical words have a matching entry in the Glossary section.

cardiac enzymes

Blood test to measure the levels of enzymes that are released into the blood when myocardial cells die. They include CK-MB, LDH, and troponin. Cardiac enzymes are measured every few hours for several days. The rise and fall of CK-MB and LDH levels occur at predictable times during a myocardial infarction and indicate when heart damage occurred. CK-MB levels begin to rise 2–8 hours after the onset of a myocardial infarction and will continue to rise until muscle damage no longer occurs, but can also indicate re-infarction. CK-MB levels start to fall 1–3 days after muscle damage has ceased. LDH levels begin to rise 12–24 hours after a myocardial infarction, peak in 2–3 days, before falling 5–14 days after muscle damage has occurred. Troponin is only found in the heart muscle and is released into the blood after a myocardial infarction. The level begins to rise in 4–6 hours and remains elevated for up to 10 days. Cardiac enzymes are often tested in conjunction with a lipid profile.

troponin	<0.3 (ng/L)		High	**angina pectoris**, heart muscle injury, **myocardial infarction**, unstable angina
			Low	normal
total CK	♂ 55–170 (U/L)	♀ 30–135 (U/L)	High	major trauma, muscle wasting diseases and conditions, **myocardial infarction**, rhabdomyelitis, skeletal muscle diseases
			Low	normal
CK-MB	<0.3 (ng/mL)		High	CK-MB is specific to heart muscle only; the higher the level or percentage of the total CK, the greater the extent of the infarction.
			Low	normal
LDH	18–33%		High	LDH is present in almost all body tissues. An elevated LDH level can be seen in some tumors and could indicate a number of diseases or conditions involving the bone marrow, heart, kidneys, or the liver. LDH levels are correlated with other lab values and are not by themselves diagnostic.
			Low	normal

Bolded and blue medical words have a matching entry in the Glossary section.

complete blood count

Group of blood tests that are performed automatically by machine to determine the number, type, and characteristics of various cells in the blood. A CBC is a common test performed to assist the physician in correlating the causes of the patient's signs and symptoms. Usually a CBC is combined with other tests for definitive diagnosis and is not usually diagnostic by itself.

			High	anabolic steroid use, carbon monoxide exposure, **cor pulmonale**, dehydration, living at high altitudes, **polycythemia vera**, pulmonary fibrosis, smoking
erythrocyte (red blood cell, RBC)	♂ 4.5–5.5 (10^6/mL)	♀ 4.0–4.9 (10^6/mL)	Low	**anemia**, bone marrow diseases, **hemorrhage**, kidney disease, malnutrition, **renal failure**, vitamin deficiencies, iron deficiency
			High	anabolic steroid use, carbon monoxide exposure, **cor pulmonale**, dehydration, living at high altitudes, **polycythemia vera**, pulmonary fibrosis, smoking
Hg	♂ 13.5–16.5 (g/dL)	♀ 12.0–15.0 (g/dL)	Low	**autoimmune diseases**, chronic disease, **Crohn's disease**, iron deficiency, **renal failure**, **systemic lupus erythematosus**, **testosterone** deficiency, thyroid hormone deficiency, vitamin deficiencies
			High	dehydration, living at high altitudes, smoking
HCT	♂ 41–50%	♀ 36–44%	Low	**anemia**, bone marrow diseases, chemotherapy, **hemorrhage**, **renal failure**, **sickle cell anemia**, vitamin deficiencies
MCV	80–100 (femtoliters)		High	alcoholism, chemotherapy, **Down syndrome**, erythropoietin therapy, **folic acid anemia**, **hypothyroidism**, immunosuppression, **jaundice**, liver disease, splenectomy. Some medications, such as AZT, can cause a false high MCV.
			Low	**anemia**, chronic disease, iron deficiency, **iron deficiency anemia**
platelet	100,000–450,000/mm³		High	bone marrow diseases, exercise (strenuous), inflammatory diseases, **myocardial infarction**, **pregnancy**, **rheumatoid arthritis**, **thrombus**
			Low	**disseminated intravascular coagulation**, drug reactions, **hemophilia**, **human immunodeficiency syndrome**, **thrombocytopenia**
leukocyte (white blood cell, WBC)	4,500–10,000 (cells/mL)		A high or low level of leukocytes depends on the type of leukocyte. Refer to the WBC differential to determine the type of leukocyte and possible disease conditions associated with it.	

complete blood count (*continued*)

WBC Differential

neutrophils	**54–62%**	High	appendicitis, bacterial infection, eclampsia, metastasis, obesity, rheumatic heart disease, smallpox, smoking, steroid use, stress
		Low	autoimmune diseases, cardiopulmonary bypass, hepatitis, hypersplenism, leukemia, rubella, systemic lupus erythematosus, viral infection, vitamin deficiencies
basophils	**0–0.75%**	High	chickenpox, hemolytic anemia, hyperestrogenemia, hypothyroidism, inflammatory diseases, splenectomy, viral infection
		Low	allergies (severe), hyperthyroidism, pregnancy, stress
eosinophils	**1–3%**	High	Addison's disease, allergies, asthma, hay fever, parasitic diseases, polycythemia vera, sarcoidosis
		Low	normal
lymphocytes	**25–33%**	High	chickenpox, chronic infection, herpes simplex, influenza, lymphatic leukemia, mononucleosis, mumps, rubella, tuberculosis, varicella, whooping cough
		Low	acquired immunodeficiency syndrome, aplastic anemia, Guillain-Barré syndrome, multiple sclerosis, myasthenia gravis, steroid use
monocytes	**3–7%**	High	endocarditis, malaria, Rocky Mountain spotted fever, typhoid fever
		Low	Can be normal, but may put the patient at risk for prolonged illnesses caused by pathogens.

lipid profile

Blood test that provides a comprehensive picture of the levels of cholesterol and triglycerides and their lipoprotein carriers in the blood: HDL, LDL, and VLDL. HDL, often called the "good cholesterol," is the one item in a lipid profile where a high number is desirable. LDL, often called the "bad cholesterol," and all of the rest of the items in a lipid profile, should be low. High levels can indicate atherosclerosis, cardiovascular disease, and an increased risk of myocardial infarction or stroke.

	optimal	borderline	high risk
total cholesterol	<200 mg/dL	200–239 mg/dL	>240 mg/dL
triglycerides	<150 mg/dL	150–199 mg/dL	>200 mg/dL
HDL	>60 mg/dL	35-45 mg/dL	<35 mg/dL
LDL	<100 mg/dL	130–159 mg/dL	>160 mg/dL
VLDL	<130 mg/dL	140–159 mg/dL	>160mg/dL
cholesterol: HDL ratio	<4:1	<5:1	<6:1

metabolic panel

Blood test that provides a comprehensive picture of the levels of protein, electrolytes, waste products, and other substances related to metabolic processes in the body.

albumin	3.9–5 (g/dL)	High	dehydration
		Low	inflammation, liver disease, malnutrition, shock
alkaline phosphatase (ALP)	33–133 (IU/L)	High	acromegaly, alcoholism, bone tumors, leukemia, liver disease, myelofibrosis, osteomalacia, Paget disease
		Low	malnutrition
ALT	13–40 (U/L)	High	alcoholism, hepatitis, mononucleosis, Reye's syndrome
		Low	normal
AST	10–34 (U/L)	High	exercise (strenuous), gangrene, hepatitis, liver disease, mononucleosis, myocardial infarction, Reye's syndrome, trauma
		Low	uremia, vitamin B$_6$ deficiency
blood urea nitrogen (BUN)	9–21 (mg/dL)	High	dehydration, heart failure, high-protein diet, renal failure
		Low	alcoholism, malnutrition, low-protein diet
calcium	8.5–10.5 (mg/dL)	High	cancer, hyperparathyroidism, Paget's disease, sarcoidosis, tuberculosis, vitamin D intake (excessive)
		Low	alcoholism, bone disease, hypoparathyroidism, malnutrition, muscle cramps, osteoporosis, renal failure
chloride	98–108 (mEq/L)	High	dehydration, metabolic acidosis, respiratory alkalosis
		Low	chronic lung disease, diarrhea (severe), emesis (excessive), emphysema
carbon dioxide	22–31 (mEq/L)	High	Cushing's syndrome, emesis (excessive), hyperaldosteronism
		Low	Addison's disease, diarrhea, ketoacidosis, kidney disease, poisoning (aspirin)
creatinine	0.7–1.4 (mg/dL)	High	acute tubular necrosis, dehydration, diabetic neuropathy, eclampsia, glomerulonephritis, muscular dystrophy, preeclampsia, renal failure
		Low	muscular dystrophy, myasthenia gravis
direct bilirubin	0–0.3 (mg/dL)	High	choledocholithiasis, cirrhosis, hepatitis
		Low	normal

metabolic panel (*continued*)			
GGT	**0–51** (U/L)	High	cholestasis, **congestive heart failure, hepatitis**, hepatotoxic drugs
		Low	normal
glucose	**70–110** (mg/dL)	High	**acromegaly, Cushing's syndrome, diabetes mellitus, hyperthyroidism,** pancreatic cancer, **pancreatitis, pheochromocytoma**
		Low	**hypopituitarism, hypothyroidism**
LDH	**56–194** (U/L)	High	cerebrovascular accident, hemolytic anemia, **hypotension**, liver disease, **muscular dystrophy, mononucleosis, myocardial infarction, pancreatitis**
		Low	**pernicious anemia**, vitamin B_{12} deficiency
phosphorus	**2.4–4.1** (mg/dL)	High	bone metastasis, hypocalcemia, **hypoparathyroidism**, liver disease, **renal failure**, sarcoidosis
		Low	**diabetic ketoacidosis, hypercalcemia, hyperinsulinism, hyperparathyroidism**
potassium	**3.6–5** (mEq/L)	High	**Addison's disease**, metabolic acidosis, red blood cell destruction, **renal failure**, respiratory acidosis
		Low	**Cushing's syndrome**, diuretic use, **emesis** (excessive), **hyperaldosteronism**
sodium	**136–143** (mEq/L)	High	burns (2nd–3rd degree), **Cushing's syndrome, diabetes insipidus, diaphoresis**, diuretic use, **hyperaldosteronism**
		Low	dehydration, **diarrhea** (severe), diuresis, **emesis** (excessive), **hypovolemia**
total bilirubin	**0.1–1.2** (mg/dL)	High	hemolytic anemia, **pernicious anemia, sickle cell anemia, transfusion reaction**
		Low	normal
total cholesterol	**100–240** (mg/dL)	High	**diabetes mellitus** (uncontrolled), **hyperlipidemia, hypothyroidism, nephrotic syndrome**
		Low	**hyperthyroidism**, liver disease, malnutrition, **pernicious anemia, septicemia**
total protein	**6.3–7.9** (g/dL)	High	chronic infection, chronic inflammation
		Low	burns (2nd–3rd degree), **glomerulonephritis, hemorrhage**, liver disease, malnutrition
uric acid	**4.1–8.8** (mg/dL)	High	alcoholism, **diabetes mellitus**, exercise (strenuous), **gout, hypoparathyroidism**, leukemia, **syndrome of nephrolithiasis**, poisoning (lead), **polycythemia vera**
		Low	**inappropriate antidiuretic hormone**

Bolded and blue medical words have a matching entry in the Glossary section.

thyroid function tests

Blood test that measures the levels of T_3, T_4, and TSH. Used to evaluate the function of the thyroid gland (which releases the hormones T_3 and T_4) and the anterior pituitary gland (which releases thyroid-stimulating hormone [TSH] to stimulate the thyroid gland). The test uses radioimmunoassay technique in which antibodies labeled with radioactive isotopes combine with the hormone and the amount of radioactivity is measured. Another value, the free thyroxine index (FTI) or T_7 is calculated from this.

T_3	**100–200** (ng/dL)	High	**Graves' disease**, thyroid cancer, **thyroiditis**
		Low	chronic disease, **hypothyroidism**, starvation
T_4	**4.5–11.2** (mcg/dL)	High	**Graves' disease**
		Low	fasting, **hypothyroidism**, malnutrition
TSH	**0.2–4.7** (μU/mL)	High	**hypothyroidism**
		Low	**hyperthyroidism**

Drug Categories

Classify Drugs by Drug Category, Therapeutic Actions, and Drug Name

Drugs are classified in several different ways, one of which is by category. Knowing the category a drug belongs to will assist you in understanding what a drug does even if you don't know the name of the drug itself.

This section provides an alphabetical listing of drug categories, along with a description of the drug action and some examples of common generic or trade name drugs in that category.

Drug Category	Description	Example
A		
ACE inhibitor drugs	Inhibit angiotensin-converting enzyme to treat hypertension and congestive heart failure	Capoten, Vasotec, Zestril
Alkylating drugs	Break DNA strands in cancerous cells by substituting an alkyl group	Cytoxan, Emcyt
Analgesic drugs	Suppress inflammation and decrease pain	acetaminophen, Bayer, Demerol, morphine, Ecotrin, Tylenol
Androgen drugs	Treat lack of production of testosterone by the testes	Androderm, Virilon

Drug Category	Description	Example
Anesthetic drugs	Topical and locally injected drugs used to prevent pain	benzocaine, lidocaine, Novocain, Pontocaine
Anesthetic gas	Inhaled gas used to produce unconsciousness, relieve anxiety, and decrease memory of surgery	nitrous oxide
Antacid drugs	Treat heartburn and peptic ulcer disease	Maalox, Mylanta
Antianxiety drugs	Treat anxiety and neurosis	Tranxene, Valium, Xanax
Antiarrhythmic drugs	Used to treat cardiac arrhythmias	Adenocard, Norpace, Rythmol, Tikosyn
Antibiotic drugs	Treat bacterial infections	amoxicillin, ampicillin, bacitracin, Bactrim, Gantrisin, Genoptic, Macrobid, neomycin, Ocuflox, Septra
Anticoagulant drugs	Prevent blood clots from forming by inhibiting the clotting factors or by inhibiting the production of vitamin K	Coumadin, heparin
Antidepressant drugs	Treat depression by prolonging the action of norepinephrine or serotonin	Paxil, Prozac, Zoloft
Antidiabetic drugs	Treat type 2 diabetes mellitus by stimulating the pancreas to produce more insulin	DiaBeta, Diabinese, Glucotrol
Antidiarrheal drugs	Slow peristalsis and increase water absorption to treat diarrhea	Imodium, Lomotil
Antiemetic drugs	Treat nausea, vomiting, and motion sickness	Antivert, Compazine, Phenergan
Antiepileptic drugs	Prevent the seizures of epilepsy	Dilantin, Tegretol
Antifungal drugs	Treat fungal infections of the skin and nails	Desenex, Lamisil AT, Lotrimin, Nizoral, Tinactin
Antihistamine drugs	Block the effect of histamine to treat allergy symptoms	Allegra, Benadryl, Claritin, Zyrtec
Antimetabolite drugs	Block folic acid required by the cancerous cells	fluorouracil, Gemzar, methotrexate
Antipruritic drugs	Decrease itching	Benadryl, Caladryl
Antipsychotic drugs	Used to treat psychosis, paranoia, and schizophrenia	Haldol, Thorazine, Zyprexa
Antitubercular drugs	Used in combination to treat tuberculosis	isoniazid (INH), Myambutol, Rifampin
Antitussive drugs	Supress the cough center in the brain to treat nonproductive coughs	dextromethorphan, Hycodan
Antiviral drugs	Treat viral infections	Aldara, Condylox, Famvir, Hivid, Valtrex, Virazole, Viroptic, Zovirax

Drug Category	Description	Example
B		
Barium	An insoluble metallic element found in the earth. Used as a radiopaque contrast dye in x-ray studies.	Baro-cat, Barosperse, Tomocat
Beta-blocker drugs	Treat angina pectoris, hypertension, or block the action of epinephrine to suppress essential familial tremor	Inderal, Lopressor, Toprol, Zebeta
Bone resorption drugs	Inhibit bone breakdown to treat osteoporosis	Boniva, Fosamax
Bronchodilator drugs	Dilate constricted airways by relaxing the smooth muscles that surround the bronchioles and bronchi	Proventil, Serevent, theophylline
C		
Calcium channel blocker drugs	Used to treat hypertension, angina pectoris, and congestive heart failure	Calan, Procardia
Chemotherapy antibiotic drugs	Inhibit an enzyme that cancerous cells need to divide	Adriamycin, bleomycin
Chemotherapy drugs	Kill rapidly dividing cancer cells	Adriamycin, Cytoxan, Taxol, vincristine
Chemotherapy enzyme drugs	Break down amino acid that cancerous cells need	Elspar, Oncaspar
COMT inhibitor drugs	Treat Parkinson's disease by inhibiting the enzyme that metabolizes the drug levodopa	Comtan, Tasmar
Corticosteroid drugs	Anti-inflammatory drugs given to suppress the immune response and decrease inflammation	Azmacort, Beconase, Decadron, Flonase, Flovent, hydrocortisone, Medrol, prednisone, Rhinocort, Solu-Medrol
D		
Decongestant drugs	Constrict blood vessels and decrease swelling of the mucous membranes of the nose and sinuses due to colds and allergies	Afrin, Dristan, Drixoral, Sudafed
Digitalis drugs	Treat congestive heart failure	digoxin, Lanoxin
Diuretic drugs	Used to block sodium from being absorbed from the renal tubule back into the blood to produce more urine	Aldactone, Hygroton, Lasix, Zaroxolyn
Drugs for alcoholism	Inhibit an enzyme that metabolizes the breakdown products of alcohol	Antabuse
Drugs for Alzheimer's disease	Inhibit the enzyme that breaks down acetylcholine in the brain	Aricept, Cognex

Drug Category	Description	Example
Drugs for benign prostatic hypertrophy	Inhibit an enzyme that causes the prostate gland to enlarge	Flomax, Proscar
Drugs for dysmenorrhea	Treat the pain associated with menstrual cramps	Motrin, Ponstel
Drugs for erectile dysfunction	Inhibit a substance that limits the flow of blood into the penis	Cialis, Levitra, Viagra
Drugs for glaucoma	Decrease the amount of aqueous humor or constrict the pupil to decrease intraocular pressure	Azopt, Betoptic
Drugs for hyperlipidemia	Treat hypercholesterolemia and hypertriglyceridemia	Lipitor, Vytorin, Zocor
Drugs for Parkinson's disease	Treat imbalance between dopamine and acetylcholine in the brain	Cogentin, levodopa, Symmetrel

E

Expectorant drugs	Reduce the thickness of sputum so that it can be coughed up	guaifenesin, Mucinex

G

Growth hormone drugs	Provide growth hormone	Humatrope, Protropin

H

H₂ blocker drugs	Block H_2 (histamine 2) receptors that trigger the release of hydrochloric acid. Used to treat peptic ulcers	Axid, Pepcid, Tagamet, Zantac
Hormonal chemotherapy drugs	Produce an opposite hormonal environment from the one that the cancer needs to reproduce	Arimidex, Femara, Lupron, Megace, tamoxifen
Hormone replacement therapy	Treat the symptoms of menopause	Estraderm, Estratest, Premarin, Prempro

I

Iodinated contrast dye	Contrast dye that contains iodine and is used in radiologic procedures	Gastrografin, Hypaque, Isovue, Omnipaque

L

Liquid nutritional supplements	Liquid formulas given through feeding tubes	Compleat, Ensure, ReSource
Laxative drugs	Treat constipation	Colace, Ex-Lax, Surfak

M

Mitosis inhibitor drugs	Cause DNA strands in the cancerous cells to break	Camptosar, VePesid

Drug Category	Description	Example
Monoclonal antibody drugs	Bind to antigens on surface of cancerous cell and destroy it	Campath, Herceptin
Muscle relaxant drugs	Relieve muscle spasm and stiffness	Flexeril, Parafon Forte, Soma
Mydriatic drugs	Dilate the pupil	atropine, Mydriacyl
N		
Nonsteroidal anti-inflammatory drugs	Suppress inflammation and decrease pain	Aleve, ibuprofen, Motrin Naprosyn
O		
Oral contraceptive drugs	Prevent ovulation so the patient does not become pregnant	Ortho-Novum, Yaz
Ovulation-stimulating drugs	Stimulate anterior pituitary gland to release hormones to stimulate ovulation in a woman with infertility	Clomid, Profasi
P		
Platelet aggregation inhibitor drugs	Prevent platelets from aggregating to form a blood clot	aspirin, Plavix, Ticlid
Platinum drugs	Create crosslinks in the DNA strands that prevent the cancerous cell from dividing	cisplatin, Paraplatin
Protease inhibitor drugs	Inhibit an enzyme the HIV virus needs to reproduce itself	Crixivan, Invirase
Proton pump inhibitor drugs	Treat peptic ulcers or gastroesophageal reflux disease	Nexium, Prilosec
Q–S		
Radioactive substances	Emit gamma rays and are used in nuclear medicine procedures	gallium-67, iodine-123, krypton-81m
Reverse transcriptase inhibitor drugs	Inhibit an enzyme the HIV virus needs to reproduce itself	Epivir, Retrovir
T		
Thrombolytic drugs	Dissolve a blood clot that is blocking blood flow through an artery	Activase

| Thyroid supplement drugs | Used to treat a lack of thyroid hormone and hypothyroidism | Cytomel, Synthroid |

Drug Category	Description	Example
U		
Urinary analgesic drugs	Exert a pain-relieving effect on the mucosa of the urinary tract	Pyridium, Urogesic
V		
Vitamin B_{12} drugs	Given by intramuscular injection or intranasally as a gel to treat vitamin B_{12} deficiency and pernicious anemia	Nascobal
W		
Weight loss drugs	Used to treat obesity, in conjunction with a reduced-calorie diet	Alli, Meridia, Xenical

Sound-Alike Medical Word Pronunciations

Medical Word, Word Part, or Abbreviation (Pronunciation)	Definition
Sound Alike	*Definition*
abduction (ab-DUK-shun)	Moving a body part (arm or leg) away from the midline of the body
adduction (ad-DUK-shun)	Moving a body part (arm or leg) toward the midline of the body
abductor (ab-DUK-tor)	Muscle that moves a body part (arm or leg) away from the midline of the body
adductor (ad-DUK-tor)	Muscle that moves a body part (arm or leg) toward the midline of the body
acetic (ah-SEE-tik)	Pertaining to acetic acid (vinegar)
acidic (ah-SID-ik)	Pertaining to an acid or having a decreased pH of the blood
ascitic (ah-SIT-ik)	Pertaining to ascites (a fluid-filled abdomen from liver disease)
acidic (ah-SID-ik)	Pertaining to an acid or having a decreased pH of the blood
acetic (ah-SEE-tik)	Pertaining to acetic acid (vinegar)
ascitic (ah-SIT-ik)	Pertaining to ascites (a fluid-filled abdomen from liver disease)
adduction (ad-DUK-shun)	Moving a body part (arm or leg) toward the midline of the body
abduction (ab-DUK-shun)	Moving a body part (arm or leg) away from the midline of the body

Bolded and blue medical words have a matching entry in the Glossary Section.

Medical Word, Word Part, or Abbreviation (Pronunciation)	Definition
Sound Alike	**Definition**
adductor (ad-DUK-tor)	Muscle that moves a body part (arm or leg) toward the midline of the body
abductor (ab-DUK-tor)	Muscle that moves a body part (arm or leg) away from the midline of the body
aden/o- (ah-DEE-noh)	Combining form that means *a gland*
adren/o- (ah-DREE-noh)	Combining form that means *adrenal gland*
adren/o- (ah-DREE-noh)	Combining form that means *adrenal gland*
aden/o- (ah-DEE-noh)	Combining form that means *a gland*
aesthetic (as-THET-ik)	English word meaning *pertaining to one who loves beautiful things*
asthenic (as-THEN-ik)	Lacking in strength and energy
affect (AF-ekt)	Outward display on the face of a person's inward emotions
effect (EE-fekt)	English word meaning *a result* or *a consequence*
afferent (AF-eh-rent)	Coming toward the center, as in nerves that carry impulses toward the spinal cord and brain
efferent (EF-eh-rent)	Going out from the center, as in nerves that carry impulses away from the spinal cord and brain
albumen (al-BYOO-men)	The white of an egg
albumin (al-BYOO-min)	Most abundant protein molecule in the blood
albumin (al-BYOO-min)	Most abundant protein molecule in the blood
albumen (al-BYOO-men)	The white of an egg
alimentary (AL-ih-MEN-tair-ee)	Pertaining to the digestive tract
elementary (EL-eh-MEN-tah-ree)	English word meaning *pertaining to basic or fundamental*
alkalosis (AL-kah-LOH-sis)	Condition of increased pH of the blood
ankylosis (ANG-kih-LOH-sis)	Condition of stiffness and fusion of the bones
ancillary (AN-sih-lair-ee)	Pertaining to providing medical support services
auxillary (awg-ZIL-yah-ree)	Pertaining to giving support or aid
axillary (AK-zih-lair-ee)	Pertaining to the armpit
ankylosis (ANG-kih-LOH-sis)	Condition of stiffness and fusion of the bones
alkalosis (AL-kah-LOH-sis)	Condition of increased pH of the blood
aphagia (ah-FAY-jee-ah)	Condition of inability to swallow
aphakia (ah-FAY-kee-ah)	Condition in which the lens of the eye has been surgically removed
aphasia (ah-FAY-zee-ah)	Condition of inability to communicate verbally or in writing

Bolded and blue medical words have a matching entry in the Glossary Section.

Medical Word, Word Part, or Abbreviation (Pronunciation)	Definition
Sound Alike	*Definition*
aphakia (ah-FAY-kee-ah)	Condition in which the lens of the eye has been surgically removed
aphagia (ah-FAY-jee-ah)	Condition of inability to swallow
aphasia (ah-FAY-zee-ah)	Condition of inability to communicate verbally or in writing
aphasia (ah-FAY-zee-ah)	Condition of inability to communicate verbally or in writing
aphagia (ah-FAY-jee-ah)	Condition of inability to swallow
aphakia (ah-FAY-kee-ah)	Condition in which the lens of the eye has been surgically removed
ascitic (ah-SIT-ik)	Pertaining to ascites (a fluid-filled abdomen from liver disease)
acetic (ah-SEE-tik)	Pertaining to acetic acid (vinegar)
acidic (ah-SID-ik)	Pertaining to an acid or having a decreased pH of the blood
asthenic (as-THEN-ik)	Lacking in strength and energy
aesthetic (as-THET-ik)	English word meaning *pertaining to one who loves beautiful things*
aura (AW-rah)	Visual or sensory sign warning of an impending seizure
aural (AW-ral)	Pertaining to the ear
aural (AW-ral)	Pertaining to the ear
aura (AW-rah)	Visual or sensory sign warning of an impending seizure
oral (OR-al)	Pertaining to the mouth
auxillary (awg-ZIL-yah-ree)	Pertaining to giving support or aid
ancillary (AN-sih-lair-ee)	Pertaining to providing medical support services
axillary (AK-zih-lair-ee)	Pertaining to the armpit
axillary (AK-zih-lair-ee)	Pertaining to the armpit
ancillary (AN-sih-lair-ee)	Pertaining to providing medical support services
auxillary (awg-ZIL-yah-ree)	Pertaining to giving support or aid
bolus (BOH-lus)	Large volume of a fluid or drug injected all at once
bullous (BUL-uhs)	Pertaining to a blister (bulla) on the skin
breath (BRETH)	The air that flows in and out of the lungs
breathe (BREETH)	The action of inhaling and exhaling air from the lungs
breathe (BREETH)	The action of inhaling and exhaling air from the lungs
breath (BRETH)	The air that flows in and out of the lungs
bullous (BUL-uhs)	Pertaining to a blister (bulla) on the skin
bolus (BOH-lus)	Large volume of a fluid or drug injected all at once
C&S (C AND S)	Abbreviation for *culture and sensitivity* (laboratory test)
CNS (C-N-S)	Abbreviation for *central nervous system*

Bolded and blue medical words have a matching entry in the Glossary Section.

Medical Word, Word Part, or Abbreviation (Pronunciation)	Definition
Sound Alike	**Definition**
calculus (KAL-kyoo-lus)	A kidney stone
	English word for a type of advanced mathematics
caliber (KAL-ih-ber)	Measurement of the diameter of the inside of a hollow tube, a bullet, or a stream of urine
calipers (KAL-ih-perz)	Instrument used to measure the thickness of skin fat
calipers (KAL-ih-perz)	Instrument used to measure the thickness of skin fat
caliber (KAL-ih-ber)	Measurement of the diameter of the inside of a hollow tube, a bullet, or a stream of urine
callous (KAL-us)	Pertaining to a callus on the skin; English word meaning *unsympathetic*
callus (KAL-us)	Thickened, hardened area on the skin due to repetitive rubbing; area of healed bone over a previous fracture site
callus (KAL-us)	Thickened, hardened area on the skin due to repetitive rubbing; area of healed bone over a previous fracture site
callous (KAL-us)	Pertaining to a callus on the skin; English word meaning *unsympathetic*
canker sore (KANG-ker SOHR)	Small ulcer on the mucosa of the oral cavity, also known as *aphthous stomatitis*
chancre (SHANG-ker)	Ulcerated, crusted skin lesion characteristic of the sexually transmitted disease syphilis
cardia (KAR-dee-ah)	Small region of the stomach where the esophagus enters
cardiac (KAR-dee-ak)	Pertaining to the heart
cardiac (KAR-dee-ak)	Pertaining to the heart
cardia (KAR-dee-ah)	Small region of the stomach where the esophagus enters
cardiac sphincter (KAR-dee-ak SFINGK-ter)	Ring of muscle at the end of the esophagus
cardiac valve (KAR-dee-ak VALV)	Structure between two chambers of the heart that opens and closes to regulate the flow of blood
cardiac valve (KAR-dee-ak VALV)	Structure between two chambers of the heart that opens and closes to regulate the flow of blood
cardiac sphincter (KAR-dee-ak SFINGK-ter)	Ring of muscle at the end of the esophagus
cari/o- (KAIR-ee-oh)	Combining form meaning *caries (tooth decay)*
kary/o- (KAIR-ee-oh)	Combining form meaning *nucleus*
carot/o- (kah-RAW-toh)	Combining form meaning *stupor; sleep*
kerat/o- (KAIR-ah-toh)	Combining form meaning *cornea (of the eye)*
	Combining form meaning *hard, fibrous protein*

Bolded and blue medical words have a matching entry in the Glossary Section.

Medical Word, Word Part, or Abbreviation (Pronunciation)	Definition
Sound Alike	**Definition**
chancre (SHANG-ker)	Ulcerated, crusted skin lesion characteristic of the sexually transmitted disease syphilis
canker sore (KANG-ker SOHR)	Small ulcer on the mucosa of the oral cavity, also known as *aphthous stomatitis*
cheil/o- (KY-loh)	Combining form meaning *lip*
kel/o- (KEE-loh)	Combining form meaning *tumor*
kilo- (KIL-oh)	Prefix meaning *one thousand*
cheilosis (ky-LOH-sis)	Condition in which the lips are dry and contain fissures
chelation (kee-LAY-shun)	Process by which toxic metals are removed from the body
chelation (kee-LAY-shun)	Process by which toxic metals are removed from the body
cheilosis (ky-LOH-sis)	Condition in which the lips are dry and contain fissures
cilia (SIL-ee-ah)	Tiny hairs that line the respiratory tract
ciliary body (SIL-ee-air-ee BAW-dee)	Layer of the eye posterior to the iris that contains muscles that change the shape of the lens
ciliary body (SIL-ee-air-ee BAW-dee)	Layer of the eye posterior to the iris that contains muscles that change the shape of the lens
cilia (SIL-ee-ah)	Tiny hairs that line the respiratory tract
CNS (C-N-S)	Abbreviation for *central nervous system*
C&S (C AND S)	Abbreviation for *culture and sensitivity* (laboratory test)
coccus (KOHK-uhs)	A bacterium with a round shape
coccyx (KOHK-siks)	Curved, fused bones at the end of the spinal column; the tailbone
coccyx (KOHK-siks)	Curved, fused bones at the end of the spinal column; the tailbone
coccus (KOHK-uhs)	A bacterium with a round shape
coma (KOH-mah)	Deep state of unconsciousness caused by trauma or disease of the brain
comedo (KOH-me-doh)	Enlarged pore filled with sebum; a blackhead
comedo (KOH-me-doh)	Enlarged pore filled with sebum; a blackhead
coma (KOH-mah)	Deep state of unconsciousness caused by trauma or disease of the brain
contraction (con-TRAK-shun)	Normal tensing and shortening of a muscle in response to a nerve impulse
contracture (con-TRAK-choor)	Abnormal, fixed position in which the muscle is permanently flexed
contracture (con-TRAK-choor)	Abnormal, fixed position in which the muscle is permanently flexed
contraction (con-TRAK-shun)	Normal tensing and shortening of a muscle in response to a nerve impulse

Bolded and blue medical words have a matching entry in the Glossary Section.

Medical Word, Word Part, or Abbreviation (Pronunciation)	Definition
Sound Alike	**Definition**
creatine kinase (KREE-ah-teen KY-nays)	Enzyme found only in skeletal muscle cells, heart cells, and brain cells. Elevated levels of CK-MB indicate a heart attack has occurred.
creatinine (kree-AT-ih-neen)	Waste product of metabolism. Increased amounts in the urine indicate kidney failure.
creatinine (kree-AT-ih-neen)	Waste product of metabolism. Increased amounts in the urine indicate kidney failure.
creatine kinase (KREE-ah-teen KY-nays)	Enzyme found only in skeletal muscle cells, heart cells, and brain cells. Elevated levels of CK-MB indicate a heart attack has occurred.
cyst/o- (SIS-toh)	Combining form meaning *bladder; fluid-filled sac;* or *semisolid cyst*
cyt/o- (SY-toh)	Combining form meaning *cell*
cyt/o- (SY-toh)	Combining form meaning *cell*
cyst/o- (SIS-toh)	Combining form meaning *bladder; fluid-filled sac;* or *semisolid cyst*
dermatome (DER-mah-tohm)	A specific area of the skin that sends sensory information through a spinal nerve
	A surgical instrument used to make a shallow, continuous cut to form a skin graft
diabetes insipidus (DY-ah-BEE-teez in-SIP-ih-dus)	Disease caused by hyposecretion of antidiuretic hormone (ADH) from the posterior pituitary gland
diabetes mellitus (DY-ah-BEE-teez MEL-ih-tus)	Disease caused by hyposecretion of insulin from the pancreas
diabetes mellitus (DY-ah-BEE-teez MEL-ih-tus)	Disease caused by hyposecretion of insulin from the pancreas
diabetes insipidus (DY-ah-BEE-teez in-SIP-ih-dus)	Disease caused by hyposecretion of antidiuretic hormone (ADH) from the posterior pituitary gland
diaphoresis (DY-ah-foh-REE-sis)	Profuse sweating of the skin
diuresis (DY-yoo-REE-sis)	Condition of excreting abnormally large amounts of urine
diaphoretic (DY-ah-foh-RET-ik)	Pertaining to having profuse sweating of the skin
diuretic (DY-yoo-RET-ik)	Drug that increases the production of urine
diarrhea (DY-ah-REE-ah)	Abnormally frequent and loose, watery stools
diuresis (DY-yoo-REE-sis)	Condition of excreting abnormally large amounts of urine
diuresis (DY-yoo-REE-sis)	Condition of excreting abnormally large amounts of urine
diaphoresis (DY-ah-foh-REE-sis)	Profuse sweating of the skin
diarrhea (DY-ah-REE-ah)	Abnormally frequent and loose, watery stools

Bolded and blue medical words have a matching entry in the Glossary Section.

Medical Word, Word Part, or Abbreviation (Pronunciation)	Definition
Sound Alike	**Definition**
diuretic (DY-yoo-RET-ik)	Drug that increases the production of urine
diaphoretic (DY-ah-foh-RET-ik)	Pertaining to having profuse sweating of the skin
dyscrasia (dis-KRAY-zee-ah)	Condition of abnormalities of the blood cells
dysphagia (dis-FAY-jee-ah)	Condition of difficult or painful eating or swallowing
dysphasia (dis-FAY-zee-ah)	Condition of difficulty speaking or understanding words
dysplasia (dis-PLAY-zee-ah) (dis-PLAY-zha)	Condition of cells that are abnormal in size, shape, or organization but not yet cancerous
dysphagia (dis-FAY-jee-ah)	Condition of difficult or painful eating or swallowing
dyscrasia (dis-KRAY-zee-ah)	Condition of abnormalities of the blood cells
dysphasia (dis-FAY-zee-ah)	Condition of difficulty speaking or understanding words
dysplasia (dis-PLAY-zee-ah) (dis-PLAY-zha)	Condition of cells that are abnormal in size, shape, or organization but not yet cancerous
dysphasia (dis-FAY-zee-ah)	Condition of difficulty speaking or understanding words
dyscrasia (dis-KRAY-zee-ah)	Condition of abnormalities of the blood cells
dysphagia (dis-FAY-jee-ah)	Condition of difficult or painful eating or swallowing
dysplasia (dis-PLAY-zee-ah) (dis-PLAY-zha)	Condition of cells that are abnormal in size, shape, or organization but not yet cancerous
dysplasia (dis-PLAY-zee-ah) (dis-PLAY-zha)	Condition of cells that are abnormal in size, shape, or organization but not yet cancerous
dyscrasia (dis-KRAY-zee-ah)	Condition of abnormalities of the blood cells
dysphagia (dis-FAY-jee-ah)	Condition of difficult or painful eating or swallowing
dysphasia (dis-FAY-zee-ah)	Condition of difficulty speaking or understanding words
ectropion (ek-TROH-pee-on)	Turning outward of the lower eyelid because of weakness in the connective tissue or muscle
entropion (en-TROH-pee-on)	Turning inward of the lower eyelid because of scar tissue or spasm of the muscle
effect (EE-fekt)	English word meaning *a result* or *a consequence*
affect (AF-ekt)	Outward display on the face of a person's inward emotions
efferent (EF-eh-rent)	Going out from the center, as in nerves that carry impulses away from the spinal cord and brain
afferent (AF-eh-rent)	Coming toward the center, as in nerves that carry impulses toward the spinal cord and brain
effusion (ee-FYOO-shun)	Collection of fluid
infusion (in-FYOO-zhun)	Action of administering intravenous fluids through a vein
elementary (EL-eh-MEN-tah-ree)	English word meaning *pertaining to basic or fundamental*
alimentary (AL-ih-MEN-tair-ee)	Pertaining to the digestive tract

Bolded and blue medical words have a matching entry in the Glossary Section.

Medical Word, Word Part, or Abbreviation (Pronunciation)	Definition
Sound Alike	*Definition*
emphysema (EM-fih-SEE-mah)	Chronic, irreversibly damaged alveoli that become large air spaces that trap air in the lungs
empyema (EM-py-EE-mah)	Localized collection of pus in the thoracic cavity
empyema (EM-py-EE-mah)	Localized collection of pus in the thoracic cavity
emphysema (EM-fih-SEE-mah)	Chronic, irreversibly damaged alveoli that become large air spaces that trap air in the lungs
endocrine (EN-doh-krin) (EN-doh-krine)	Glands and organs that release hormones directly into the blood
exocrine (EK-soh-krin) (EK-soh-krine)	Glands that release substances through ducts (not directly into the blood)
entropion (en-TROH-pee-on)	Turning inward of the lower eyelid because of scar tissue or spasm of the muscle
ectropion (ek-TROH-pee-on)	Turning outward of the lower eyelid because of weakness in the connective tissue or muscle
esotropia (ES-oh-TROH-pee-ah)	Deviation of one or both eyes toward the midline. Also known as *cross-eye*.
exotropia (EKS-oh-TROH-pee-ah)	Deviation of one or both eyes laterally. Also known as *wall-eye*.
eversion (ee-VER-zhun)	Turning a body part outward
inversion (in-VER-zhun)	Turning a body part inward
exocrine (EK-soh-krin) (EK-soh-krine)	Glands that release substances through ducts (not directly into the blood)
endocrine (EN-doh-krin) (EN-doh-krine)	Glands and organs that release hormones directly into the blood
exotropia (EKS-oh-TROH-pee-ah)	Deviation of one or both eyes laterally. Also known as *wall-eye*.
esotropia (ES-oh-TROH-pee-ah)	Deviation of one or both eyes toward the midline. Also known as *cross-eye*.
facial (FAY-shal)	Pertaining to the face
fascial (FASH-ee-al)	Pertaining to the fascia
fascial (FASH-ee-al)	Pertaining to the fascia
facial (FAY-shal)	Pertaining to the face
fecal (FEE-kal)	Pertaining to the feces or stool
thecal (THEE-kal)	Pertaining to the thecum, a sheath around certain anatomical structures
genu valgum (JEE-noo VAL-gum)	Congenital deformity known as *knock-knee*
genu varum (JEE-noo VAR-um)	Congenital deformity known as *bowleg*

Bolded and blue medical words have a matching entry in the Glossary Section.

Medical Word, Word Part, or Abbreviation (Pronunciation)	Definition
Sound Alike	**Definition**
genu varum (JEE-noo VAR-um)	Congenital deformity known as *bowleg*
genu valgum (JEE-noo VAL-gum)	Congenital deformity known as *knock-knee*
glands (GLANZ)	Organs of the endocrine system that secrete hormones directly into the blood
glans (GLANZ)	Part of the Latin phrase *glans penis*; the tip of the penis of the male
glans (GLANZ)	Part of the Latin phrase *glans penis*; the tip of the penis of the male
glands (GLANZ)	Organs of the endocrine system that secrete hormones directly into the blood
globins (GLOH-binz)	Chains of protein molecules in hemoglobin
globulin (GLAWB-yoo-lin)	Protein molecule that makes up immunoglobulins
globulin (GLAWB-yoo-lin)	Protein molecule that makes up immunoglobulins
globins (GLOH-binz)	Chains of protein molecules in hemoglobin
glucagon (GLOO-kah-gawn)	Hormone secreted by alpha cells in the islets of Langerhans in the pancreas to break down glycogen into glucose.
glycogen (GLY-koh-jen)	A form of glucose that is stored in the liver and skeletal muscles
glycogen (GLY-koh-jen)	A form of glucose that is stored in the liver and skeletal muscles
glucagon (GLOO-kah-gawn)	Hormone secreted by alpha cells in the islets of Langerhans in the pancreas to break down glycogen into glucose.
gtt. (g-t-t)	Abbreviation for *drops (of a drug)*
GTT (G-T-T)	Abbreviation for *glucose tolerance test*
GTT (G-T-T)	Abbreviation for *glucose tolerance test*
gtt. (g-t-t)	Abbreviation for *drops (of a drug)*
H&P (H AND P)	Abbreviation for *history and physical (examination)*
HNP (H-N-P)	Abbreviation for *herniated nucleus pulposus*
hematoma (HEE-mah-TOH-mah)	An elevated, localized collection of blood under the skin
hepatoma (HEP-ah-TOH-mah)	A cancerous tumor of the liver
hemostasis (HEE-moh-STAY-sis)	The cessation of bleeding after the formation of a blood clot
homeostasis (HOH-mee-oh-STAY-sis)	A state of equilibrium of the internal environment of the body
hepatoma (HEP-ah-TOH-mah)	A cancerous tumor of the liver
hematoma (HEE-mah-TOH-mah)	An elevated, localized collection of blood under the skin

Bolded and blue medical words have a matching entry in the Glossary Section.

Medical Word, Word Part, or Abbreviation (Pronunciation)	Definition
Sound Alike	Definition
HNP (H-N-P)	Abbreviation for *herniated nucleus pulposus*
H&P (H AND P)	Abbreviation for *history and physical (examination)*
homeostasis (HOH-mee-oh-STAY-sis)	A state of equilibrium of the internal environment of the body
hemostasis (HEE-moh-STAY-sis)	The cessation of bleeding after the formation of a blood clot
humeral (HYOO-mer-al)	Pertaining to the bone of the upper arm
humoral (HYOO-mor-al)	Pertaining to immunity (resistance) to infection that comes from antibodies in the blood
humerus (HYOO-mer-us)	The bone of the upper arm
humorous (HYOO-mor-us)	English word meaning *funny*
humoral (HYOO-mor-al)	Pertaining to immunity (resistance) to infection that comes from antibodies in the blood
humeral (HYOO-mer-al)	Pertaining to the bone of the upper arm
humorous (HYOO-mor-us)	English word meaning *funny*
humerus (HYOO-mer-us)	The bone of the upper arm
ileum (IL-ee-um)	Third part of the small intestine
ilium (IL-ee-um)	Superior flaring part of the hip bone of the pelvis
ileus (IL-ee-us)	Abnormal absence of contractions of the small intestine
ileus (IL-ee-us)	Abnormal absence of contractions of the small intestine
ileum (IL-ee-um)	Third part of the small intestine
ilium (IL-ee-um)	Superior flaring part of the hip bone of the pelvis
ilium (IL-ee-um)	Superior flaring part of the hip bone of the pelvis
ileum (IL-ee-um)	Third part of the small intestine
ileus (IL-ee-us)	Abnormal absence of contractions of the small intestine
in vivo (in VEE-voh)	Latin phrase meaning *in life* or *in a living organism*
in vitro (in-VEE-troh)	Latin phrase meaning *in a test tube*
in vitro (in-VEE-troh)	Latin phrase meaning *in a test tube*
in vivo (in VEE-voh)	Latin phrase meaning *in life* or *in a living organism*
infusion (in-FYOO-zhun)	Action of administering intravenous fluids through a vein
effusion (ee-FYOO-shun)	Collection of fluid
inter- (IN-ter)	Prefix meaning *between*
intra- (IN-trah)	Prefix meaning *within*
intra- (IN-trah)	Prefix meaning *within*
inter- (IN-ter)	Prefix meaning *between*
inversion (in-VER-zhun)	Turning a body part inward
eversion (ee-VER-zhun)	Turning a body part outward

Bolded and blue medical words have a matching entry in the Glossary Section.

Medical Word, Word Part, or Abbreviation (Pronunciation)	**Definition**
Sound Alike	*Definition*
kary/o- (KAIR-ee-oh)	Combining form meaning *nucleus*
cari/o- (KAIR-ee-oh)	Combining form meaning *caries (tooth decay)*
kel/o- (KEE-loh)	Combining form meaning *tumor*
cheil/o- (KIGH-loh)	Combining form meaning *lip*
kilo- (KIL-oh)	Prefix meaning *one thousand*
kerat/o- (KAIR-ah-toh)	Combining form meaning *cornea (of the eye)*
	Combining form meaning *hard, fibrous protein*
carot/o- (kah-RAW-toh)	Combining form meaning *stupor; sleep*
kilo- (KIL-oh)	Prefix meaning *one thousand*
cheil/o- (KY-loh)	Combining form meaning *lip*
kel/o- (KEE-loh)	Combining form meaning *tumor*
labial (LAY-bee-al)	Pertaining to the labia of the female genital system
labile (LAY-bile)	Pertaining to an emotion that is unstable or prone to change
labile (LAY-bile)	Pertaining to an emotion that is unstable or prone to change
labial (LAY-bee-al)	Pertaining to the labia of the female genital system
lice (LYS)	Parasitic infection known as pediculosis
lyse (LYZ)	To break apart into separate components
lymph (LIMF)	Fluid that flows through lymphatic vessels and lymph nodes
lymphs (LIMFS)	Abbreviation meaning *lymphocytes*
lymphs (LIMFS)	Abbreviation meaning *lymphocytes*
lymph (LIMF)	Fluid that flows through lymphatic vessels and lymph nodes
lyse (LYZ)	To break apart into separate components
lice (LYS)	Parasitic infection known as pediculosis
macula (MAK-yoo-lah)	Dark yellow-orange area on the retina that contains the fovea (area of greatest visual acuity)
macule (MAK-yool)	Pigmented brown or black spot on the skin
macule (MAK-yool)	Pigmented brown or black spot on the skin
macula (MAK-yoo-lah)	Dark yellow-orange area on the retina that contains the fovea (area of greatest visual acuity)
malleolus (mah-LEE-oh-lus)	Bony projection on the distal tibia or the distal fibula
malleus (MAL-ee-us)	First bone in the middle ear cavity
malleus (MAL-ee-us)	First bone in the middle ear cavity
malleolus (mah-LEE-oh-lus)	Bony projection on the distal tibia or the distal fibula
mastication (MAS-tih-KAY-shun)	Process of chewing food
masturbation (MAS-tur-BAY-shun)	Process of sexual self-stimulation
masturbation (MAS-tur-BAY-shun)	Process of sexual self-stimulation
mastication (MAS-tih-KAY-shun)	Process of chewing food

Bolded and blue medical words have a matching entry in the Glossary Section.

Medical Word, Word Part, or Abbreviation (Pronunciation)	Definition
Sound Alike	**Definition**
meiosis (my-OH-sis)	Process by which a spermatocyte or ovum reduces the number of chromosomes in its nucleus by half to create gametes
miosis (my-OH-sis)	Contraction of the iris muscle to decrease the size of the pupil in the eye
mitosis (my-TOH-sis)	Process of cellular division
mycosis (my-KOH-sis)	Condition of a fungus infection on the skin or in the body
melanin (MEL-ah-nin)	Dark brown or black pigment produced by melanocytes in the skin
melatonin (MEL-ah-TOH-nin)	Hormone secreted by the pineal gland that controls the wake–sleep cycle
melatonin (MEL-ah-TOH-nin)	Hormone secreted by the pineal gland that controls the wake–sleep cycle
melanin (MEL-ah-nin)	Dark brown or black pigment produced by melanocytes in the skin
metr/o- (MET-roh)	Combining form meaning *measurement*
metr/o- (MEE-troh)	Combining form meaning *uterus*
mets (METS)	Slang for *metastases*
	Unit of measurement used during a cardiac treadmill stress test
miosis (my-OH-sis)	Contraction of the iris muscle to decrease the size of the pupil in the eye
meiosis (my-OH-sis)	Process by which a spermatocyte or ovum reduces the number of chromosomes in its nucleus by half to create gametes
mitosis (my-TOH-sis)	Process of cellular division
mycosis (my-KOH-sis)	Condition of a fungus infection on the skin or in the body
mitosis (my-TOH-sis)	Process of cellular division
meiosis (my-OH-sis)	Process by which a spermatocyte or ovum reduces the number of chromosomes in its nucleus by half to create gametes
miosis (my-OH-sis)	Contraction of the iris muscle to decrease the size of the pupil in the eye
mycosis (my-KOH-sis)	Condition of a fungus infection on the skin or in the body
mono (MAWN-oh)	Slang for *mononucleosis*
monos (MAWN-ohz)	Abbreviation meaning *monocytes*
monos (MAWN-ohz)	Abbreviation meaning *monocytes*
mono (MAWN-oh)	Slang for *mononucleosis*
mucosa (myoo-KOH-sah)	Latin word that means *mucous membrane*
mucous (MYOO-kus)	Pertaining to a membrane that secretes mucus
mucus (MYOO-kus)	A secretion from a mucous membrane

Bolded and blue medical words have a matching entry in the Glossary Section.

Medical Word, Word Part, or Abbreviation (Pronunciation)	Definition
Sound Alike	**Definition**
mucous (MYOO-kus)	Pertaining to a membrane that secretes mucus
mucosa (myoo-KOH-sah)	Latin word that means *mucous membrane*
mucus (MYOO-kus)	A secretion from a mucous membrane
mucus (MYOO-kus)	A secretion from a mucous membrane
mucosa (myoo-KOH-sah)	Latin word that means *mucous membrane*
mucous (MYOO-kus)	Pertaining to a membrane that secretes mucus
myc/o- (MY-koh)	Combining form meaning *fungus*
myel/o- (MY-eh-loh)	Combining form meaning *bone marrow; spinal cord; myelin*
my/o- (MY-oh)	Combining form meaning *muscle*
mycosis (my-KOH-sis)	Condition of a fungus infection on the skin or in the body
meiosis (my-OH-sis)	Process by which a spermatocyte or ovum reduces the number of chromosomes in its nucleus by half to create gametes
miosis (my-OH-sis)	Contraction of the iris muscle to decrease the size of the pupil in the eye
mitosis (my-TOH-sis)	Process of cellular division
myel/o- (MY-eh-loh)	Combining form meaning *bone marrow; spinal cord; myelin*
myc/o- (MY-koh)	Combining form meaning *fungus*
my/o- (MY-oh)	Combining form meaning *muscle*
myeloma (MY-eh-LOH-mah)	Tumor of the bone marrow that produces cancerous cells and antibodies
myoma (my-OH-mah)	Benign tumor of the muscle
my/o- (MY-oh)	Combining form meaning *muscle*
myc/o- (MY-koh)	Combining form meaning *fungus*
myel/o- (MY-eh-loh)	Combining form meaning *bone marrow; spinal cord; myelin*
myoma (my-OH-mah)	Benign tumor of the muscle
myeloma (MY-eh-LOH-mah)	Tumor of the bone marrow that produces cancerous cells and antibodies
nephropathy (neh-FRAWP-ah-thee)	Degenerative scarring of the nephrons of the kidneys
neuropathy (nyoo-RAWP-ah-thee)	Decreased or abnormal sensation in the extremities because of nerve damage
neuropathy (nyoo-RAWP-ah-thee)	Decreased or abnormal sensation in the extremities because of nerve damage
nephropathy (neh-FRAWP-ah-thee)	Degenerative scarring of the nephrons of the kidneys
oral (OR-al)	Pertaining to the mouth
aural (AW-ral)	Pertaining to the ear

Bolded and blue medical words have a matching entry in the Glossary Section.

Medical Word, Word Part, or Abbreviation (Pronunciation)	Definition
Sound Alike	**Definition**
palpation (pal-PAY-shun)	Using the fingers to press on a body part to detect any abnormality or tenderness
palpitation (PAL-pih-TAY-shun)	Uncomfortable sensation in the chest during a premature contraction of the heart
palpitation (PAL-pih-TAY-shun)	Uncomfortable sensation in the chest during a premature contraction of the heart
palpation (pal-PAY-shun)	Using the fingers to press on a body part to detect any abnormality or tenderness
pelvis (PEL-vis)	The hip bones as well as the sacrum and coccyx of the spinal column
	Large, funnel-shaped cavity in each kidney that collects urine
perineal (PAIR-ih-NEE-al)	Pertaining to the perineum (area of skin between the vulva and the anus)
peritoneal (PAIR-ih-toh-NEE-al)	Pertaining to the peritoneum (membrane that lines the abdominopelvic cavity)
peroneal (PAIR-oh-NEE-al)	Pertaining to the fibula (lower leg bone)
perineum (PAIR-ih-NEE-um)	Area of skin between the edge of the vulva and the anus
peritoneum (PAIR-ih-toh-NEE-um)	Membrane that lines the abdominopelvic cavity
peritoneal (PAIR-ih-toh-NEE-al)	Pertaining to the peritoneum (membrane that lines the abdominopelvic cavity)
perineal (PAIR-ih-NEE-al)	Pertaining to the perineum (area of skin between the vulva and the anus)
peroneal (PAIR-oh-NEE-al)	Pertaining to the fibula (lower leg bone)
peritoneum (PAIR-ih-toh-NEE-um)	Membrane that lines the abdominopelvic cavity
perineum (PAIR-ih-NEE-um)	Area of skin between the edge of the vulva and the anus
peroneal (PAIR-oh-NEE-al)	Pertaining to the fibula (lower leg bone)
perineal (PAIR-ih-NEE-al)	Pertaining to the perineum (area of skin between the vulva and the anus)
peritoneal (PAIR-ih-toh-NEE-al)	Pertaining to the peritoneum (membrane that lines the abdominopelvic cavity)
plain (PLAYN)	Type of x-ray taken without the use of a contrast material
plane (PLAYN)	Imaginary flat surface that can be used anatomically to divide the body into anterior/posterior sections, right/left sections, and top/bottom sections
plane (PLAYN)	Imaginary flat surface that can be used anatomically to divide the body into anterior/posterior sections, right/left sections, and top/bottom sections
plain (PLAYN)	Type of x-ray taken without the use of a contrast material

Bolded and blue medical words have a matching entry in the Glossary Section.

Medical Word, Word Part, or Abbreviation (Pronunciation)	Definition
Sound Alike	**Definition**
pleural (PLOOR-al)	Pertaining to the pleura (serous membrane around the lungs)
plural (PLOOR-al)	English word meaning *more than one*
pleuritis (ploo-RY-tis)	Inflammation of the pleura (serous membrane around the lungs)
pruritus (proo-RY-tus)	Condition of itching
plural (PLOOR-al)	English word meaning *more than one*
pleural (PLOOR-al)	Pertaining to the pleura (serous membrane around the lungs)
prostate (PRAWS-tayt)	Gland that surrounds the urethra in men
prostrate (PRAWS-trayt)	Lying in a face-down position
prostatic (praws-TAT-ik)	Pertaining to the prostate gland
prosthetic (praws-THET-ik)	Pertaining to a prosthesis, an orthopedic device such as an artificial leg
prosthetic (praws-THET-ik)	Pertaining to a prosthesis, an orthopedic device such as an artificial leg
prostatic (praws-TAT-ik)	Pertaining to the prostate gland
prostrate (PRAWS-trayt)	Lying in a face-down position
prostate (PRAWS-tayt)	Gland that surrounds the urethra in men
pruritus (proo-RY-tus)	Condition of itching
pleuritis (ploo-RY-tis)	Inflammation of the pleura (serous membrane around the lungs)
rectum (REK-tum)	Straight part of the distal large intestine
rectus (REK-tus)	Latin word that means *straight (skeletal) muscle*
rectus (REK-tus)	Latin word that means *straight (skeletal) muscle*
rectum (REK-tum)	Straight part of the distal large intestine
reflex (REE-fleks)	Involuntary automatic response of the muscular–nervous pathway
reflux (REE-fluks)	Backward flow of fluid, most often from the stomach into the esophagus
reflux (REE-fluks)	Backward flow of fluid, most often from the stomach into the esophagus
reflex (REE-fleks)	Involuntary automatic response of the muscular–nervous pathway
rem (REM)	Abbreviation meaning *unit of measurement of radiation exposure*
REM (R-E-M)	Abbreviation meaning *rapid eye movements (during sleep)*
rod (ROD)	Bacterium with a rectangular shape
rods (RODZ)	Light-sensitive cells in the retina that detect black and white images

Bolded and blue medical words have a matching entry in the Glossary Section.

Medical Word, Word Part, or Abbreviation (Pronunciation)	Definition
Sound Alike	*Definition*
rods (RODZ)	Light-sensitive cells in the retina that detect black and white images
rod (ROD)	Bacterium with a rectangular shape
scirrhous (SKIR-us)	Pertaining to a cancer in the form of a hard tumor
serous (SEER-us)	Pertaining to a membrane that secretes a clear, watery fluid
serous (SEER-us)	Pertaining to a membrane that secretes a clear, watery fluid
scirrhous (SKIR-uhs)	Pertaining to a cancer in the form of a hard tumor
stoma (STOH-mah)	A surgically created opening in the abdomen
stomach (STUM-uk)	Organ of digestion between the esophagus and duodenum
stomatitis (stoh-mah-TY-tis)	Inflammation of the oral mucosa of the mouth
stomach (STUM-uk)	Organ of digestion between the esophagus and duodenum
stoma (STOH-mah)	A surgically created opening in the abdomen
stomatitis (stoh-mah-TY-tis)	Inflammation of the oral mucosa of the mouth
stomatitis (stoh-mah-TY-tis)	Inflammation of the oral mucosa of the mouth
stoma (STOH-mah)	A surgically created opening in the abdomen
stomach (STUM-uk)	Organ of digestion between the esophagus and duodenum
thecal (THEE-kal)	Pertaining to the thecum, a sheath around certain anatomical structures
fecal (FEE-kal)	Pertaining to the feces or stool
urea (yoo-REE-ah)	Waste product of metabolism. Increased amounts in the urine can indicate kidney failure.
uvea (YOO-vee-ah)	Collective word for the iris, choroid, and ciliary body of the eye
ureter (YOO-ree-ter) (yoo-REE-ter)	Tube that carries urine from the kidney to the bladder
urethra (yoo-REE-thrah)	Tube that carries urine from the bladder to the outside of the body
urethra (yoo-REE-thrah)	Tube that carries urine from the bladder to the outside of the body
ureter (YOO-ree-ter) (yoo-REE-ter)	Tube that carries urine from the kidney to the bladder
uvea (YOO-vee-ah)	Collective word for the iris, choroid, and ciliary body of the eye
urea (yoo-REE-ah)	Waste product of metabolism. Increased amounts in the urine can indicate kidney failure.

Bolded and blue medical words have a matching entry in the Glossary Section.

Medical Word, Word Part, or Abbreviation (Pronunciation)	Definition
Sound Alike	**Definition**
vesical (VES-ih-kal)	Pertaining to the bladder
vesicle (VES-ih-kl)	Skin lesion with a pointed top that is filled with clear fluid
vesicle (VES-ih-kl)	Skin lesion with a pointed top that is filled with clear fluid
vesical (VES-ih-kal)	Pertaining to the bladder
vial (VY-al)	Small glass bottle with a rubber stopper top that contains a liquid or powdered drug
vile (VYL)	English word meaning *foul or filthy*
vile (VYL)	English word meaning *foul or filthy*
vial (VY-al)	Small glass bottle with a rubber stopper top that contains a liquid or powdered drug

SECTION 9

Tables and Illustrated Figures

The tables and illustrated figures in this section demonstrate human anatomy in an easy-to-view format.

The realistic human photographs with their overlaid medical illustrations accurately and beautifully depict the anatomical details of the various body systems. This section contains two parts.

PART A: TABLES

This section contains two tables. The first has an alphabetical listing of the bones with their locations. Then, there is a table listing the endocrine glands and their hormones.

PART B: FULL-COLOR ILLUSTRATED FIGURES OF BODY SYSTEMS

This section contains full-color illustrations of the body systems with anatomical labels.

The authors wish to express their sincere thanks to medical illustrator Anita Impagliazzo for the use of her unique anatomical medical illustrations that first appeared in the textbook *Medical Language* (Prentice Hall, 2007).

PART A: TABLES

Bones		
Name	**#**	**Location**
calcaneus	2	heels
capitate	2	wrists
cervical vertebra	7	neck
clavicle	2	shoulders
coccyx	1	tailbone
cuboid	2	ankles
distal phalanx	20	fingers and toes
ethmoid	1	cranium
femur	2	legs
fibula	2	legs
frontal	1	cranium
hamate	2	wrists
humerus	2	arms
hyoid	1	throat
ilium (part of the os coxae)		pelvis
incus	2	ears
inferior nasal concha	2	face
intermediate cuneiform	2	ankles
intermediate phalanx	16	fingers and toes
ischium (part of the os coxae)		pelvis
lacrimal	2	face
lateral cuneiform	2	ankles
lumbar vertebra	5	lower back
lunate	2	wrists
malleus	2	ears
mandible	1	face
maxilla	2	face
medial cuneiform	2	ankles
metacarpal	10	palms
metatarsal	10	feet
nasal	2	face
navicular	2	ankles
occipital	1	cranium
os coxae (fused ilium, ischium, and pubis)	2	pelvis
palatine	2	face
parietal	2	cranium
patella	2	legs
pisiform	2	wrists
proximal phalanx	20	fingers and toes
pubis (part of the os coxae)		pelvis

Name	#	Location
radius	2	arms
rib	24	chest
sacrum	1	lower back
scaphoid	2	wrists
scapula	2	shoulders
sphenoid	1	cranium
stapes	2	ears
sternum	1	chest
talus	2	ankles
temporal	2	cranium
thoracic vertebra	12	upper back
tibia	2	legs
trapezium	2	wrists
trapezoid	2	wrists
triquetrum	2	wrists
ulna	2	arms
vomer	1	face
zygomatic	2	face

Endocrine Glands and Hormones

Gland	Hormone
Pituitary Gland	
anterior lobe (adenohypophysis)	adrenocorticotropic hormone follicle-stimulating hormone growth hormone luteinizing hormone melanocyte-stimulating hormone prolactin thyroid-stimulating hormone
posterior lobe (neurohypophysis)	antidiuretic hormone oxytocin
Pineal Body	
	melatonin
Thyroid Gland	
	calcitonin thyroxine triiodothyronine
Parathyroid Glands	
	parathyroid hormone
Thymus	
	thymosins
Pancreas	
	glugacon insulin somatostatin
Adrenal Glands	
adrenal cortex	aldosterone androgens cortisol
adrenal medulla	epinephrine norepinephrine
Ovaries	
	estradiol progesterone
Testes	
	testosterone

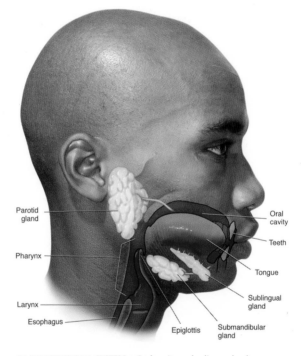

Parotid gland

Oral cavity

Teeth

Pharynx

Tongue

Sublingual gland

Larynx

Esophagus

Epiglottis

Submandibular gland

GASTROINTESTINAL SYSTEM ■ Oral cavity and salivary glands

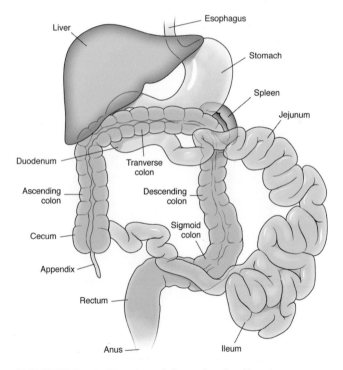

GASTROINTESTINAL SYSTEM ■ Stomach, liver, and small and large intestines

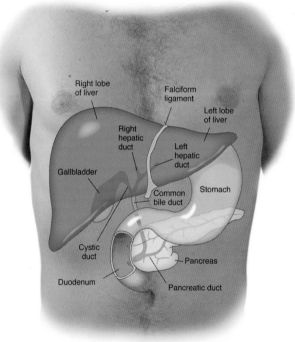

GASTROINTESTINAL SYSTEM ■ Liver, gallbladder, biliary tree, and pancreas

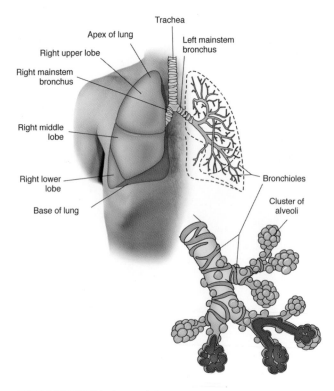

RESPIRATORY SYSTEM ■ Lung and air passageways

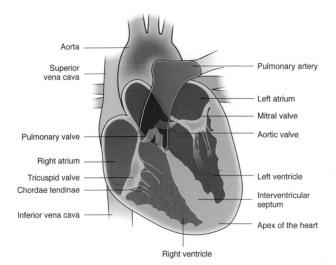

Aorta

Superior
vena cava

Pulmonary valve

Right atrium

Tricuspid valve

Chordae tendinae

Inferior vena cava

Pulmonary artery

Left atrium

Mitral valve

Aortic valve

Left ventricle

Interventricular
septum

Apex of the heart

Right ventricle

CARDIOVASCULAR SYSTEM ■ Heart structures and great vessels

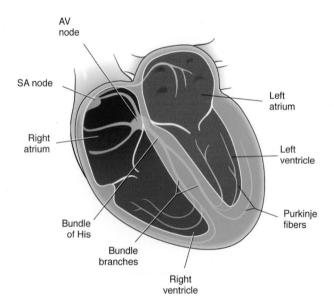

AV node

SA node

Right atrium

Left atrium

Left ventricle

Bundle of His

Bundle branches

Right ventricle

Purkinje fibers

CARDIOVASCULAR SYSTEM ■ Conduction system of the heart

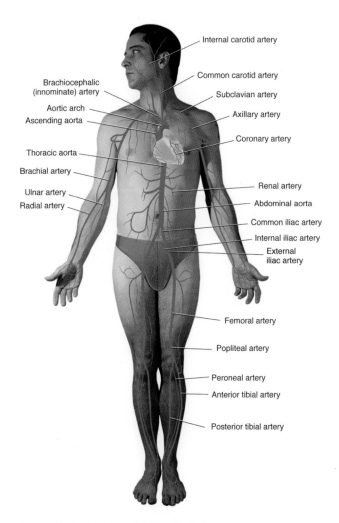

Internal carotid artery

Common carotid artery

Subclavian artery

Axillary artery

Coronary artery

Brachiocephalic (innominate) artery

Aortic arch

Ascending aorta

Thoracic aorta

Brachial artery

Ulnar artery

Radial artery

Renal artery

Abdominal aorta

Common iliac artery

Internal iliac artery

External iliac artery

Femoral artery

Popliteal artery

Peroneal artery

Anterior tibial artery

Posterior tibial artery

CARDIOVASCULAR SYSTEM ■ Arteries of the body

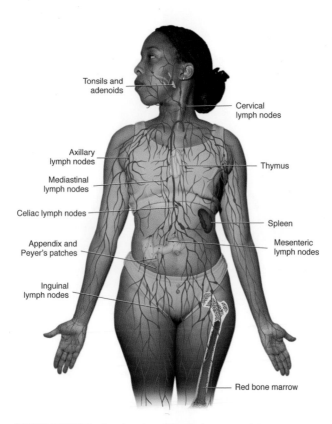

Tonsils and
adenoids

Cervical
lymph nodes

Axillary
lymph nodes

Thymus

Mediastinal
lymph nodes

Celiac lymph nodes

Spleen

Appendix and
Peyer's patches

Mesenteric
lymph nodes

Inguinal
lymph nodes

Red bone marrow

LYMPHATIC SYSTEM ■ Lymph nodes and lymphatic organs and tissues

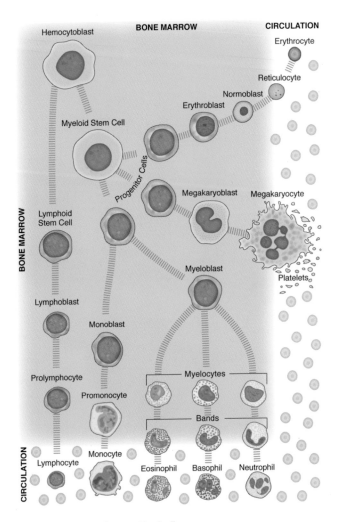

BLOOD ■ Immature and mature blood cells

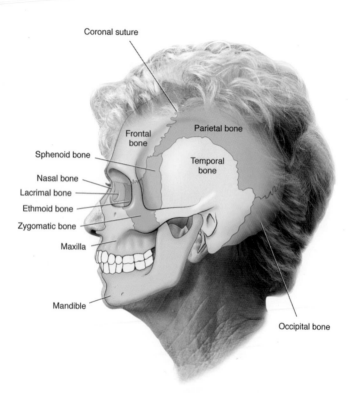

Coronal suture

Parietal bone

Frontal bone

Sphenoid bone

Temporal bone

Nasal bone

Lacrimal bone

Ethmoid bone

Zygomatic bone

Maxilla

Mandible

Occipital bone

SKELETAL SYSTEM ■ Bones of the face and cranium

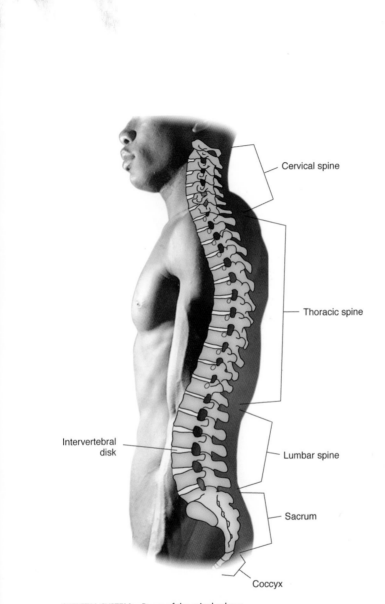

Cervical spine

Thoracic spine

Intervertebral disk

Lumbar spine

Sacrum

Coccyx

SKELETAL SYSTEM ■ Bones of the spinal column

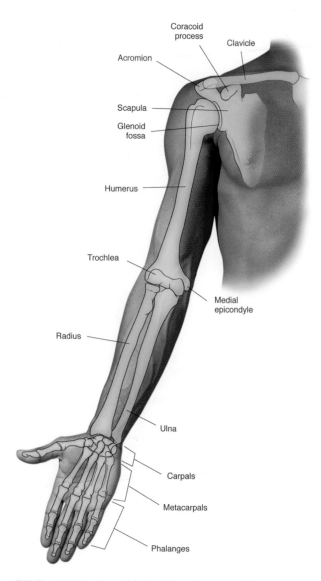

SKELETAL SYSTEM ■ Bones of the shoulder and upper extremity

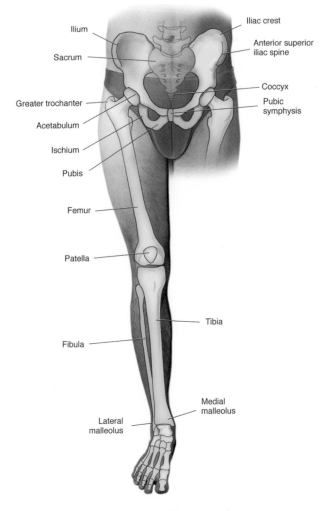

Ilium

Sacrum

Greater trochanter

Acetabulum

Ischium

Pubis

Femur

Patella

Fibula

Lateral
malleolus

Iliac crest

Anterior superior
iliac spine

Coccyx

Pubic
symphysis

Tibia

Medial
malleolus

SKELETAL SYSTEM ■ Bones of the hip and lower extremity

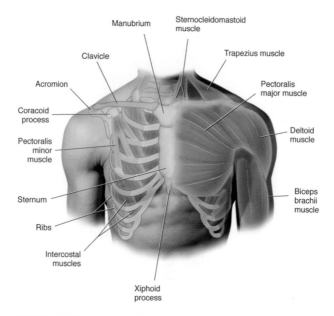

Manubrium

Sternocleidomastoid muscle

Clavicle

Trapezius muscle

Acromion

Pectoralis major muscle

Coracoid process

Pectoralis minor muscle

Deltoid muscle

Sternum

Biceps brachii muscle

Ribs

Intercostal muscles

Xiphoid process

SKELETAL SYSTEM ■ Muscles of the shoulder and chest
MUSCULAR SYSTEM ■ Bones of the spinal column

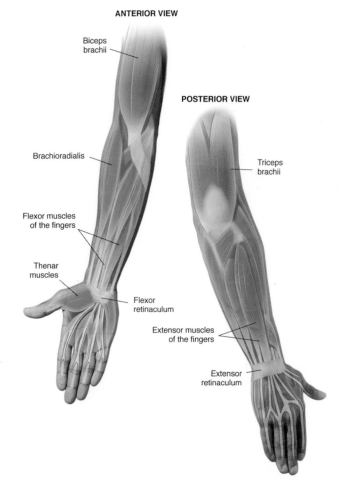

ANTERIOR VIEW

Biceps
brachii

POSTERIOR VIEW

Brachioradialis

Triceps
brachii

Flexor muscles
of the fingers

Thenar
muscles

Flexor
retinaculum

Extensor muscles
of the fingers

Extensor
retinaculum

MUSCULAR SYSTEM ■ Muscles of the upper extremity

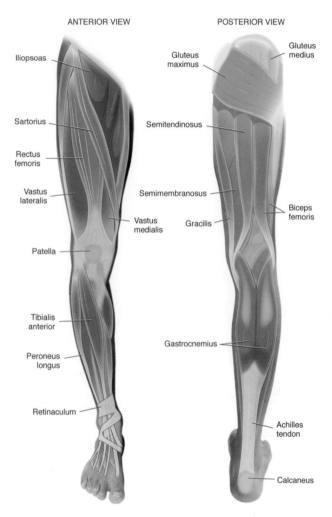

ANTERIOR VIEW

POSTERIOR VIEW

Iliopsoas

Sartorius

Rectus
femoris

Vastus
lateralis

Vastus
medialis

Patella

Tibialis
anterior

Peroneus
longus

Retinaculum

Gluteus
maximus

Gluteus
medius

Semitendinosus

Semimembranosus

Gracilis

Biceps
femoris

Gastrocnemius

Achilles
tendon

Calcaneus

MUSCULAR SYSTEM ■ Muscles of the lower extremity

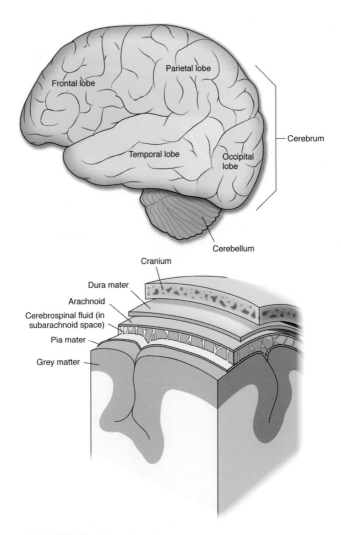

Frontal lobe

Parietal lobe

Temporal lobe

Occipital lobe

Cerebrum

Cerebellum

Cranium

Dura mater

Arachnoid

Cerebrospinal fluid (in subarachnoid space)

Pia mater

Grey matter

NERVOUS SYSTEM ■ Brain and meninges

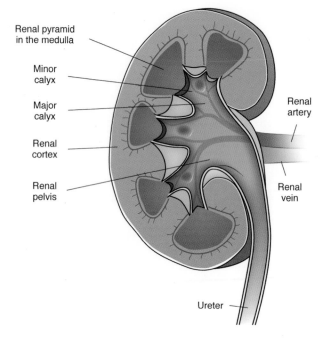

Renal pyramid
in the medulla

Minor
calyx

Major
calyx

Renal
cortex

Renal
pelvis

Renal
artery

Renal
vein

Ureter

URINARY SYSTEM ■ Kidney and ueter

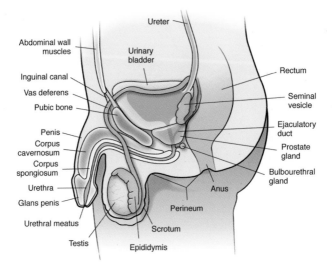

Ureter

Abdominal wall
muscles

Urinary
bladder

Inguinal canal

Vas deferens

Pubic bone

Penis

Corpus
cavernosum

Corpus
spongiosum

Urethra

Glans penis

Urethral meatus

Testis

Epididymis

Scrotum

Perineum

Anus

Rectum

Seminal
vesicle

Ejaculatory
duct

Prostate
gland

Bulbourethral
gland

MALE GENITOURINARY SYSTEM ■ Male external and internal genitalia
and urinary system

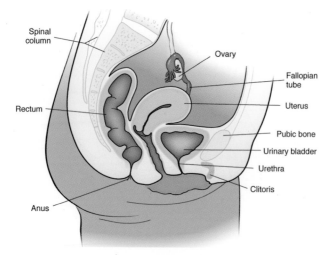

Spinal column

Ovary

Fallopian tube

Rectum

Uterus

Pubic bone

Urinary bladder

Urethra

Clitoris

Anus

FEMALE GENITAL AND REPRODUCTIVE SYSTEM ■ Female pelvic cavity and internal genitalia

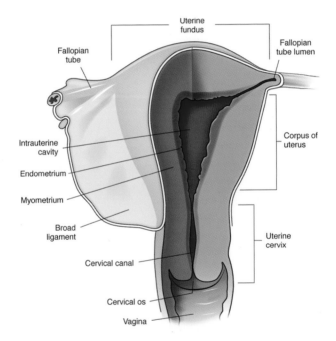

Uterine fundus

Fallopian tube

Fallopian tube lumen

Intrauterine cavity

Endometrium

Myometrium

Broad ligament

Cervical canal

Cervical os

Vagina

Corpus of uterus

Uterine cervix

FEMALE GENITAL AND REPRODUCTIVE SYSTEM ■ Uterus and vagina

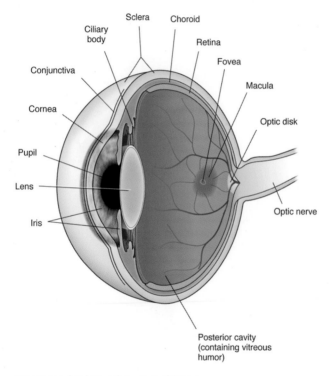

Sclera
Ciliary body
Conjunctiva
Cornea
Pupil
Lens
Iris
Choroid
Retina
Fovea
Macula
Optic disk
Optic nerve
Posterior cavity (containing vitreous humor)

EYE ■ External and internal structures of the eye

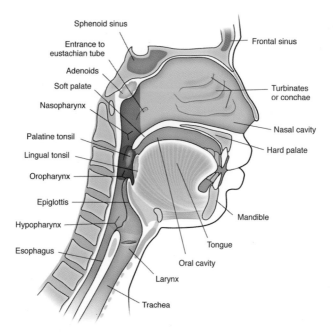

EARS, NOSE AND THROAT SYSTEM ■ Nose, oral cavity, and throat

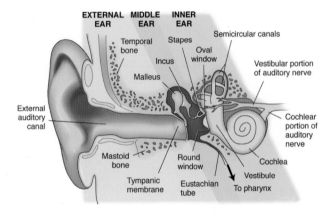

EARS, NOSE AND THROAT SYSTEM ■ External and internal structures of the ear